ISCCM Manual of Critical Care Nursing

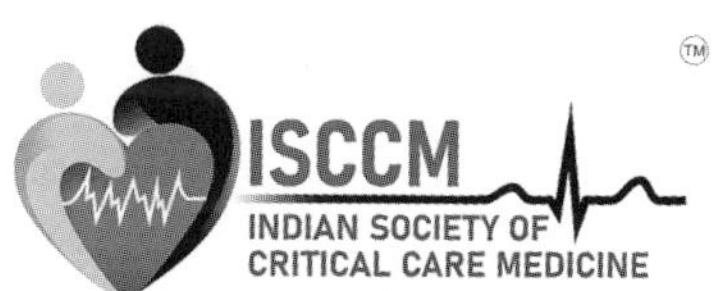

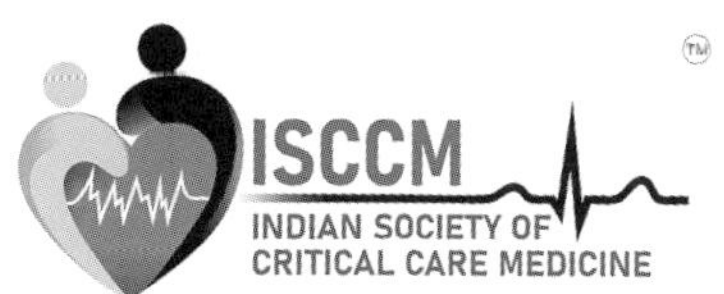

ISCCM Manual of Critical Care Nursing

Editors

Ranvir Singh Tyagi
MD FICCM FCCM
Director
Department of Anesthesia and Critical Care Medicine
Synergy Plus Hospital and Galaxy Hospital
Agra, Uttar Pradesh, India

Susruta Bandyopadhyay
MD (Medicine) Diploma in Cardiology
Director
Department of Critical Care
Manipal Hospitals Broadway
Kolkata, West Bengal, India

Sheila Nainan Myatra
MD FCCM FICCM
Professor of Critical Care Medicine
Department of Anesthesiology
Critical Care and Pain
Tata Memorial Hospital
Mumbai, Maharashtra, India
Immediate Past President, ISCCM
Chair, Intensive and Critical Care Medicine Committee
World Federation of Societies of Anaesthesiologists (WFSA)

Babu K Abraham
MD MRCP (UK) Fellowship in Critical Care Medicine (University of Toronto) FICCM
Senior Consultant
Department of Critical Care Medicine
Apollo Hospitals
Chennai, Tamil Nadu, India

Sumit Ray
MD FICCM
Medical Director and Head
Department of Critical Care Medicine
Holy Family Hospital
New Delhi, India

Foreword
JV Divatia

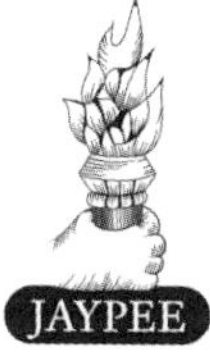

JAYPEE BROTHERS MEDICAL PUBLISHERS
The Health Sciences Publisher
New Delhi | London

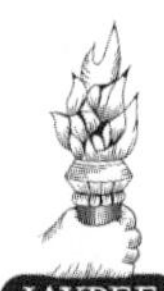

Jaypee Brothers Medical Publishers (P) Ltd

Headquarters
EMCA House
23/23-B, Ansari Road, Daryaganj
New Delhi 110 002, India
Landline: +91-11-23272143, +91-11-23272703
+91-11-23282021, +91-11-23245672
E-mail: jaypee@jaypeebrothers.com

Corporate Office
Jaypee Brothers Medical Publishers (P) Ltd.
4838/24, Ansari Road, Daryaganj
New Delhi 110 002, India
Phone: +91-11-43574357
Fax: +91-11-43574314
E-mail: jaypee@jaypeebrothers.com

Overseas Office
JP Medical Ltd.
83, Victoria Street, London
SW1H 0HW (UK)
Phone: +44-20 3170 8910
E-mail: info@jpmedpub.com

EU GPSR Authorised Representative
Logos Europe, 9 rue Nicolas Poussin
17000, La Rochelle, France
Phone: +33 (0) 6 67 93 73 78
E-mail: Contact@logoseurope.eu

Website: www.jaypeebrothers.com
Website: www.jaypeedigital.com

Inquiries for bulk sales may be solicited at: jaypee@jaypeebrothers.com

ISCCM Manual of Critical Care Nursing

First Edition: **2025**

ISBN: 978-93-5696-503-4

Printed in India by: Rahul Print O Pack

Contributors

Agnideb Bhattacharjee MBBS MD
Specialist
Department of Critical Care Medicine
Tata Main Hospital
Jamshedpur, Jharkhand, India

Ajith Kumar AK MBBS MD DNB EDIC FRCP
Lead Consultant
Department of Critical Care
Aster Whitefield Hospital
Bengaluru, Karnataka, India

Alisha Chaudhury MD IDCCM
Consultant
Department of Critical Care
SUM Ultimate Medicare
Bhubaneswar, Odisha, India

Amit Das
MD (Anesthesiology) FNB (Critical Care Medicine)
Consultant (Critical Care)
Manipal Hospitals
Kolkata, West Bengal, India

Amit Kumar Sharma MBBS MD
Associate Specialist
Department of Critical Care Medicine
Tata Main Hospital
Jamshedpur, Jharkhand, India

Anand Srivastava MBBS MD (Anesthesia) IDCCM
Consultant
Department of Critical Care
Kokilaben Dhirubhai Ambani Hospital
Mumbai, Maharashtra, India

Anand Vinaykumar Joshi
MBBS DNB (Gen Med) FRCP (Lon) FNB (Critical Care) EDIC FCICM (Australia & NZ) PGCC in Echo (Uni Melb)
Intensivist and Physician
Gaman Hospitals, Hyderabad, Telangana, India
Intensive Care Unit, Campbelltown Hospital
Sydney, Australia
Intensive Care Unit, SVPH, Toowoomba
Queensland, Australia
Intensive Care Unit, Mater Private Hospital
Townsville, Queensland, Australia

Anish Joshi
MD IDCCM FNB FCCCM FCCP
Critical Care Specialist
Narayana Health
Ahmedabad, Gujarat, India

Ankur Bhavsar DA IFCCM EDIC
Head, Critical Care
Department of Critical Care
Spandan Multispecialty Hospital
Vadodara, Gujarat, India

Anoopjit Kaur MSc (Nursing Critical Care)
Assistant Professor
Dayanand Medical College and Hospital
Ludhiana, Punjab, India

Arindam Kar
MD DNB FNBE EDICM FCCP FCCM FICCM EPHM
Additional Director
Department of Critical Care
Sir HN Reliance Foundation Hospital
and Research Center
Mumbai, Maharashtra, India

Ashutosh Bhardwaj
MD IDCCM FICCM EDIC FIECMO
Director and Senior Consultant
Department of Critical Care Medicine
Dharamshila Narayana Superspeciality Hospital
New Delhi, India

Asif Ahmed
MBBS DNB (Gold Medal) IDCCM FICCM
Consultant and Head
Department of Critical Care Medicine
Tata Main Hospital
Jamshedpur, Jharkhand, India

Bharat G Jagiasi MD IDCCM FICCM
Director
Department of Critical Care
Kokilaben Dhirubhai Ambani Hospital
Mumbai, Maharashtra, India

Bikram K Gupta
MBBS MD PDCC EDIC FICCM FACEE
Professor
Division of Critical Care Medicine
Department of Anesthesiology
Institute of Medical Sciences
Banaras Hindu University
Varanasi, Uttar Pradesh, India

Chandrashish Chakravarty
MD (AIIMS, Delhi) MRCP (UK) FRCP (Edin) EDIC EDRM FCCM (Miami FL USA)
Senior Consultant
Department of Critical Care
Manipal Hospital
Kolkata, West Bengal, India

Deven Juneja DNB FNB EDIC
Director
Institute of Critical Care Medicine
Max Super Speciality Hospital
New Delhi, India

Devi Prasad Samaddar MD FICCM FICA
Director (Medical Affairs, Administration Critical Care, Quality, Academics)
Ruby General Hospital
Kolkata, West Bengal, India

Dharmajivan Samantaray
MBBS DNB (Anesthesia) IDCC
Associate Clinical Director
Care Hospital
Bhubaneswar, Odisha, India

Dharmendra Kumar Ojha
BSc (Alternative Medicine) GNM IDCCN PGDHHM MBA (Hospital Administration)
In-charge
ICU Nursing Staff
Shri Ram Murti Smarak Institute of Medical Sciences (SRMS-IMS)
Bareilly, Uttar Pradesh, India

Diptanjan Ray
MBBS MD (Anesthesia) PDT (Critical Care Medicine)
Senior Resident
Department of Critical Care Medicine
Manipal Hospitals Broadway
Kolkata, West Bengal, India

Diptimala Agarwal
Diploma in Anesthesiology FICCM PGDHA
Chief (Critical Care Services)
Department of Anesthesia and Critical Care
Shanti Ved Institute of Medical Sciences
Agra, Uttar Pradesh, India

Durgesh Satalkar
MD IDCCM IFCCM EDIC
Senior Consultant
Department of Critical Care Medicine
Yashoda Hospital
Hyderabad, Telangana, India

Ganesh KM DNB FNB
Consultant
Department of Critical Care Medicine
Fortis Hospital
Bengaluru, Karnataka, India

Ganshyam Jagathkar
MBBS MD FNB FICCM MBA
Director
Department of Critical Care
Medicover Hospitals
Hyderabad, Telangana, India
Vice President, ISCCM (2024–2025)

Gunjan Chanchalani
MD FNB IFCCM EDIC
Director
Department of Critical Care Medicine
Wockhardt Hospitals
Mumbai, Maharashtra, India

Inderpreet Kaur
MSc (Nursing) NPCCM
Advance Nurse Practitioner in Critical Care
Department of Critical Care Medicine
Dayanand Medical College and Hospital
Ludhiana, Punjab, India

Kanwalpreet Sodhi
DA DNB IDCCM EDIC FICCM
Director and Head
Department of Critical Care
Deep Hospital
Ludhiana, Punjab, India

Kapil Sharad Borawake
DNB (Medicine) IDCCM FICCM
Director (Critical Care)
Sahyadri Super Specialty Hospital
Pune Consultant (Critical Care)
Prayag Hospital
Deccan Gymkhana
Pune, Maharashtra, India

Lalit Gupta MD
Professor
Anesthesia
Internal Medicine Critical Care
Maulana Azad Medical College
New Delhi, India

Lalit Singh MD FICCM
Professor and Head
Department of Respiratory and Critical Care
Shri Ram Murti Smarak Institute of Medical Sciences (SRMS-IMS)
Bareilly, Uttar Pradesh, India

Manender Kumar
MD (Anesthesiology) PDCC (Cardiac Anesthesia and Critical Care) FTEE
Additional Director
Department of Cardiac Anesthesia
Fortis Hospital
Ludhiana, Punjab, India

Manish Munjal MD FICCM FCCM
Medical Director
Department of Anesthesia and Critical Care
Priyanka Hospital and Cardiac Centre
Jaipur, Rajasthan, India

Manoj K Singh MD DNB FNB EDIC FICCM
Senior Consultant
Department of Chest and Critical Care
Zydus Hospital and Research Centre
Ahmedabad, Gujarat, India

Mary Kutty Babu RNRM GNM PB BSN MBA
Nursing Superintendent
Tata Main Hospital
Jamshedpur, Jharkhand, India

Nandhakishore Jampala DA IDCCM EDIC
Head
Department of Critical Care
Pulse Heart Center
Hyderabad, Telangana, India

Nilesh Dnyaneshwar Chile
GNM (Nursing) ACLS and BLS (AHA)
ICU In-charge Nurse
Sahyadri Hospital
Pune, Maharashtra, India

Nisha Bhojnagarwala
MBBS MD (Anesthesia) FNB (Critical Care)
Consultant
Department of Critical Care
Manipal Hospital
Kolkata, West Bengal, India

Nupur Karan MD DM (Neuroanesthesia)
Associate Professor
Department of Anesthesiology
All India Institute of Medical Sciences
Raipur, Chhattisgarh, India

Parshotam Lal Gautam MD DNB MNAMS FICCM
Professor and Head
Department of Critical Care Medicine
Dayanand Medical College and Hospital
Ludhiana, Punjab, India

Parul Samadder RN MSc PhD MHA
Director (Nursing)
Ruby General Hospital
Kolkata, West Bengal, India

Pradeep Michael D'Costa
DNB (Gen Med) Certificate in Critical Care ISCCM
ICU In-charge
KEM Hospital, Pune
Lead Intensivist Physician
Sahyadri Hospital
Pune, Maharashtra, India

Pragyan Kumar Routray
MBBS MD (Internal Medicine) IDCCM
Head
Department of Critical Care
Care Hospital
Bhubaneswar, Odisha, India

Prakash Shastri MD FRCA FICCM
Chairman, Institute of Critical Care Medicine
Department of Care Medicine
Sir Ganga Ram Hospital
New Delhi, India

Pramod Sood
MD (Pulmonary Medicine) IDCCM FNB (Critical Care Medicine) FICCM
Professor and Head
Department of Critical Care Medicine
Geetanjali Medical College
Udaipur, Rajasthan, India

Prashant Nasa MD FNB EDIC
Specialist
Institute of Critical Care Medicine
Max Super Speciality Hospital
New Delhi, India

Preetam Ranjan Sil MBBS MD (Medicine)
Consultant
Department of Critical Care
Manipal Hospital
Kolkata, West Bengal, India

Preeti Singh MSc (Nursing)
Coordinator, Trauma Center
Nursing Officer
Institute of Medical Sciences
Banaras Hindu University
Varanasi, Uttar Pradesh, India

Quadri SM MBBS CTCCM IDCCM FCCS
Consultant
Department of Critical Care Medicine
Dharamshila Narayana Superspeciality Hospital
New Delhi, India

Rahul Anil Pandit
MD FCICM FJFICM EDIC FICCM FCCP DA
Chair, Critical Care and EMS
Sir HN Reliance Foundation Hospital and Research Centre and All Other Reliance Healthcare Initiatives
Mumbai, Maharashtra, India

Rajarshi Roy MBBS MD
Consultant
Department of Critical Care
Manipal Hospitals
Kolkata, West Bengal, India

Rakesh Panchal MD FNB
Consultant
Department of Critical Care
SMVS Swaminarayan Hospital
Gandhinagar, Gujarat, India

Rakhee Baruah MBBS MD IDCCM
Head of Department Anesthesia and Senior Consultant
Department of Critical Care Medicine
Health City Hospital
Guwahati, Assam, India

Ranajit Chatterjee
MBBS MRCPI FRCPI DA EDIC FIACM
CMO SAG, Head Critical Care
Anesthesia, Internal Medicine, Critical Care
Swami Dayanand Hospital
New Delhi, India

Ranvir Singh Tyagi MD FICCM FCCM
Director
Department of Anesthesia and Critical Care Medicine
Synergy Plus Hospital and Galaxy Hospital
Agra, Uttar Pradesh, India
President Elect, ISCCM

Reshu Gupta Khanikar MBBS DA IDCCM
Senior Consultant
Department of Critical Care Medicine
Health City Hospital
Guwahati, Assam, India

Ritesh Shah MD IDCCM FICCM FIECMO
Director
Department of Critical Care
Shreeji Hospital and ICU
Vitals Multispecialty Hospital
Smt Jayaben Mody Hospital
Bharuch, Gujarat, India

Rohit Kumar Patnaik
MD DM (Critical Care Medicine) ESICM Fellowship in Severe Infections (Rome, Italy)
Specialist Critical Care Medicine
Medeor 24x7 Hospital
Abu Dhabi, UAE

Ronak Patel MBBS CTCCM IDCCM
Consultant Intensivist
Department of Critical Care
Shreeji Hospital and ICU
Vadodara, Gujarat, India

Rubina Khullar Mahajan MD EDIC IFCCM PDF
Associate Professor
Department of Critical Care Medicine
Dayanand Medical College and Hospital
Ludhiana, Punjab, India

Sachin Tambhare MBBS CTCCM
IDCCM Student
Department of Critical Care
Aditya Birla Memorial Hospital
Pune, Maharashtra, India

Sananda Chakraborty
BSc (Nursing) MSc (Medical Surgical Nursing)
Senior Nursing Supervisor
Department of Critical Care Medicine
Tata Medical Center
Kolkata, West Bengal, India

Sanjith Saseedharan Saroja
IDCCM EDIC FNNCC (ISRAEL) FICCM
Director
Department of Critical Care
SL Raheja Hospital—a Fortis Associate
Mumbai, Maharashtra, India

Saswati Sinha MD (Medicine) IDCCM EDIC
Senior Consultant
Department of Critical Care
Manipal Hospitals
Kolkata, West Bengal, India

Seema S Tekwani MD MHA
Associate Professor of Medicine
Division of Pulmonary, Allergy
Critical Care and Sleep Medicine
Emory University
Atlanta, GA, USA

Sharmili Sinha MD DNB EDIC FICCM FCCM
Senior Consultant
Department of Critical Care
Apollo Hospitals
Bhubaneswar, Odisha, India

Shrikant Suhas Sahasrabudhe
MD (Chest) IDCCM TDD
Head
Department of Critical Care
Medicine and Pulmonology
Senior Consultant Intensivist and Pulmonologist
KIMS Manavata Hospital
Nashik, Maharashtra, India

Shwetha Ram Chandankhede
MBBS MD IDCCM FICCM
Senior Consultant
Department of Critical Care Medicine
Virinchi Hospitals
Hyderabad, Telangana, India

Shyam Sunder Tipparaju MD FICCM
Director
Department of Critical Care Medicine
Virinchi Hospitals
Hyderabad, Telangana, India

Smita Singh MBBS
Senior Registrar
Department of Critical Care Medicine
Tata Main Hospital
Jamshedpur, Jharkhand, India

Snigdhadeb Ghosh
MBBS MD DrNB (PDT) Critical Care
DrNB PDT
Department of Critical Care
Manipal Hospitals
Kolkata, West Bengal, India

Subramani Kandasamy
MD (Anesthesia) DA FRCA CST FANZCA EDIC FICCM
Senior Professor
Department of Critical Care Medicine
Surgical Intensive Care Unit
Christian Medical College
Vellore, Tamil Nadu, India

Sudipta Mukherjee
MBBS MD IDCCM FNB EDICM FOAPM
Senior Consultant and Head
Department of Critical Care Medicine
Tata Medical Center
Kolkata, West Bengal, India

Susruta Bandyopadhyay MD Dip Card
Director
Department of Critical Care
Manipal Hospitals Broadway
Kolkata, West Bengal, India

Swagata Tripathy
MBBS MD DNB IDCC EDIC FSNCC (Hon) FICCM Fellow Neuroanesthesia, Walton Centre, Liverpool
Professor
Department of Anesthesiology and Critical Care
All India Institute of Medical Sciences
Bhubaneswar, Odisha, India

Swapnabharati Moharana MBBS MD (PGIMER)
Senior Resident
Assistant Professor
Postgraduate Institute of Medical Education and Research
Chandigarh, India

Swapnil Thulung MSc Nursing (Critical Care)
General Manager
Hospital Operations
Victor Hospital
Goa, India

Swarna Deepak Kuragayala
MD MRCP (UK) EDIC IDCCM IFCCM FIDM
Senior Consultant
Department of Critical Care Medicine
Professor of General Medicine
Apollo Health City and Apollo Institute of Medical Sciences and Research
Hyderabad, Telangana, India

Tapas Kumar Sahoo
MD FNB FICCM FCCP EDIC MBA Canadian Critical Care Fellowship
Associate Director and Head
Department of Critical Care
Medanta Hospital
Ranchi, Jharkhand, India

Urvi Shukla
MBBS MD DNB (Anesthesia) Eric FICCM
Director, Intensive Care Unit
Department of Critical Care
Aditya Birla Memorial Hospital
Pune, Maharashtra, India

Vitrag Shah
MD FNB (Critical Care) EDIC
Physician and Intensivist
Vitrag Hosptial
Surat, Gujarat, India

Vivek Badada DNB IDCCM FCC
Associate Professor
Department of Anesthesia and Critical Care
FH Medical College
Agra, Uttar Pradesh, India

Vivek Dave MD IDCCM EDIC FCCP
Head, Critical Care Unit
ISCCM Course Coordinator
Narayana Health
Ahmedabad, Gujarat, India

Yogesh Lakkas MD (Medicine)
Professor of Medicine and In-charge, ICU
JIIU's Indian Institute of Medical Science and Research
Jalna, Maharashtra, India

Foreword

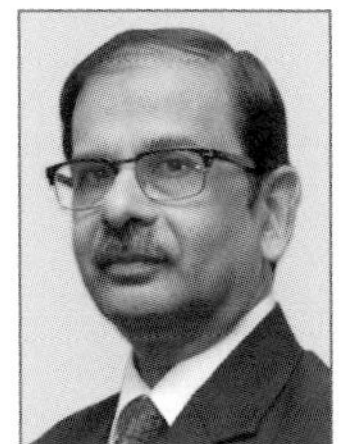

It gives me great pleasure to write a foreword for the book *ISCCM Manual of Critical Care Nursing* by the Indian Society of Critical Care Medicine (ISCCM). This book stands as a testament to the commitment of the ISCCM to critical care education.

The critical care nurse plays a vital role in the intensive care unit (ICU), where patients require constant monitoring and specialized care. Their role is crucial for stabilizing critically ill patients, saving lives and supporting families during an acute illness. The simplified, concise, and comprehensive way in which the chapters have been written makes the manual an essential tool for every critical care nurse. This manual will serve as an excellent guide to the nurses, enhancing their knowledge during their day-to-day working at the bedside in ICU.

In this manual, the editors have brought together an impressive group of authors including doctors and nurses. This book bridges a crucial gap in critical care education by harnessing the combined knowledge and wisdom of critical care physicians and nurses. It provides comprehensive coverage of most of the important aspects of critical care nursing. A wide range of topics have been included addressing various body systems, monitoring, and organ support. A range of general nursing topics including, but not limited to, airway management, sedation, nutrition, blood and fluid therapy have been covered in a lucid manner with illustrations to aid a better understanding. The manual also includes important content for nurses such as infection control, soft skills, disaster management, brain death, and organ donation among many others.

This manual is a labor of love to improve the quality of critical care nursing. It will undoubtedly enhance the knowledge and capabilities not only of the nurses, but also of anyone who reads it. This will undoubtedly benefit our ICU patients, their families, and healthcare systems. I congratulate the editors and authors on this outstanding service to critical care.

JV Divatia
MD FICCM
Head (Critical Care)
Lilavati Hospital and Research Centre
Mumbai, Maharashtra, India
Immediate Past President, Indian Society of Anaesthesiologists
Vice-Chancellor, College of the Indian Society of Anaesthesiologists
Past Editor-in-Chief, Indian Journal of Anaesthesia
Past President, Indian Society of Critical Care Medicine

Preface

It gives us great pleasure to bring forth this *ISCCM Manual of Critical Care Nursing*. The Indian Society of Critical Care Medicine (ISCCM) has a long legacy of educating doctors and nurses in the various aspects of critical care medicine. This book is the latest milestone in that aspect. As the name implies, this book is a manual, intended for the critical care nurses as well as the students of critical care nursing. It has been designed to be carried out and be used as a manual in day-to-day nursing. The manual contains several sections concentrating on various aspects such as initial assessment and stabilization, monitoring, general nursing care, systemic illnesses, etc. All the chapters have been kept brief and to the point. The authors have endeavored to give clear-cut instructions about how a nurse in the critical care department should act in different clinical situations. Some novel chapters have been included, keeping in mind the actual responsibilities of a nurse in an intensive care unit. Illustrations, graphics, tables, and flowcharts have been used frequently to make the book lucid. The brevity of the chapters has not compromised the quality of the information provided. Hence, the book can also be used as a basic textbook of critical care nursing. The contributors have been chosen from both physician/intensivists and critical care nurses. We want the book to be an excellent companion to all the nurses working in the intensive care units.

Ranvir Singh Tyagi
Susruta Bandyopadhyay
Sheila Nainan Myatra
Babu K Abraham
Sumit Ray

Acknowledgments

The idea of this book was conceived in the college board. We designed this book as a sequel to *ISCCM Manual for Critical Care Nursing* edited by Drs Prakash Shastri, BK Rao, and Shirish Prayag. That book has been the textbook for students of the Indian Diploma of Critical Care Nursing till date. We acknowledge the guidance by Dr Prakash Shastri, even while publishing the present book. We acknowledge the contributions from all the authors, who carved time out of their busy schedules to write their chapters. We are indebted to Dr JV Divatia for kindly writing the foreword. We remain grateful to Ms Ruby Sharma and Mr Akhilesh Saxena of M/s Jaypee Brothers Medical Publishers (P) Ltd, New Delhi, India, for extending utmost cooperation in publishing this book in the shortest possible time. We acknowledge the help from Drs Snigdhadeb Ghosh, Diptanjan Ray, and Zareen Kauser for spending long hours on editing and proofreading. Last, we are indebted to the ISCCM College Board, the Chancellor, Dr Pradip Kumar Bhattacharya, and the Vice Chancellor, Dr Sumit Ray, for their help and guidance.

Contents

SECTION 1: An Introduction to Critical Care Nursing

Section Editor: *Prakash Shastri*

1. **Intensive Care Unit Nursing: How is it Different?** 3
   Prakash Shastri
2. **Initial Nursing Assessment of a Patient Admitted to the Intensive Care Unit** 5
   Asif Ahmed, Mary Kutty Babu, Smita Singh, Agnideb Bhattacharjee
3. **Intensive Care Unit Rounds (FAST HUG BIDS) and Beyond** 12
   Pradeep Michael D'Costa, Nilesh Dnyaneshwar Chile
4. **Resuscitation of an Acutely Ill Patient** 27
   Nisha Bhojnagarwala, Preetam Ranjan Sil

SECTION 2: Monitoring

Section Editor: *Saswati Sinha*

5. **Bedside Monitoring: Oxygen, Carbon Dioxide, Blood Sugar, and Temperature** 35
   Rajarshi Roy, Snigdhadeb Ghosh
6. **Electrocardiogram and Arrhythmias** 45
   Shrikant Suhas Sahasrabudhe, Yogesh Lakkas
7. **Arterial Blood Gas Analysis and Electrolyte Imbalances** 56
   Deven Juneja, Prashant Nasa
8. **Hemodynamic Monitoring** 66
   Saswati Sinha, Amit Das

SECTION 3: Organ Support

Section Editor: *Pragyan Kumar Routray*

9. **High-flow Nasal Oxygen and Noninvasive Ventilation** 79
   Manoj K Singh, Rakesh Panchal
10. **Mechanical Ventilation Simplified** 88
    Pragyan Kumar Routray, Dharmajivan Samantaray
11. **Renal Replacement Therapy** 98
    Ranajit Chatterjee, Lalit Gupta

12. **The Role of Nurses in the Care of Extracorporeal Membrane Oxygenation Patients** 101
Rahul Anil Pandit, Arindam Kar

SECTION 4: Systems

Section Editor: *Reshu Gupta Khanikar*

13. **Cardiac Critical Care** 107
Ritesh Shah, Ankur Bhavsar, Vitrag Shah, Ronak Patel

14. **Critical Care Neurology and Neurosurgery** 116
Urvi Shukla, Sachin Tambhare

15. **Pulmonary Critical Care Nursing** 123
Sharmili Sinha, Alisha Chaudhury

16. **Emergencies in Gastroenterology** 130
Reshu Gupta Khanikar, Rakhee Baruah

17. **Care of a Patient Undergoing Major Surgery** 144
Vivek Dave, Anish Joshi

18. **Endocrine Emergencies** 149
Gunjan Chanchalani, Seema S Tekwani

19. **Trauma and Burns** 157
Ashutosh Bhardwaj, Quadri SM

SECTION 5: General Nursing

Section Editor: *Asif Ahmed*

20. **Airway Management** 165
Ranvir Singh Tyagi

21. **Oral and Eye Care in Critically Ill Patients** 172
Lalit Singh, Dharmendra Kumar Ojha

22. **Delirium and Sedation in Intensive Care Unit** 177
Swapnabharati Moharana, Swagata Tripathy

23. **Bedsore and Pressure Injuries** 184
Durgesh Satalkar

24. **Physiotherapy and Mobilization** 193
Parshotam Lal Gautam, Rubina Khullar Mahajan, Anoopjit Kaur

25. **Transferring a Critically Ill Patient** 201
Manish Munjal, Bikram K Gupta, Preeti Singh

26. **Nutrition** 207
Sanjith Saseedharan Saroja

27. **Defibrillation, Cardioversion, and Transcutaneous Pacing** 213
Shyam Sunder Tipparaju, Shwetha Ram Chandankhede

28. **Injections and Infusions** 223
Rohit Kumar Patnaik, Nupur Karan, Tapas Kumar Sahoo

29. **Transfusion Medicine** 233
Chandrashish Chakravarty

30. **Intravenous Fluid Therapy in Intensive Care Nursing** 237
Anand Vinaykumar Joshi

31. **Setting Up Trays** 250
Sananda Chakraborty, Sudipta Mukherjee

32. **Alarm Fatigue and Burn Out** 256
Susruta Bandyopadhyay, Diptanjan Ray

33. **Sample Collection** 260
Kanwalpreet Sodhi, Manender Kumar

34. **Nursing Care of the Terminally Ill** 268
Nandhakishore Jampala, Ganshyam Jagathkar

SECTION 6: Infection

Section Editor: *Kapil Sharad Borawake*

35. **Infection Control** 277
Kapil Sharad Borawake, Swarna Deepak Kuragayala

36. **Needlestick Injury** 283
Asif Ahmed, Amit Kumar Sharma

37. **Sterilization, Disinfection, and Waste Disposal** 288
Pramod Sood, Inderpreet Kaur

SECTION 7: Soft Skills

Section Editor: *Ajith Kumar AK*

38. **Communication for Nurses** 295
Ganesh KM, Ajith Kumar AK

39. **Documentation in Intensive Care Unit: Nursing Guideline** 300
Swapnil Thulung

40. **Nursing Standards and Quality Indicators** 308
Devi Prasad Samaddar, Parul Samadder

SECTION 8: Disaster Management

Section Editor: *Subramani Kandasamy*

41. Disaster Management 323
Subramani Kandasamy

SECTION 9: Brain Death and Organ Donation

Section Editor: *Bharat G Jagiasi*

42. Brain Death 331
Bharat G Jagiasi, Anand Srivastava

SECTION 10: Formulas and Scores

Section Editor: *Diptimala Agarwal*

43. Formulas and Scores Used in Intensive Care Unit 339
Diptimala Agarwal, Vivek Badada

Index 347

SECTION 1

An Introduction to Critical Care Nursing

Section Editor: *Prakash Shastri*

1. **Intensive Care Unit Nursing: How is it Different?**
   Prakash Shastri
2. **Initial Nursing Assessment of a Patient Admitted to the Intensive Care Unit**
   Asif Ahmed, Mary Kutty Babu, Smita Singh, Agnideb Bhattacharjee
3. **Intensive Care Unit Rounds (FAST HUG BIDS) and Beyond**
   Pradeep Michael D'Costa, Nilesh Dnyaneshwar Chile
4. **Resuscitation of an Acutely Ill Patient**
   Nisha Bhojnagarwala, Preetam Ranjan Sil

CHAPTER 1

Intensive Care Unit Nursing: How is it Different?

Prakash Shastri

INTRODUCTION

The intensive care unit (ICU) nurses are looked at with awe by their colleagues in the hospital because of the self-assurance which they carry themselves and being forthright in their statements. How does this come naturally to them is the question asked. One of the many reasons is that they have acquired knowledge during their early years in the ICU, which along with the inherent empathy that they have, empowers them to make decisions on their feet.

The difference in the ICU is that health care personnel are working under a constant threat to life. The stress levels are high and responses need to be immediate. Maintaining the high standard of intensive care is always a great challenge, and the nursing staff is the mainstay in achieving that goal.

Many issues in the critical care will require prompt corrective actions. The critical nurses will need to understand the importance of speed and promptness.

Most of the critical care units will employ much more gadgets than in the rest of the hospital. The nurses who work in critical care units must be more tech savvy. It is compulsory for all nurses working in a critical care unit to be well acquainted with all the instruments and gadgets in the ICU.

In addition to conventional nursing responsibilities, much of the clinical decision today is being decentralized to a skilled nursing staff. Thus, what we see today is the expanded role of nurses who take ownership in patient management besides implementing the ICU protocols.

The *seven Cs of critical care nursing* are as follows:

1. Compassion (toward the patient)
2. Communication (with the patient, the patient's relatives, and with the physicians)
3. Consideration (toward the patient, the patient's family)
4. Comfort (to the patient)
5. Carefulness (avoid causing harm)
6. Consistency (the high level of care to be provided 24 hours a day)
7. Closure (limitation and withdrawal of treatment, when it is futile)

EXPANDED ROLE OF NURSES

Drugs Therapy

Inotropes, vasodilators, sedatives, analgesics, insulin, heparin, and many other drugs are given by continuous intravenous (IV) infusion. The patients in the ICU need constant adjustment of these life-saving drugs. Adjustments of dose delivery and infusion rates is decided by nursing staff, based on clinical and laboratory data.

Weaning from Mechanical Ventilation

The weaning process from the ventilator of a ventilated patient (e.g., adjusting ventilatory rates and pressures) can be carried out by the nursing staff using weaning protocols, blood gas values, and bedside monitoring. They also keep a watch on the changes in the status of a ventilated patient and are the first to notice and react in emergency situations.

Infection Control

The entire gamut of processes and protocols involving infection control in the ICU revolves around the nurse. ICU is the place which handles most of the patients with serious infections. It is also one of the places which needs stringent infection control. The critical care nurses are an integral part of the infection control team of any hospital.

Organizing Communications with Other Health Care Teams

The nursing staff serves as a bridge between several teams that contribute to patient management, as well as dealing with their friends and relatives. Although it is difficult to quantify the effect of this role on patient outcome, most experienced intensivists value this aspect of their contribution highly. The nurses also play a major role in the end-of-life care. From looking into the patient's comfort to giving emotional support to the family members, the nurses are also in the team, which primes the patients' relatives for organ donation.

Ward Rounds and Continuity of Care

One of the most notable aspects of ICU is the comprehensive ward round each day when one shift hands over to the next shift. The half-life of major decisions regarding seriously ill patients is approximately 24 hours, whereas for patients in general wards it is approximately 3–4 days. The nursing staff and others involved in a patient's management formulate a strategy for the next 24 hours in these ward rounds. This is a framework around which fine-tuning can occur, depending on changes in the patient's condition and the findings on laboratory tests. Detailed handovers with a short- and long-term plan are essential for continuity and optimal management of the patient, especially by senior medical staff.

Communication Between the Various Specialists

The nurses play a major role in the communication between various specialties who become involved in the treatment of a particular patient. The specialists often do not visit the patient at the same time. It is the job of the critical care nurses to maintain the liaison between various specialties.

Relatives and Friends

The relations of the patient are more comfortable with the nurses, who explain the condition of the patient in an honest and forthright manner. They admit that many aspects of the patient's disease process are, as yet, unknown. An explanation of the possible time course of the patient's illness is conveyed. It is important to inform relatives of such possibilities, so that they can arrange their schedules regarding sleep, work, and other responsibilities.

Intensive care unit nurses are in demand the world over leading to high attrition rates for nurses. It is imperative on the part of senior medical and nursing staff to "break in" the new entrants and ensure that standards are maintained. Ultimately working effectively in an ICU is all about team work and bonhomie. The newcomers have to feel that they are part of a family and proud members of it.

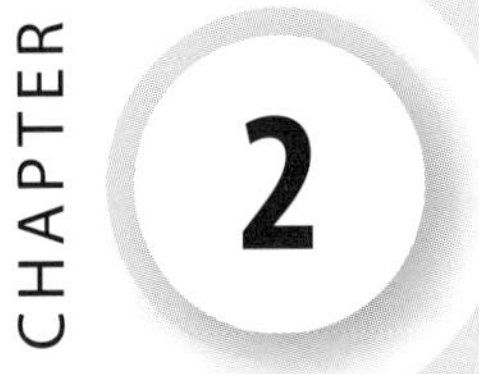

Initial Nursing Assessment of a Patient Admitted to the Intensive Care Unit

Asif Ahmed, Mary Kutty Babu, Smita Singh, Agnideb Bhattacharjee

INTRODUCTION

The initial assessment of a patient admitted to the intensive care unit (ICU) is a crucial and important step in the management of seriously ill patients. Though the initial assessment is multidisciplinary and involves intensivists, other specialists, and nurses, but the comprehensive and systematic approach of the ICU nurses, who are at the forefront, lays the foundation for good patient care and management and includes stabilization, monitoring, and planning of subsequent treatment. ICU nurses are specialized professionals who are well trained to handle complex patients and situations, including performing detailed patient assessment, administering medicines and treatment, identifying potential problems and complications, with necessary and timely interventions, coordinating and collaborating with other members of the healthcare team, and also providing emotional support to the patients.

There are multiple benefits of the initial assessment, when performed by the ICU nurses in a well-structured and systematic format, which includes:

- Early identification of the life-threatening situation on admission to the unit, where immediate resuscitation would help in stabilization of the patient
- Assessment of the severity of the disease
- Prioritization of the treatment and interventions
- Setting up of the baseline status of patients, as a reference for monitoring trend and progress
- Facilitating effective communication with the health-care team
- Preventing errors
- Improving patient safety
- Improving psychological support to patients and relatives, adding to better customer satisfaction

PREPARATION OF THE UNIT FOR RECEIVING THE PATIENT IN INTENSIVE CARE UNIT

The preparation of the unit for receiving the patient in an ICU aids in smooth transfer of the patient in the ICU, so that subsequent assessment and treatment can then be provided seamlessly. The unit includes the ICU bed, table, locker, and medical equipment like ventilator, monitor, suction unit, oxygen delivery unit, infusion pumps, and more, as required for safe and optimum patient management.

It includes:

- Prior protocolized cleaning and disinfection of the unit including all furniture and equipment
- Keeping all equipment like monitors, ventilators, crash carts checked, and in readiness for immediate usage; it should also include setting of the alarm limits on the devices.

- Checking of all medicines and consumables, as would be required for patient care for both resuscitation and subsequent care
- Availability of trained nurses for receiving the serious patients
- Ensuring a comfortable environment of the unit with adequate temperature and humidity control
- Ensuring good infection control practices like availability of hand sanitizers at the bedside and proper biomedical waste disposal provisions

RECEIVING THE PATIENT IN INTENSIVE CARE UNIT WITH PROPER HANDOVER

A proper *handover* at the time of receiving the patient in ICU gives relevant and important information about the patient, which also adds on to the initial assessment and appreciation of the patient's condition. Handover is a two-way communication process between a nurse, who gives or provides the patient details, and an ICU nurse, who takes over the patient, including both verbal as well as written information. It should include patient's past and current clinical condition including vital signs, relevant medical history including allergies, reason for admission to hospital and ICU, injuries if any, treatment received and planned for, diagnostics performed and planned for, investigation reports, visit and advise of treating doctors, or any other issue which could impact patient's stay in the ICU.

The above parameters should be proper documented and maintained in relevant record with legible signatures of the nurses, as it serves in providing complete details and information of the patient as part of the assessment and management approach.

INITIAL ASSESSMENT—SYSTEMATIC APPROACH

The first round of initial assessment by the ICU nurse is done to analyze the immediate patient-related concerns and need-based treatment and support. This is normally done both by the doctor and the nurse and can provide the double-check of missing key findings.

Initial assessment could be both subjective as well as objective, where the latter is more precise and preferred. ABCDE bundle approach is commonly practiced all across as an objective mode of assessment.

ABCDE bundle:

- *Airway:* To assess airway patency and its protection if necessary
- *Breathing:* To evaluate the respiratory parameters including oxygen saturation
- *Circulation:* To assess heart rate (HR), blood pressure, and perfusion
- *Disability:* To evaluate the neurological status [Glasgow Coma Scale (GCS) or Full Outline of UnResponsiveness (FOUR) score]
- *Exposure:* To assess temperature and evaluate for injuries or features of infection

Resuscitation: The ABC resuscitation model should be applied on all new admissions to the ICU and all nurses should follow the prescribed sequence of assessment and need-based intervention.

1. *Airway:* Signs of airway compromise are:
   a. Stridor
   b. Wheezing
   c. Snoring
   d. Gurgling sounds
   e. Use of accessory muscles
   f. Suprasternal retractions
   g. Cyanosis

Altered mental status with a reduced GCS score of <8 require airway protection by intubation.

Oxygen therapy to be administered as needed.

2. *Breathing:* Respiratory parameters to monitor are as follows:
   a. *Respiratory rate (RR):* Tachypnea (>24 breaths/min) indicates respiratory distress while bradypnea (<10 breaths/min) suggests impending respiratory failure.
   b. *Oxygen saturation:* Peripheral oxygen saturation (SpO_2) <90% requires urgent intervention.
   c. *Chest expansion and symmetry* should be checked for signs of pneumothorax, collapse, or effusion.
   d. *Arterial blood gases (ABGs):* ABGs determine the acid–base balance, oxygenation, and ventilation status.
   e. *Chest auscultation:* To assess for abnormal lung sounds (e.g., crackles in pulmonary edema, wheezing in bronchospasm, and absent breath sounds in pneumothorax)

   Respiratory support:
   a. Oxygen therapy (nasal cannula, non-rebreather mask, or ventilator support)
   b. Noninvasive ventilation (NIV), which includes continuous positive airway pressure (CPAP) or bilevel positive airway pressure (BiPAP)
   c. Invasive mechanical ventilation
   d. Bronchodilators and steroids in patients with obstructive airway diseases
3. *Circulation:* Cardiovascular parameters to monitor are as follows:
   a. *HR:* Tachycardia (>100 beats/min) may indicate shock, sepsis, or arrhythmias, while bradycardia (<50 beats/min) suggests heart block or impending arrest.
   b. *BP:* Hypotension (<90/60 mm Hg) may indicate shock and immediate fluid resuscitation and vasopressors should be provided.
   c. *Capillary refill time:* A prolonged refill of >3 seconds suggests poor perfusion.
   d. Central venous pressure (CVP) trend line can help in assessing the fluid status, where other modalities are not available.

   Cardiac examination:
   a. *Auscultation:* Murmurs may indicate valvular heart disease while muffled heart sounds could be due to pericardial effusion.
   b. Electrocardiogram (ECG) is required to detect ischemia, arrhythmias, and conduction abnormalities.

   Cardiovascular support:
   a. *Fluid resuscitation:* Administer IV fluids to restore blood volume and perfusion.
   b. *Vasopressor support:* Initiate vasopressors (e.g., norepinephrine) to support blood pressure.
   c. *Inotropic support:* Initiate inotropes (e.g., dobutamine) to support cardiac function.
4. *Disability:* Neurological status assessment is essential particularly in unconscious or post-trauma patients.

   Consciousness to be assessed using the GCS:
   a. *Mild brain injury:* GCS 13–15
   b. *Moderate brain injury:* GCS 9–12
   c. *Severe brain injury:* GCS ≤8 (consider intubation)

A FOUR scale can also be used for the neurological assessment.

Pupillary examination:
a. Fixed and dilated pupils suggest severe brain injury or herniation.

b. Unequal pupils (anisocoria) indicate raised intracranial pressure.
c. Decerebrate or decorticate posturing indicate damage to the brain stem.

Motor and sensory functions should be evaluated for all patients.

Other interventions:

a. Head-end elevation of the bed to 30° if increased intracranial pressure is suspected
b. Seizure prophylaxis
c. Antiedema medications
d. Blood glucose testing as hypoglycemia can mimic neurological impairment.

5. *Exposure:*
    a. *Temperature management:* Purpose is to assess and maintain normothermia (36–38°C).
    b. *Infection control:* Implementation of infection control measures, such as use of antibiotics, source control, and prevention of nosocomial infections.
    c. *Interventions:* Care of wound and pressure points, along with prevention of pressure sore, is important.

HEAD-TO-TOE ASSESSMENT (SECONDARY ASSESSMENT IN STABLE PATIENTS)

After life-threatening conditions are addressed, a comprehensive head-to-toe assessment ensures that all of the body systems are evaluated.

Head and neck:

- GCS
- Signs of trauma
- Assessment for stroke

Chest and respiratory system:

- Work of breathing and use of accessory muscles
- Auscultation for abnormalities

Cardiovascular system:

- Peripheral edema, peripheral pulses, and capillary refill time
- Signs of fluid overload
- Signs of heart failure

Abdomen and gastrointestinal system:

- Palpation for distension, tenderness, or rigidity
- Bowel sounds, vomiting, or gastrointestinal bleeding

Renal and urinary system:

- Monitoring of urine output (>0.5 mL/kg/h)
- Signs of dehydration

Musculoskeletal system:

- Motor power and movement of all limbs
- Presence of fractures or other injuries

FOCUSED ASSESSMENT BASED ON THE PATIENT CONDITION

In addition to systematic assessments, nurses must perform focused assessments depending on the patient's condition.

Cardiac assessment for acute coronary syndrome or heart failure:

- Chest pain (with relevant history)
- ECG
- Troponin and B-type natriuretic peptide (BNP) levels

Neurological assessment for stroke, head injury, and seizures:

- Assess reflexes
- Monitor for seizures
- Scoring systems

Respiratory assessment for pneumonia and obstructive diseases:

- Evaluation of oxygen requirement and support
- Monitoring for respiratory failure

LABORATORY AND IMAGING INVESTIGATIONS

All should be aware of the role of comprehensive laboratory and imaging modalities for proper diagnosis. Previous and new reports should be reviewed during the initial assessment and decision should be taken for doing repeat or fresh tests. It includes complete blood count, ABG, electrolytes, renal and liver function tests, inflammatory markers and cultures, and imaging studies like chest X-ray, ultrasound study, computed tomography (CT) scan or magnetic resonance imaging (MRI) scan.

It is important that all above assessments are done objectively and uniformly across the *unit*, based on a *checklist* with proper documentation and record.

The plan of treatment and intervention should be decided based on the above comprehensive assessment.

Various other tools like Early Warning Score (EWS), New Early Warning Score (NEWS), and Modified Early Warning Score (MEWS) are also available and can be applied in the unit, as per protocol.

COMMUNICATION

Effective communication by nurses in the ICU is of paramount importance as part of the initial assessment and subsequent management of patients. Communication could be among healthcare personnels, or it could be between healthcare personnel and patient or patients' relatives, where in both modes are essential initial activities, based on which further actions are initiated or implemented. ICU nurses being at the forefront and with high patient contact time are key to the above.

- Communication between healthcare personnels, both verbal as well as written, is important for effective collaboration, and safe patient management thereby minimizing errors and unwanted complications, leading to unfavorable outcome. A robust communication system including a handover process during the time of admission is very important and it adds value to the initial assessment of seriously ill patients in the ICU. Use of communication tools like ISBAR (Identify, Situation, Background, Assessment, Recommendation) reinforced with a *checkback* method at the bedside provides a structured and standardized format for use in the ICU. Language-related barrier should be addressed, key information sharing should be prioritized, and handover should happen in a quiet and less crowded area.
- Communication with patients and patients' relatives provides emotional and psychological support, by laying down the seeds of trust and prevents volatile situations in the unit. It also adds to the credibility of the unit and healthcare providers and improved customer satisfaction. Use of various soft skills and communication tools like AIDET, BLAST, SPIKES, and many more can bring about uniformity and standardization in the unit, along with of ease of training and monitoring compliance. Patient confidentiality and privacy should be strictly adhered to, at all times.

DOCUMENTATION

Documentation involves recording of the details of the patient, the condition, the diagnosis, and the treatment plans either manually or electronically. It benefits the other healthcare staff as a means of communication, as a record for subsequent follow-up, and for future reference including the medicolegal requirement.

It should be clear, precise, easy to understand, with important details in completeness, and in chronological order. There could be various formats for documentation, but it needs to be customized to the local requirements of the unit for best results.

Some of the documentation formats are:

- *Admission and discharge register:* Name, Age, Address, Hospital ID number, Date of Admission, Provisional diagnosis, Area from where the patient was shifted in, Medicolegal status, details of documents, and valuables with patient and ownership
- *Initial nursing assessment sheet (immediately after admission):* History, clinical details, current status with vital signs, objective assessment tools like ABCDE tool including head-to-toe assessment or EWS details, and intervention or treatment plan.
- *Continuous nursing assessment sheet:* Nursing care plan which includes subsequent assessment, monitoring, investigation reports, changes in condition, diagnosis, and treatment.
- *Daily monitoring tools:* EWS, MEWS, NEWS, or vital signs chart, as per the unit's protocol for continuous monitoring, appreciation of a change or deterioration in condition followed by the corrective action taken.
- *Intake-output chart:* Details of intake with different constituents, and the output in different forms
- *Diabetic chart:* Details of glycemic control with insulin therapy and monitoring of blood sugar levels.
- *Treatment card:* Details of medicines and drugs prescribed, dosage, frequency, and route of administration which should be countersigned by both the doctors and nurses.
- *Ventilator chart:* Includes details of oxygen and respiratory support with oxygen consumption details and patient related parameters
- *Activity chart:* Details of the different procedures performed which will be required for communication, record keeping, and capturing in the hospital billing system
- *Shift handover register:* Relevant details of patient and all associated activities as mentioned above

Documentation should be done as per standard formats created for each unit, tailored to their requirement, and notably included in the *standard operating procedure*. Every unit should train their staff to ensure compliance to the documentation requirement with constant training, monitoring, audit, with follow-up and review. Care should be taken to comply to the medicolegal requirements like entry of correct details and facts, avoidance of alterations, date and time, and proper signature with name and details.

CHALLENGES DURING INITIAL ASSESSMENT

The initial assessment by nurses is also fraught with challenges, which are encountered very commonly by all:

- A busy ICU with large number of admissions and cycling in a day would leave little time for a comprehensive and detailed assessment by the nurses, more so, if majority of patients require immediate and rapid interventions.
- Shortage of nurses in the unit would also pose a challenge for the initial assessment, which is both time- and labor-intensive.
- Work stress and excessive load may lead to decreased assessment accuracy with possibility of errors.

- Communication and language barrier could be a major factor for inadequate assessment, misdiagnosis, and incorrect interventions.
- A detailed assessment might not be possible in patients who are comatose or in altered sensorium.
- Absence of past medical records and history, improper handover, and lack of assessment facilities at certain centers could be a major challenge.

OVERCOMING THE CHALLENGES

To improve the working of the unit, it is important to overcome the challenges faced:

- Use of standardized assessment tools like the ABCDE approach would make the assessment more objective and easier to perform.
- Continuous training and monitoring the skills with constant feedback, would improve both awareness and the compliance.
- Taking care of the weakest link and mentorship programs can mitigate the performance-related issues.
- Effective communication with proper handover would ensure job completeness and minimize errors.
- Inculcation of a positive work atmosphere with good interpersonal relationship and teamwork can mitigate the work-related stress and inefficiency.
- Triaging and prioritization of patients in the unit can also aid in performing the patient-related work including the initial assessment.

CONCLUSION

The initial assessment of patients admitted to the ICU forms one of the cornerstones of the critical care nursing, which requires knowledge, expertise, vigilance along with empathy. Having understood the benefits of the initial assessment, like early detection of conditions demanding urgent interventions, planning treatment, monitoring, setting up baseline values with risk assessments, ensuring good communication and handover, it is imperative that this good practice is adopted by all as a step toward the improvement of the unit and better patient care and customer satisfaction.

FURTHER READING

1. Baid H, Creed F, Hargreaves J. Systematic assessment. Oxford Handbook of Critical Care Nursing, 2nd edition. Oxford: Oxford University Press; 2016.
2. Cathala X, Moorley C. Performing an A-G patient assessment: a step-by-step guide. Nurs Times. 2020;116(1):53-5.
3. Devlin JW, Skrobik Y, Gélinas C, Needham DM, Slooter AJC, Pandharipande PP, et al. Clinical practice guidelines for the prevention and management of pain, agitation/sedation, delirium, immobility, and sleep disruption in adult patients in the ICU. Crit Care Med. 2018;46(9):e825-e873.
4. Hill K. Essential critical care skills. Nurs Times. 2021;117(12):35-8.
5. Hodde NM, Engelberg RA, Treece PD, Steinberg KP, Curtis JR. Factors associated with nurse assessment of the quality of dying and death in the intensive care unit. Crit Care Med. 2004;32(8):1648-53.
6. Huygh J, Peeters Y, Bernards J, Malbrain ML. Hemodynamic monitoring in the critically ill: an overview of current cardiac output monitoring methods. F1000Res. 2016;5:F1000 Faculty Rev-2855.
7. Massey D, Chaboyer W, Anderson V. What factors influence ward nurses' recognition of and response to patient deterioration? An integrative review of literature. Nurs Open. 2016;4(1):6-23.
8. Thim T, Krarup NH, Grove EL, Rohde CV, Løfgren B. Initial assessment and treatment with the Airway, Breathing, Circulation, Disability, Exposure (ABCDE) approach. Int J Gen Med; 2012;5:117-21.
9. Toney-Butler TJ, Unison-Pace WJ. Nursing Admission Assessment and Examination. In: StatPearls. Treasure Island (FL): StatPearls Publishing; 2025.

CHAPTER 3

Intensive Care Unit Rounds (FAST HUG BIDS) and Beyond

Pradeep Michael D'Costa, Nilesh Dnyaneshwar Chile

INTRODUCTION

Critically ill patients require very close monitoring and care in the intensive care unit (ICU).

A large number of ICU personnel, including doctors, nurses, technicians, physiotherapists, and other supportive care workers are in constant contact with these patients.

There is a big heterogeneity in this group right from their understanding of the disease process to the "picking up of changes in the patients' parameters".

Hence, the importance of following protocols becomes extremely important in this group.

Taking "rounds" is a very important tool for this monitoring process.

Although it may sound simple, an ICU patient's round is a very complex one and can be a very time consuming one as well.

The purpose of this chapter is to simplify a method which can be easily used to improve general care of these patients.

It is important to stick to a checklist while taking the daily rounds of any ICU patient. Many of the points mentioned here as a checklist are adapted from the landmark article by JL Vincent in 2005 which describes a process called "FAST HUG" approach. Here, FAST HUG is a mnemonic to remember all the points of the checklist.

Subsequent additions to this approach were done in 2017 and the mnemonic changed to FAST HUGS BID.

Additional points were added for this approach in a surgical/complicated patient.

FAST HUG MAIDENS has also been described.

The FAST HUG components:
- F—Feeding
- A—Analgesia
- S—Sedation
- T—Thromboembolic prevention
- H—Head of bed elevation
- U—Stress ulcer prophylaxis
- G—Glucose control
- S—Spontaneous breathing trials
- B—Bowel movement
- I—Indwelling catheter
- D—De-escalation (of antibiotics)

In our practice, we have expanded the algorithm to include a few more points. So, the mnemonic now is as follows:

The FAST HUG components:
- F—Feeding
- A—Analgesia
- S—Sedation
- T—Thromboembolic prevention

Temperature monitoring
Tubes
H—Head of bed elevation
Hemodynamics
U—Stress ulcer prophylaxis
Urine output
- G—Glucose control
- S—Spontaneous breathing trials

Special bundles
- B—Bowel movement
- I—Indwelling catheter

Imbalances
D—De-escalation (of antibiotics)
Directed and decisive communication

APPLICATION OF THE PROTOCOL

Table 1 explains the salient features of the checklist.

TABLE 1: The components of FAST HUG BID.

Practice point	*Rationale*	*Comments*
	F for feeding	
• Institute a feeding plan as soon as feasible	Any patient >48 hours in ICU is considered a candidate for malnutrition	
• Make a quick assessment of the nutritional status of the patient	Use screening tools like SGA (subjective global assessment), MNA (mini nutrition assessment) NRS (nutritional risk screening), MUST (malnutrition universal screening tool) or modified NUTRIC (nutrition risk in the critically ill) scores. Else use history and clinical assessment like bodyweight, skinfold thickness, muscle mass, etc.	Reduction in muscle mass is associated with a prolongation of stay, and also more complications (infective, thrombotic)
• Start feeding as early as possible, enteral is the preferred route	Either oral or tube feeding should be instituted as early as possible, usually within 24–48 hours of admission	Studies show a reduction in infectious complications as well as length of ICU stay with early enteral nutrition
• Confirmation of tube placement is a prerequisite before tube feeding is commenced	• Confirmation may be done by either clinical methods (auscultation), checking the pH of the aspirate (whether the pH is <5.5), radiological methods like X-ray, ultrasound prior to feeding • A good suggested practice is also to check for tube "coiling" in oral cavity during rounds, as well as food particles in the oral cavity	An endobronchial insertion of the feeding tube is a very high risk of aspiration, infections, and collapsed lung **Figs. 1 and 2** show the proper position and wrong positions of the nasogastric tube
• Use great caution while administering parenteral nutrition	• A proper hand hygiene method, insertion port infection control policies, connection, labeling policies must be adhered to strictly • A dedicated separate line (either central or peripheral) must be used for PN infusions preferably • If peripheral lines are used, regular checks for phlebitis and changes if needed must be done	Improper handling can lead to life-threatening complications related to PN, like sepsis Thrombophlebitis is common and must be watched for **(Fig. 3)** As many solutions contain carbohydrates, lipids, monitoring is required for blood sugar and lipids and liver function

Contd...

Contd...

Practice point	*Rationale*	*Comments*
	A for analgesia	
• Perform a good pain assessment at bedside	• Assess pain by many methods, conscious patient may be asked subjectively about pain • Use various scales like VDS (verbal description scale) (pain thermometer) **(Fig. 4)** Visual analogical scale (VAS) **(Fig. 5)** Numerical rating scale (NRS) may be used	• Pain is not always easy to assess in the critically ill patient (many times ventilated) • It should be kept in mind that the patient may be very sensitive to pain during suctioning of an ET tube, dressing, position change, etc.
• Perform pain assessment by both subjective and other methods	Look for clinical findings like facial grimaces, movements, other expressions as well as physiological parameters (heart rate changes, respiratory rate changes)	*"PQRSTUV" mnemonic may be used:* P—Provocative/palliative factors Q—Quality of pain R—Region/area affected S—Severity T—Timing (continuous/ occasional) U—Understand, look for previous incidents V—Values of treatment
• Try nonpharmacologic methods first	• Music, sound therapy • Relaxation therapy • Cold therapy • Massage therapy may be tried	These therapies try to cure the sensory pain pathways as well as the perceptive pathways of emotion, affection, and cognition
• Pharmacologic therapies may be tried	• Opioids are the first line for non-neuropathic pains • Ketamine infusions, acetaminophen, gabapentin, NSAIDs, and regional anesthesia may be used	Use these approaches always with protocolized pain assessments at regular intervals
• Ensure adequate analgesia	May try either continuous infusions or boluses	• Avoid excessive analgesia which may lead to unwanted side effects like delirium or respiratory depression! • Oversedation may also increase the risks of venous thrombosis, polyneuropathy, reduced intestinal mobility, and increase the cost of stay and duration

Contd...

Contd...

Practice point	***Rationale***	***Comments***
	S for sedation	
• Use a structured tool to assess level of sedation and agitation	• Assess both the depth and quality of sedation • RASS—Richmond agitation sedation scale can be used **(Table 2)**	• RASS scale has shown to reduce the dose of sedatives as well as length of mechanical ventilation • Higher methods like frontalis electromyogram, lower esophageal contractility, continuous EEG, and evoked potentials (sensory/auditory) are not easily available
• Get the level of sedation right	• One should try for a light sedation (unless the clinical condition demands more deepening of sedation) • Intermittent bolus or continuous infusion may be used to achieve this level • An attempt should be made for daily interruption of sedation (unless contraindicated) to assess the patient both neurologically and for chances of weaning from ventilator	May use CCC mnemonic: C—Calm C—Comfortable C—Collaborative To determine appropriate sedation levels
• Use pharmacologic agents judiciously and smartly	Various medications like benzodiazepines (midazolam, diazepam, lorazepam), propofol, ketamine, remifentanil, fentanyl, and dexmedetomidine may be considered based on the patients clinical status	Some guidelines recommend: • Midazolam for short-term sedation • Lorazepam for long-term sedation • Propofol for those requiring intermittent awakenings
	T for thromboprophylaxis	
• First assess the risk of deep vein thrombosis	The most commonly used score is the Wells score **(Table 3)**	Probability of developing thrombotic complications can be computed
• Decide the type of thromboprophylaxis	• Mechanical thrombo-prophylaxis is only recommended alone when contraindications exist to anticoagulation (platelets <50,000 or high risk of bleed or in acute hemorrhagic strokes, etc.)	The benefit of thromboprophylaxis must always be weighed against the risk of bleeding

Contd...

Contd...

Practice point	***Rationale***	***Comments***
	• Intermittent pneumatic compression devices are preferred over graded stockings **(Fig. 6)** • LMWH is usually preferred over unfractionated heparin (UFH) for pharmacological prophylaxis • UFH is preferred in patients with severe renal insufficiency	
	T for temperature monitoring	
Pick up variations in temperature and act fast. Core temperature monitoring is preferred in patients with serious temperature-related problems	• Reduce temperature by drug cooling or physical cooling measures (ice packs, cooling blankets, and water baths)	High persistent fever (>38°C) is associated with increased risk of mortality
	• Hypothermia (<32°C) also should be picked up early and acted upon by warmers, blankets, etc.	Hypothermia, if prolonged, may cause arrhythmias, coagulopathy and may interfere with neurological reflexes
	T for tubes	
An ICU patient requires close monitoring for all possible tubes/drains	• Commonly used tubes include endotracheal tubes, nasogastric tubes, feeding gastrostomy tubes, urine catheters, drainage tubes, intercostal drain tubes, surgical and postoperative drains • Daily of tube positions, drain positions, quality, days, local examinations must be done • Dressings must be inspected, changed and monitored very closely • Clear instructions on tube fixation points (ETT tie), tube durations (days), local infection signs must be noted and brought to the notice of the treating team	• Tube dislodgement, tube malposition (ETT dislodgement, accidental drain removals) are a major cause of increased duration of stay, cost, and morbidity **(Fig. 7)** • Inadequate care of these tubes can be a major cause of infections and nosocomial sepsis
	H for head of bed elevation/position	
Position patients appropriately in the ICU	• Head end of the bed should be elevated at 45° as an important part of the VAP prevention bundle of care	• Many studies have shown incidence of VAP, bed sores to be higher in patients who did not get proper positioning or position changes

Contd...

Contd...

Practice point	***Rationale***	***Comments***
	• 2 hourly position changes from supine position to lateral is considered by many as a standard of care • Prone positioning may be done in critically ill patients with ARDS (special care to be taken for the pressure points on the face and the chest of a prone patient) • Rotatory beds may be used where available beneficial in patients with lung pathologies	• Attempts must be made to keep the thorax of patient also elevated at 45° as critically ill patients when sedated may involuntarily slip down along the bed
	H for hemodynamics	
Keep a close watch on hemodynamic parameters is the key to good outcomes	• At the bedside close watch should be made for basal parameters particularly the sudden changes • Trends in parameters should be actively picked up and brought to the notice • Arrhythmias many a time are picked up at the bedside and may change outcomes drastically (e.g., patient in ventricular tachycardia, if missed, may lose his/her life)	Multiple methods and modalities are available at bedside like NIBP, invasive arterial pressures, point of care ultrasound, etc. for monitoring
	U is for stress ulcer prevention	
Use stress ulcer prophylaxis when recommended	• H_2-receptor antagonists, proton pump inhibitors, are the commonly used prophylactic medications Sucralfate is not commonly used for this purpose • An enteral PPI is preferred over a parenteral one Commonly used PPIs are pantoprazole, lansoprazole, and omeprazole • No recommendations of a PPI over a H_2-receptor blocker	Certain groups of critically ill patients are at an increased risk of stress ulcers especially those on ventilator (>48 hours), preexisting peptic ulcer disease, steroid therapy, coagulopathies (platelet count <50,000, INR >1.5, aPTT >2 times normal), patients in shock, patients with GI bleeds in past 1 year, burns >35% BSA They require close attention
	U for urine output	
Accurate and timely documentation of urine output in the ICU is an important part of monitoring	• Measure the urine output on an hourly basis in the ICU	• Urine output can help identify patients of AKI

Contd...

Contd...

Practice point	***Rationale***	***Comments***
	• Reduction or increase in output may be observed every few hours and appropriate action taken. The minimum adequate urine output is taken as 0.5 mL/kg bodyweight	• Care must be taken to accurately measure and report output, many times the healthcare workers given this responsibility require to be overseen to prevent errors in quantification
G for glycemic control		
• Correctly measure the blood sugar level with appropriate equipment	Measure the blood sugar level at bedside either by the glucometer or conventional blood sugar testing in the laboratory	• A very stringent blood sugar control has been associated with adverse out comes (CBG <110 mg/dL) • Many guidelines recommend keeping sugar levels below 180 mg/dL
• Correctly use glucometer at bedside	Be familiar with correct procedure to do the blood sugar level at bedside by glucometer **(Fig. 8)**	• Use the sides of fingers for testing • Do not squeeze the finger as that can create false results • Do not use expired strips • Calibrate the glucometer at regular intervals
• Use appropriate monitoring to maintain sugar control • See the reference number 17 for further reading	• Use unit-specific protocols to monitor and control sugars • Sliding scales are not recommended, readymade nomograms may be referred to with fixed duration sugar monitoring (at intervals of 1–2 hours, pre-meal monitoring) • Insulin requirements may be calculated on a daily basis to get an idea of increasing or reducing requirements • Good dietary instructions must be given to avoid errors and difficulty in sugar management	• Caution must be taken in patients who are already on antidiabetic medications, both oral hypoglycemic agents and insulins (rapidly acting, long acting, basal) • Stopping or switching these agents must be made after a close review of overall condition, liver, renal function tests and sepsis • Patients on sympathomimetic drugs should be closely monitored as they may have wide variations in sugar levels (use of pressor agents) • Nutritional supplements must be chosen carefully based on their glycemic indices
S for spontaneous breathing trial		
Assess closely for a possibility of liberation from mechanical ventilation	• Use either SBT-PS (spontaneous breathing trial with pressure support) or SBT-TP (spontaneous breathing trial with T piece)	• SBT-PS—lower pressure support <10 cm water ± PEEP • SBT-TP—disconnect ventilator and put on T piece with/without oxygen

Contd...

Contd...

Practice point	***Rationale***	***Comments***
	• Use appropriate oxygen delivery device (mask, NIV, high-flow oxygen)	
	S for special care bundles	
Try to implement care bundles to improve outcomes of the critically ill patient	• Antibiotic care bundle • VAP bundle [ventilator-associated pneumonia bundle: notably elevation of the head end **(Fig. 9)**] • CLABSI bundle (central line-associated bloodstream infection) • CAUTI bundle (catheter-associated urinary tract infection bundle) • Sepsis bundle (surviving sepsis guidelines)	• Following care bundles attempts to standardize quality of care and also prevent mishaps and nosocomial infections in the ICU • Quality control and audits of units can be conducted based on adherence to these bundles and appropriate corrective measures taken based on results
	B for bowel movement	
Monitor for regular bowel movements	• Appropriate care must be given to the bowel especially if the patient is sedated • Appropriate laxatives may be used as per the clinical situation • Excessive bowel movement should also be looked for and measures taken to correct • Look for gaseous bowel distension or ileus before finalizing the feeding schedule	• Constipation and diarrhea are often overlooked entities in the ICU
	I for indwelling lines/catheters	
Remove indwelling lines/venous catheters as soon as feasible	• Daily assessment of all indwelling lines/catheters must be made • Note should be made about number of days, local reactions, as well as technical difficulties during insertion process • Removal of all such indwelling catheters/lines must be made at regular intervals by the treating team and removal attempted as soon as possible	Indwelling catheters/lines are a major source of nosocomial sepsis, and should be removed as quickly as possible

Contd...

Contd...

Practice point	***Rationale***	***Comments***
	I for imbalances	
• Watch out closely for imbalances in homeostasis and act swiftly to correct the same	• Daily or multiple daily reviews must be done for abnormal laboratory values (electrolytes, special laboratory like cultures), values must be brought to notice of treating team and acted upon fast • A proper handover among all team members at end of duty hours to be given to prevent delays in getting reports or errors in transport of samples to appropriate laboratory	• Time delays between the collection of the blood, transport to laboratory, running of the test, and reporting can occur and must be prevented • Samples must be sent in prescribed containers only to prevent delays (EDTA, fluoride bulb) • Certain tests which have a longer turnover time like cultures, some PCR assays must be followed and acted upon
• Fluid charting must be done properly	Correctly chart fluid balances including all intake of oral and IV medication, feeding quantities, medication quantities, as well as losses of fluids, including urine, stool, insensible losses with appropriate considerations for fever, procedures, etc.	Good fluid management is crucial in overall outcome. Remember 5 R's with fluids: 1. R—Resuscitation 2. R—Routine maintenance 3. R—Replacement 4. R—Redistribution 5. R—Reassessment
	D for drug de-escalation	
• De-escalate antibiotics at the earliest	• A close watch on improvement in clinical condition and septic focus must be made • All attempts must be made to de-escalate antibiotics as early as possible or narrow spectrum based on the diagnosis • Usual duration of antibiotics is 7–10 days, unless ongoing septic focus or a multidrug-resistant infection or a disease process requiring longer duration (endocarditis, pyelonephritis) • Days of antibiotic use may be charted on the ICU sheet as a ready reckoner	• Improper duration and inadequate duration of antibiotics are one of the most common causes of drug resistance in the critical care unit • Antibiotic stewardship programs are required to be strictly followed by the team
	D for direct and decisive communication	
Good effective communication among all team members at all times is the key to success of a unit	• Follow all rules of good communication, both verbal and written for better patient care	Good communication among all team members is the key to a safe and strong ICU

Contd...

Contd...

Practice point	***Rationale***	***Comments***
	• *Communication among all team members:* Doctor, nurse, patient, allied staff, medical administration, and allied departments must be clear, precise, accurate, and to the point • Clear transparent communications for consents for patient care, procedures, and operations must be done • Written communications to be documented for critical decisions, procedures, and carried forward among all duty shifts	

(AKI: acute kidney injury; ARDS: acute respiratory distress syndrome; aPTT: activated partial thromboplastin time; BSA: body surface area; ETT: endotracheal tube; GI: gastrointestinal; ICU: intensive care unit; INR: international normalized ratio; LMWH: low molecular weight heparin; NIBP: noninvasive blood pressure; NIV: noninvasive ventilation; NSAIDs: nonsteroidal anti-inflammatory drugs; PCR: polymerase chain reaction; PEEP: positive end-expiratory pressure; PN: parenteral nutrition; PPI: proton pump inhibitor)

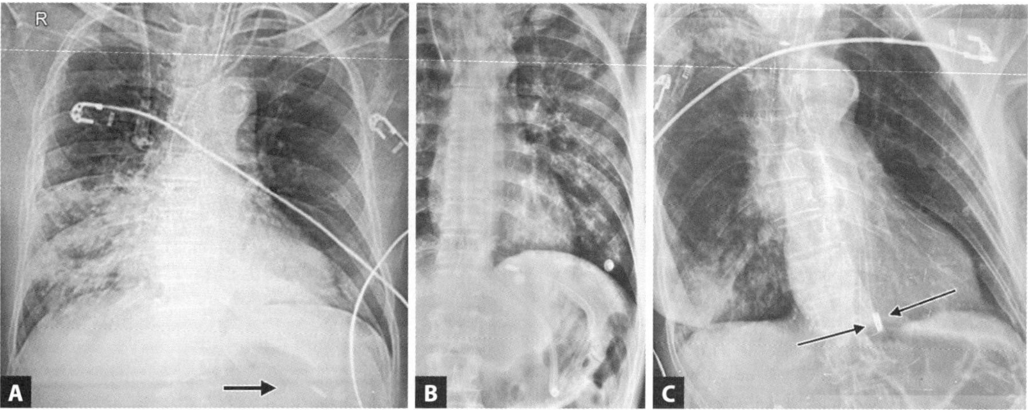

Figs. 1A to C: (A) Nasogastric tube in situ;(B) Nasogastric tube in stomach (subdiaphragmatic); and (C) Nasogastric tube malposition.

CONCLUSION

Components of the above article must be considered by all team members attending patients.

It is a good practice to run through all the points every time one comes in contact with the patient.

The protocol has been modified from the original protocol by Dr JL Vincent, and subsequently the FAST HUGS BID protocol which has been described.

We feel this approach would cover most of the points in the ICU which lead to errors and indeed improve success and quality of carer.

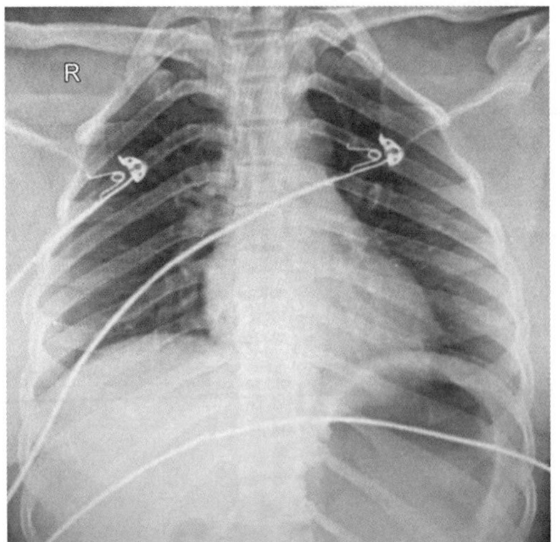

Fig. 2: Cautions with nasogastric tube with gastric dilatation.

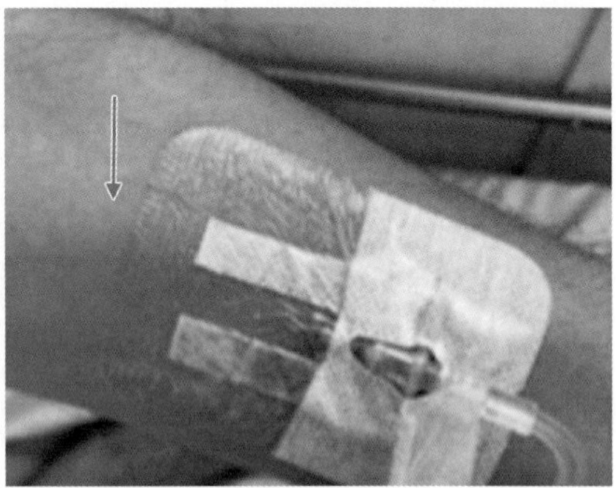

Fig. 3: Thrombophlebitis after TPN. (TPN: total parenteral nutrition)

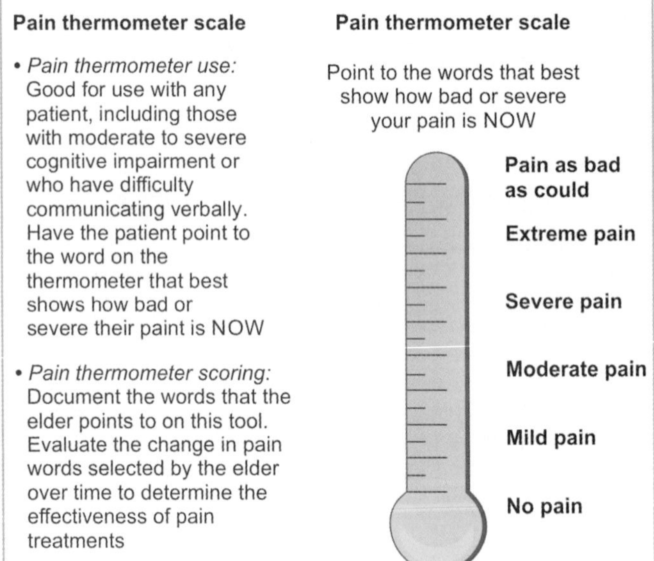

Fig. 4: Pain thermometer/VDS. (VDS: verbal description scale)

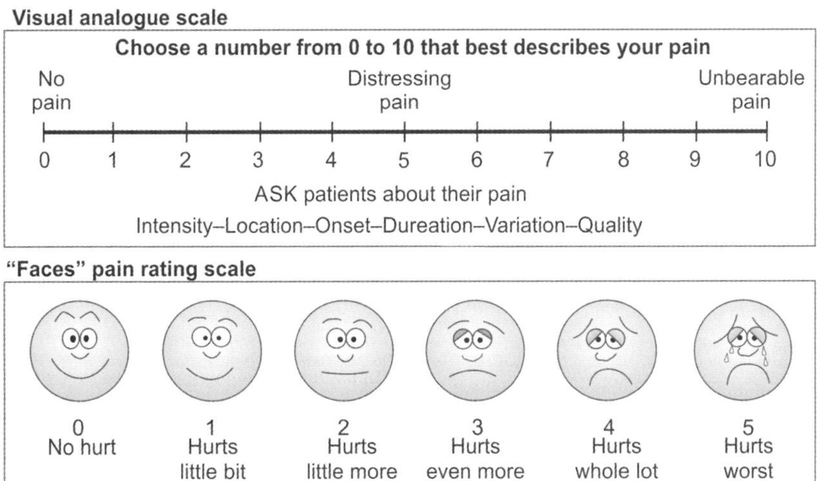

Fig. 5: VAS (visual analog scale).

TABLE 2: Richmond agitation sedation scale (RASS).

Score	***Term***	***Description***	
+4	Combative	Overtly combative, violent, immediate danger to staff	
+3	Very agitated	Pulls or removes tube(s) or catheter(s), aggressive	
+2	Agitated	Frequent nonpurposeful movement, fights ventilator	
+1	Restless	Anxious but movements not aggressively vigorous	
0	Alert and calm		
−1	Drowsy	Not fully alert but has sustained awakening (eye opening/eye contact) to *voice* (≥10 seconds)	Verbal stimulation
−2	Light sedation	Briefly awakens to *voice* with eye contact (<10 seconds)	
−3	Moderate sedation	Movement or eye opening to *voice* (but no eye contact)	
−4	Deep sedation	No response to voice but movement or eye opening to *physical* stimulation	Physical stimulation
−5	Unarousable	No response to *voice* or *physical* stimulation	

Note:
Levels −1 to −5 denote 5 levels of sedation.
Levels +1 to +4 describe increasing levels of agitation.
RASS level 0 is "alert and calm".

TABLE 3: Wells criteria.

Wells criteria for the prediction of deep vein thrombosis (DVT)[a]:	
Clinical characteristic	***Score***
Active cancer (patient either receiving treatment for cancer within the previous 6 months or currently receiving palliative treatment)	1
Paralysis, paresis, or recent cast immobilization of the lower extremities	1
Recently bedridden for ≥3 days, or major surgery within the previous 12 weeks requiring general or regional anesthesia	1
Localized tenderness along the distribution of the deep venous system	1
Entire leg swelling	1
Calf swelling at least 3 cm larger than that on the asymptomatic side (measured 10 cm below tibial tuberosity)	1
Pitting edema confined to the symptomatic leg	1
Collateral superficial veins (nonvaricose)	1
Previously documented deep vein thrombosis	1
Alternative diagnosis at least as likely as deep vein thrombosis	–2

Note: [a]Wells scoring system for DVT: –2 to 0: low probability, 1–2 points: moderate probability, 3– 8 points: high probability

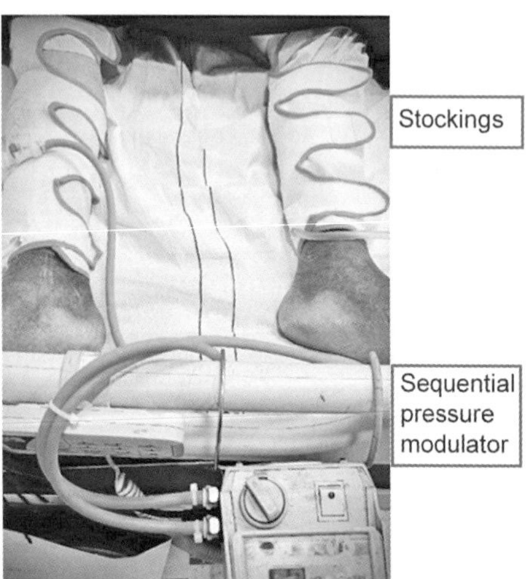

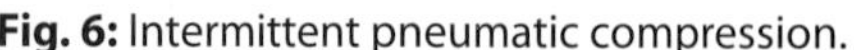

Fig. 6: Intermittent pneumatic compression.

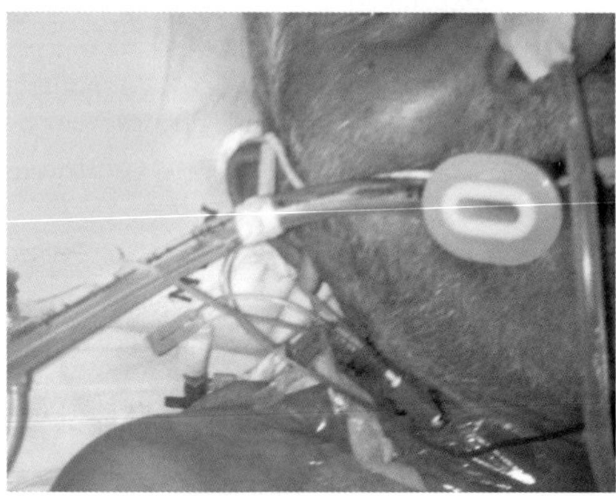

Fig. 7: Dislodged ETT. (ETT: endotracheal tube)

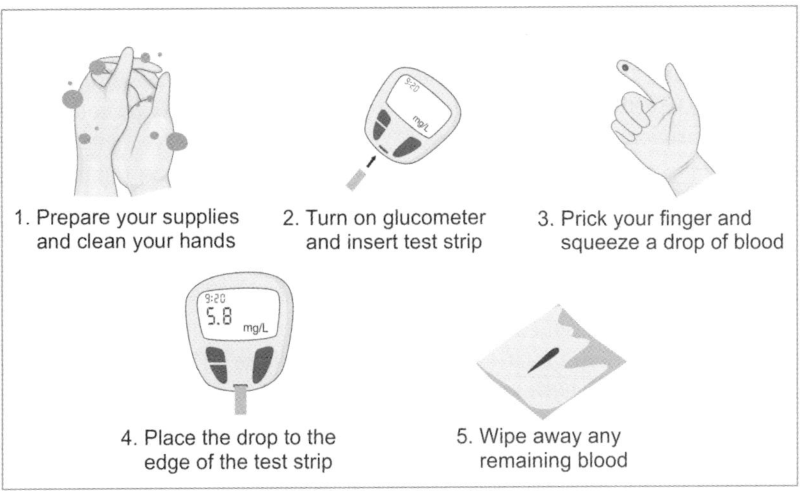

Fig. 8: Use of glucometer.

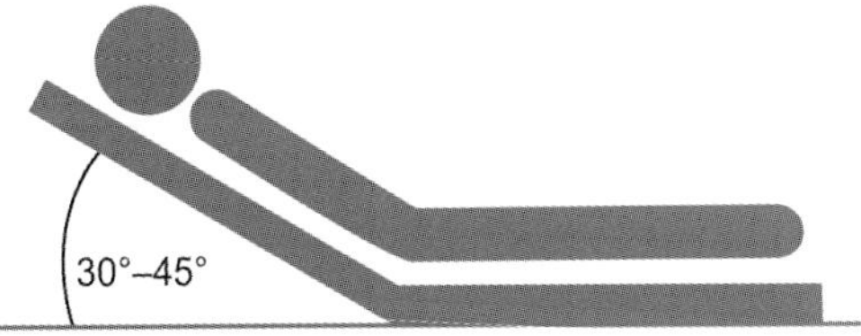

Fig. 9: Head of bed elevation.

Some additional points have been added keeping the scenario and functioning of ICUs in our country.

FURTHER READING

1. Al-Shamaly HS. Patterns of communicating care and caring in the intensive care unit. Nursing Open. 2022;9:277-98.
2. Bird SB, Dickson EW. Clinically significant changes in pain along the visual analog scale. Ann Emerg Med. 2001;38(6):639-43.
3. Chauhan D, Varma S, Dani M, Fertleman MB, Koizia LJ. Nasogastric Tube Feeding in Older Patients: A Review of Current Practice and Challenges Faced. Curr Gerontol Geriatr Res. 2021;2021:6650675.
4. Clayton S, Petrungaro J, Starr F, Mbekeani K, Sriram K, Khorasani A, et al. Implementation of an evidence-based stress ulcer prophylaxis protocol in the ICU. Crit Care. 2006;10 (Suppl 1):P222.
5. De Waele JJ, Schouten J, Beovic B, Tabah A, Leone M. Antimicrobial de-escalation as part of antimicrobial stewardship in intensive care: no simple answers to simple questions—a viewpoint of experts. Intensive Care Med. 2020;46:236-44.
6. Ellia M. The 'MUST' report. Nutritional screening for adults: a multidisciplinary responsibility. Redditch: BAPEN; 2003.
7. Goldhill DR, Badacsonyi A, Goldhill AA, Waldmann C. A prospective observational study of ICU patient position and frequency of turning. Anaesthesia. 2008;63:509-15.
8. Hamdan M, Puckett Y. (2023). Total Parenteral Nutrition. Available from https://www.ncbi.nlm.nih.gov/books/NBK559036/. [Last accessed February, 2025]
9. Helms J, Middeldorp S, Spyropoulos AC. Thromboprophylaxis in critical care. Intensive Care Med. 2022;49:75-8.
10. Honarmand K, Sirimaturos M, Hirshberg EL, Bircher NG, Agus MSD, Carpenter DL, et al. Society of Critical Care Medicine Guidelines on Glycemic Control for Critically Ill Children and Adults 2024. Crit Care Med. 2024;52(4):e161-81.

11. Jin K, Murugan R, Sileanu FE, Foldes E, Priyanka P, Clermont G, et al. Intensive Monitoring of Urine Output is Associated With Increased Detection of Acute Kidney Injury and Improved Outcomes. Chest. 2017;152(5):972-9.
12. Kondrup J. Nutritional risk screening (NRS 2002): a new method based on an analysis of controlled clinical trials. Clin Nutr. 2003;22:321-36.
13. Leoni MLG, Moschini E, Beretta M, Zanello M, Nolli M. The modified NUTRIC score (mNUTRIC) is associated with increased 28-day mortality in critically ill COVID-19 patients: Internal validation of a prediction model. Clin Nutr ESPEN. 2022;48:202-9.
14. Meng L, Wang C, Liu X, Bi Y, Zhu K, Yue Y, et al. Temperature management in the intensive care unit: a practical survey from China. Libyan J Med. 2023;18:1.
15. Metheny NA, Frantz RA. Head-of-bed elevation in critically ill patients: a review. Crit Care Nurse. 2013;33(3):53-66; quiz 67.
16. Mezidi M, Yonis H, Chauvelot L, Danjou W, Dhelft F, Bazzani A, et al. Pressure support and positive end-expiratory pressure versus T-piece during spontaneous breathing trial in difficult weaning from mechanical ventilation: study protocol for the SBT-ICU study. Trials. 2022;23:993.
17. Neme D, Aweke Z, Micho H, Mola S, Jemal B, Regasa T. Evidence-Based Guideline for Adult Sedation, Pain Assessment, and Analgesia in a Low Resource Setting Intensive Care Unit: Review Article. Int J Gen Med. 2020;13:1445-52.
18. Nordness MF, Hayhurst CJ, Pandharipande P. Current Perspectives on the Assessment and Management of Pain in the Intensive Care Unit. J Pain Res. 2021;14:1733-44.
19. Silveira PC, Ip IK, Goldhaber SZ, Piazza G, Benson CB, Khorasani R. Performance of Wells Score for Deep Vein Thrombosis in the Inpatient Setting. JAMA Intern Med. 2015;175(7):1112-7.
20. Singer P, Blaser AR, Berger MM, Calder PC, Casaer M, Hiesmayr M, et al. ESPEN practical and partially revised guideline: Clinical nutrition in the intensive care unit. Clin Nutr. 2023;42:1671-89.

CHAPTER 4

Resuscitation of an Acutely Ill Patient

Nisha Bhojnagarwala, Preetam Ranjan Sil

INTRODUCTION

Resuscitation means reviving a patient from a death-like situation or from unconsciousness. Although we have excellent protocols for a pulseless patient [Acute Cardiopulmonary Life Support (ACLS)], the scope of resuscitation is much broader. Often it is the critical care nurse who first receives a patient and hence it is the nurse who starts the process of resuscitation. Here we will discuss the resuscitations of:

- A pulseless patient
- A patient in severe shock
- A patient with acute respiratory distress
- An unconscious patient

The other resuscitations like patients of trauma will be discussed in the respective chapters.

INITIAL APPROACH TO A CRITICAL PATIENT

- It is essential to use ABCD approach to assess and treat the patient. This means checking the Airway, Breathing, Circulation, and Disability (neurological defect).
- Always ask for the help while handling an unstable patient.
- Do complete initial assessment and reassessment regularly.
- Stabilize a patient with life-threatening problem before moving to next step.
- Attach patient to monitor and observe the vitals like peripheral oxygen saturation (SpO_2), electrocardiogram (ECG), respiratory rate, and blood pressure (BP).
- Insert intravenous (IV) cannula and send blood sample for arterial blood gas and chemistry analysis, check the capillary blood glucose.

IDENTIFYING AN UNSTABLE PATIENT

Most of the critically ill patients are easily identifiable as unstable. They may be pulseless, not breathing, or taking agonal breaths or tachypneic, with hypotension, or unconscious. Sometimes using scores like National Early Warning Score (NEWS) or Modified Early Warning Score (MEWS) will help in identifying the unstable patient. The calculators for such scores are available online.

Modified Early Warning Score is given in **Table 1**.

A Pulseless Patient

A pulseless patient who is not breathing should be treated as per ACLS protocol. Although we mention as a pulseless patient, there may be patients with severe bradycardia, serious tachyarrhythmias (like ventricular tachycardia), and respiratory arrest. The full ACLS protocol is beyond the scope of this manual. It is offered as a course. A basic flowchart for cardiopulmonary resuscitation (CPR) is given in **Flowchart 1**.

TABLE 1: Modified Early Warning Score.

Score	*3*	*2*	*1*	*0*	*1*	*2*	*3*
Systolic blood pressure (mm Hg)	<70	71–80	81–100	101–199		≥200	
Heart rate (beats/min)		<40	41–50	51–100	101–110	11–129	≥130
Respiratory rate (breaths/min		<9		9–14	15–20	21–29	≥30
Temperature (°C)		<35		35–38.4		>38.5	
Level of consciousness				Alert	Reacting to voice	Reacting to pain	Unresponsive

A Patient in Shock

Shock basically means a lack of tissue perfusion and oxygenation. It is usually but not always found in a patient with hypotension. Hypotension conventionally means a BP <90/60 mm Hg. One needs to look for skin color and temperature of the extremities. Cold, clammy extremities are due to peripheral vasoconstriction that redirects blood to vital organs during hypotension. Cyanotic and mottled appearance is late feature of shock. Warm hyperemic skin does not rule out shock as may be present in distributive shock (to be described later).

Assessment of circulation:

- Assess capillary refill time. Apply firm pressure to a nail in a finger or toe for 10 seconds so as to blanch it and then release the pressure. If the time taken for the normal color to reappear is >3 seconds, it indicates poor peripheral perfusion.
- Assess pulse rate as younger patients develop severe tachycardia before developing hypotension in late stages of shock.
- Measure BP. Hypotension is present in majority of patients with shock. In early stages of shock, patients can be normotensive or hypertensive.
- Assess arterial blood gas for metabolic acidosis and high lactate levels.
- Assess urine volume.
- Record 12 lead ECG to see for life-threatening arrhythmias or acute coronary syndrome.
- Look for obvious source of bleeding.
- Arrange echocardiogram and ultrasonography to identify the etiology.
- Chest X-ray should be done especially in trauma patient to rule out tension pneumothorax.
- Establish 14–18 G IV cannula for resuscitation with IV fluid in patient with shock. Peripheral IV access is preferred over central venous access for large-volume fluid resuscitation.
- Patients suspected of having anaphylactic shock, e.g., facial and angioedema, urticaria, history of exposure to allergens, should receive immediately injection of epinephrine (1:1000) 0.5 mg intramuscularly in anterolateral aspect of thigh.
- Start a vasopressor agent (usually norepinephrine) if the BP remains low, to stabilize the BP, while the work up and the fluid resuscitation are continuing.

The common types of shock are as follows:

- *Hypovolemic shock:* This means the hypotension is due to a loss of fluids from the body. This may be due to causes like diarrhea, vomiting, burns, excess diuresis, etc. The treatment is mainly infusion of fluids. Crystalloid fluids like normal

Flowchart 1: Cardiopulmonary resuscitation (CPR).

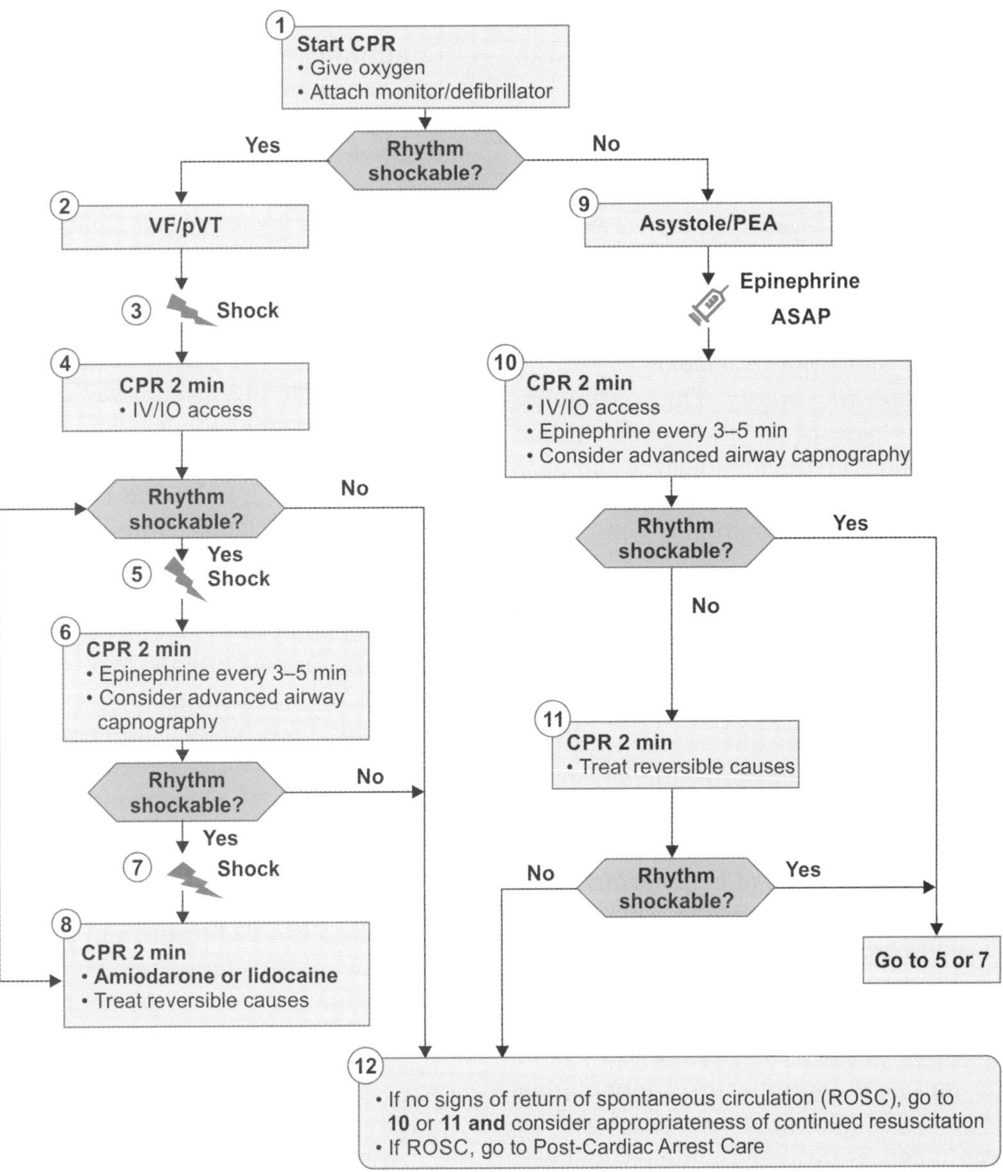

(IO: intraosseous; IV: intravenous; PEA: pulseless electrical activity; pVT: pulseless ventricular tachycardia; VF: ventricular fibrillation)

Source: ©2020 American Heart Association

saline, lactated Ringer, or balanced crystalloids are favored.

- *Hemorrhagic shock:* This is also a type of hypovolemic shock, where there is blood loss instead of fluid loss. The replacement of blood loss is by transfusion of packed red cell (PRBC), with or without other blood products. Till the PRBC arrives crystalloids are to be transfused in critically ill patients, the dictum being it is the low volume which kills rather than low hemoglobin. In patients with acute hemorrhagic shock, a hypotensive approach, where the target BP is kept lower than normal has been shown to reduce mortality.

- *Distributive shock:* Here although there is no significant fluid loss, the fluid in the body is redistributed and shunted away from the vital organs. The typical example is septic shock. Anaphylactic shock and shock secondary to spinal injury are other examples. These patients also need initial resuscitation with crystalloids.
- *Cardiogenic shock:* The pathology in this type of shock is poor cardiac function. The usual etiology is coronary artery disease, however other causes like cardiomyopathy, myocarditis, and valvular heart disease may also be there.
- *Obstructive shock:* The shock is due to some obstruction in the circulatory pathway. Examples are pericardial tamponade or massive pulmonary embolism.

The general principles of resuscitating a patient in shock are correction of volume status, vasopressors like norepinephrine, and inotropes like dobutamine. All patients of shock except those of cardiogenic shock will need initial fluid infusion. Till the fluid infusion corrects the hypotension or if the shock persists even after the infusions, vasopressors are used to maintain the BP. If the cardiac output is poor in spite of the above two measures inotropes like dobutamine are used. The etiology of the shock has to be determined. Particularly, cardiogenic shock patients should be identified early as usually they should not receive IV fluids. This can be done by bedside echocardiography.

A Patient with Acute Respiratory Distress

It may be due to:

- Hypoxemia is secondary to usually pulmonary or cardiac diseases
- Hypercapnia is secondary to usually pulmonary diseases
- Conditions where there is neither hypoxemia nor hypercapnia, e.g., severe metabolic acidosis.

While the management of a respiratory distress involves a proper diagnosis, and specific therapy, the initial resuscitation can be done by the following steps:

1. *Airway:* If the patient is unconscious but pulse present, look for any paradoxical movement of chest and abdomen or stridor which suggests airway obstruction. Exclude the tongue falling back in unconscious patients. The airway can be kept patent by clearing secretions, using airway maneuver, oropharyngeal/nasopharyngeal airway, or placement of advance airway. Airway can be opened by using maneuvers like head tilt and chin lift. Some patients may require endotracheal intubation.
2. *Breathing:* Look for signs of respiratory distress like sweating, tachypnea, nasal flaring, retractions, working of accessory muscles of respiration, and paradoxical breathing. Assess for rate of breathing. Normal respiratory rate is 12–20 breaths/min. Rate above 22 breaths/min is called tachypnea. Assess for pattern and depth of breathing. Watch for bilateral chest expansion. Chest expansion may be diminished on the side of pneumothorax.
3. Check oxygen saturation level. Initially a pulse oximeter should be used and also an arterial sample is to be sent for blood gas analysis. Note that the pulse rate counted by the pulse oximeter should match the actual pulse rate of the patient as measured manually or by the ECG monitor. If the two pulse rates vary widely, the pulse oximetry is improper. Oximeters which show pulse waves can be checked for proper contour of the pulse waves to validate the oximetric measurement.

4. All hypoxemic patients are to be given oxygen (for details of oxygen therapy see Chapter 20).
5. Patients remaining hypoxemic after oxygen therapy or hypercapnic patients require further assistance like noninvasive or invasive ventilators.

RESUSCITATING AN UNCONSCIOUS PATIENT

- Assess consciousness level of patient by using Glasgow Coma Scale score **(Table 2)** or assessing level of responsiveness by using *A*lert, *V*erbal, *P*ain, *U*nresponsive score.
- Assess pupillary size and reaction.
- Assess brain stem reflexes in deeply comatose patient.
- Asymmetric findings on physical examination such as unilateral dilated pupil and asymmetric motor responses should be rapidly evaluated for structural diseases of brain.
- Computed tomography (CT) brain should be done in all patients suspected of having structural causes of coma.
- Patients with abrupt onset of history are more likely to have structural causes like stroke, seizure, or a cardiac event and gradual onset of course is more suggestive of metabolic or toxicologic processes.
- Measure blood glucose routinely in all patients with decreased level of consciousness.
- Thiamine should be given to all patients at risk of nutritional deficiency like chronic alcoholics, malnourished patients, bariatric surgery patients.
- Review medication history of the patient.
- In patient suspected of toxin ingestion get toxicologic screening done.
- Send routine blood investigations including electrolytes.
- The basic resuscitation like maintaining the airway, monitoring BP and pulse rate, and oxygenation to be done for all comatose patients.

TABLE 2: Glasgow Coma Scale.

Component tested	*Score*
Eye response	
Eyes open spontaneously	4
Eye opening to verbal command	3
Eye opening to pain	2
No eye opening	1
Motor response	
Obeys command	6
Localizes pain	5
Withdraws from pain	4
Flexion response to pain	3
Extension response to pain	2
No motor response	1
Verbal response	
Oriented	5
Confused	4
Inappropriate words	3
Incomprehensible sounds	2
No verbal response	1

FURTHER READING

1. American Heart Association. Advanced Cardiovascular Life Support Instructor Manual. Dallas: American Heart Association; 2020.
2. Kollef MH, Isakow W, Burks AC, Despotovic VN. The Washington Manual of Critical Care, 3rd edition. Philadelphia: Lippincott Williams & Wilkins 2017.
3. Kowalski A, Brandis D. Shock Resuscitation. In: StatPearls [Internet]. Treasure Island (FL): StatPearls Publishing; 2025.
4. Resuscitation Council UK. Available from https://www.resus.org.uk [Last accessed February 2025].
5. Stevens RD, Cadena RS, Pineda J. Emergency Neurological Life Support: Approach to the Patient with Coma. Neurocrit Care. 2015;23 Suppl 2:S69-75.

SECTION

2

Monitoring

Section Editor: *Saswati Sinha*

5. **Bedside Monitoring: Oxygen, Carbon Dioxide, Blood Sugar, and Temperature**
   Rajarshi Roy, Snigdhadeb Ghosh
6. **Electrocardiogram and Arrhythmias**
   Shrikant Suhas Sahasrabudhe, Yogesh Lakkas
7. **Arterial Blood Gas Analysis and Electrolyte Imbalances**
   Deven Juneja, Prashant Nasa
8. **Hemodynamic Monitoring**
   Saswati Sinha, Amit Das

CHAPTER 5

Bedside Monitoring: Oxygen, Carbon Dioxide, Blood Sugar, and Temperature

Rajarshi Roy, Snigdhadeb Ghosh

BEDSIDE OXYGEN MONITORING (PULSE OXIMETRY)

Introduction

It is noninvasive method of measuring hemoglobin saturation with oxygen using a light signal transmitted through tissue.

Principle

- Pulse oximeter estimates oxygen saturation (SpO_2) from differential absorption of red and infrared light in tissues
- *Beer-Lambert law:* Relates concentration of solute to intensity of light transmitted through the solution
- Oxyhemoglobin absorbs more infrared light (940 nm).
- Deoxyhemoglobin absorbs more red light (660 nm).

Physics

- *Combines two technologies*:
  1. *Spectrophotometer:* Measures oxyhemoglobin saturation **(Fig. 1)**

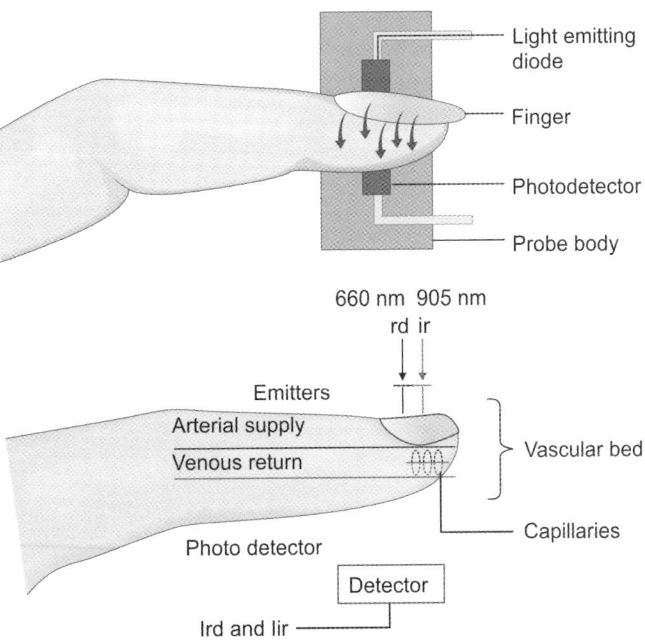

Fig. 1: Spectrophotometer.

2. *Optical plethysmography:* Measures pulsatile changes in arterial blood volume at sensor site

- Differentiation between arterial blood and other components by determining change in transmitted light caused by pulsatile flow of arterial blood.

Types of Pulse Oximetry

Transmission pulse oximetry:

- Most common type
- Light beam transmitted through a vascular bed and detected on the opposite side of that bed **(Fig. 2)**

Reflectance pulse oximetry:

- Relies on light reflected back from blood **(Fig. 3)**
- Probe has both the LED and photodiode on same side.

Disadvantages:

- Can be errors due to light reflected from skin
- Vasoconstriction may overestimate SpO_2.
- *CO-oximetry: Gold standard* for measuring SaO_2.

Traditional blood gas analyzer capable of measuring:

- Concentration of oxyhemoglobin
- Reduced hemoglobin
- Carboxyhemoglobin
- Methemoglobin
- *Transcutaneous oximetry:*
    - Two wavelengths of light used to measure quantity of oxygenated and deoxygenated blood **(Fig. 4)**.
    - Measure SaO_2 instead of SpO_2.

Results displayed:

- Percentage saturation of hemoglobin
- Arterial pulse waveform
- Heart rate
- *Variables:*
    - Fractional O_2 saturation (% HbO_2 or FO_2Hb) is ratio of oxyhemoglobin to sum of all hemoglobin species present

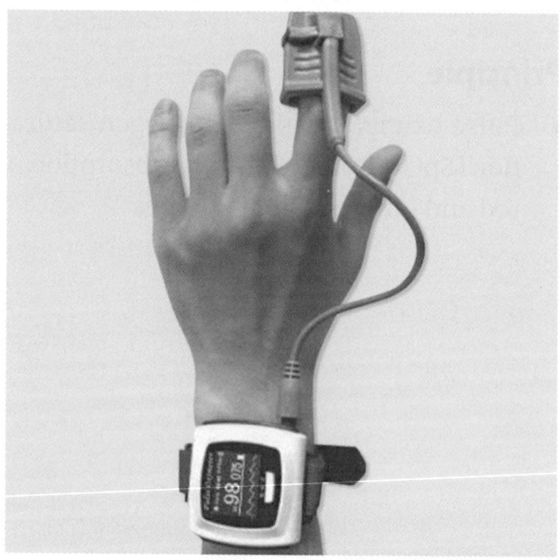

Fig. 3: Reflectance pulse oximetry.

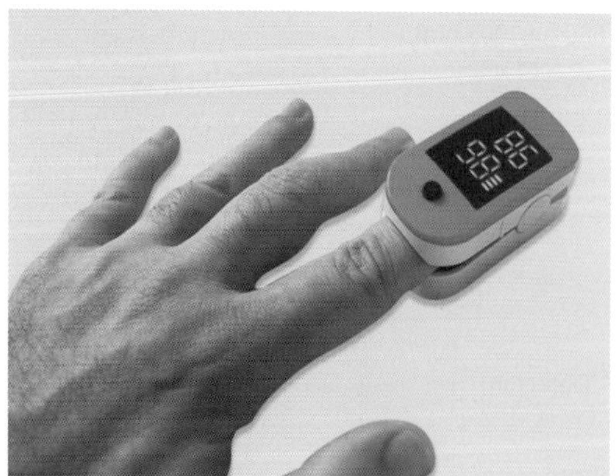

Fig. 2: Transmission pulse oximetry.

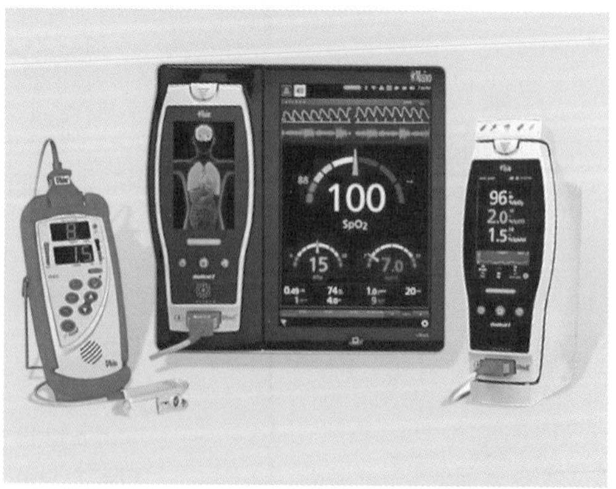

Fig. 4: The results being displayed.

- $O_2Hb\,\% = HbO_2/(HbO_2 + Hb + metHb + COHb)$
- Functional O_2 saturation (SaO_2) is ratio of oxyhemoglobin to all functional hemoglobin

$$SaO_2 = HbO_2/HbO_2 + Hb$$

SpO_2	The saturation of oxygen as per pulse oximeter
SaO_2	The amount of oxygen in arterial blood
PaO_2	The partial pressure of oxygen in arterial blood

Follow these steps to make sure the pulse oximeter gives the correct reading:

- Remove any nail polish or false nails.
- Hand warming is an essential part.
- Make sure you have been resting for 5 minutes before taking the reading.
- Do not press or apply any pressure while you are taking the reading.
- Be careful to identify which one is heart rate (HR) and which one is SpO_2.

Sites of application:
- Finger, toe
- Ear
- Cheek, forehead
- Tongue, pharynx, esophagus
- Thenar, hypothenar eminence, palm, wrist
- Lower calf, ankle, foot
- Penis

Uses of Pulse Oximetry

- Assess patients with acutely worsening symptoms, especially shortness of breath
- Allows lowest safe oxygen flow
- Avoids hyperoxia
- Looks for exercise-related dyspnea
- Identification of the cause of underlying lung disease (with SpO_2 <92%)
- Titrating the rate of flow of oxygen in patients on long-term oxygen therapy—the target is resting and ambulatory pulse oximetry around 88–92%
- Evaluate patients with severe disease such as cyanosis, or cor pulmonale for possible respiratory insufficiency/failure
- Titrating home oxygen therapy during exacerbation of any underlying lung disease— chronic obstructive pulmonary disease (COPD), asthma, interstitial lung diseases, pulmonary fibrosis, etc.
- Pulse oximetry also indicates hypovolemia and cardiac output status
- Amplitude of pulse oximetry waveform indicates adequacy of cardiopulmonary resuscitation (CPR)

Advantages

- Light weight and compact
- Accurate, noninvasive fast response time
- Not affected by other gases/vapors
- Tone modulation with change in saturation
- Continuous measurement displayed
- *Determines respiratory and circulatory variables:*
  - If blood pressure (BP) is low and pulse signal is good, patient is vasodilated with good CO
  - If BP and pulse signal are low, patient has low CO.

Recent advances:
- *Multi-wavelength pulse oximeters:* Eight wavelength pulse oximeters capable of measuring several species of Hb
- *Reflectance pulse oximetry:* Useful if poor signal transmission during hypoperfusion
- Newer pulse oximeter can also real time cardiac output status

Limitations/Disadvantages

- Pulse oximeter cannot detect hypotension or hypertension.
- Does not detect hypoventilation and hypercarbia with reduction in SpO_2:

Especially if patient is receiving supplemental O_2.

- *The measurements are incorrect in:*
  - *Sickle cell anemia:*
    - High amounts of fetal Hb
    - Low saturation levels: SpO_2 below 60%
  - *Dark-skinned people:*
    - *Dyes:* Methylene blue, indocyanine green
    - *Nail polish:* Poor peripheral pulsations
  - *Methemoglobinemia:* Carbon monoxide poisoning

Interference

- *Optical interference:* Due to stray light like sunlight/fluorescent light/OR light/infrared (IR) radiant warmers causing inaccurate readings
- *Electrical interference:* Due to electrocautery
- *Motion artefacts:* In shivering/Parkinson's
- Erratic performance in dysrhythmias
- May not function in patients on intra-aortic balloon pump (IABP) patients

BEDSIDE TEMPERATURE MONITORING

Introduction

- Normal body temperature is approximately 37°C (98.6°F) and ranges from 36.0 to 37.5°C (96.8 to 99.5°F), although this varies with the time of day (low in the early morning and peaks late evening) and the method of measurement.
- All critically ill patients should have core temperature monitoring.

Temperature Monitoring in Intensive Care Unit

- Advanced age of the patient
- Long-duration stay in intensive care unit (ICU) setup
- Large shift of body fluid
- Blood transfusion
- Several comorbidity
- Many high-risk postoperative cases
- Effect of different medication (antibiotics, sedative drugs)
- High frequency of infection (septicemia, septic shock, and hypovolemic shock)
- Many patients are in noninvasive ventilation (NIV), ventilatory support for long duration.

Uses

- To estimate mean body temperature
- To estimate total body heat content
- Prevent overheating and hypothermia
- Rough measure of peripheral perfusion and cardiac output

Hypothermia

Different types of hypothermia are described in **Table 1**.

Classification of Fever

Classification of fever is given in **Table 2.**

Temperature Monitoring Sites

Peripheral temperature monitoring method:

- Skin (frontal)
- Oral or sublingual
- Axilla
- Temporal artery

Core temperature monitoring method:

- *Semi-invasive method*:
  - Rectal temperature
  - Bladder temperature
- *Invasive method*:
  - Tracheal
  - Pulmonary artery
  - Distal esophagus
  - Tympanic membrane
  - Nasopharynx

TABLE 1: Different types of hypothermia.

Mild	*Moderate*	*Severe*
32–35°C (90–95°F)	28–32°C (82–90°F)	<28°C or <82°F
Shivering	Loss of compensatory shivering	Muscle rigidity without shivering
Increased metabolism	Decreased metabolism	
Vasoconstriction	Decreased cerebral blood flow	Loss of thermoregulation
Mild tachycardia	Diuresis	Vasodilation
	Extravasation of fluids	Decreased HR, SV, CO
	Hypovolemia	Decreased cardiac conduction
		Increased cardiac irritability
		Slowing of nerve conduction
		Suspended cerebral activity

(CO: cardiac output; HR: heart rate; SV: stroke volume)

TABLE 2: Classification of fever.

Grade	*Celsius*	*Fahrenheit*
Low grade	37.2–37.8	99–100
Moderate	37.8–39.4	100–103
High grade	39.4–40.5	103–105
Hyperpyrexia	>40.5	>106

Types of thermometer:
- Mercury thermometer
- Electrical thermometer:
  - Thermistor
  - Thermocouple
- Deep tissue thermometers
- Infrared monitors
- Liquid crystal thermometry

Peripheral Temperature Monitoring

- Considerably lower than core temperature
- Forehead temperature 2°C lower than core temperature **(Fig. 5)**
- It indicates the peripheral perfusion and cardiac output.

Oral and Axillary Temperature

- Most readily available temperature monitoring method in hospital **(Fig. 6)**
- Easy to perform
- Not reliable method of core temperature monitoring
- Axillary temperature is 0.5–1°C lesser than oral temperature.
- Oral temperature is 0.5–1°C lesser than the rectal temperature.

Core Temperature Monitoring Method

Urinary bladder:
- It is considered as intermediate temperature **(Fig. 7)**
- Difficult to place the thermal probe
- Temperature altered by urinary flow

Rectal temperature:
- It is considered as intermediate temperature **(Fig. 8)**
- It is affected by lavage, stools
- There is slow response to change in core temperature

Tympanic membrane temperature:
- Difficult to position due to curvature of aural canal **(Fig. 9)**
- Good reflection of core temperature
- Measures brain temperature as tympanic membrane is close to intracranial area
- Minimal lag time
- Risk chances of tympanic membrane perforation

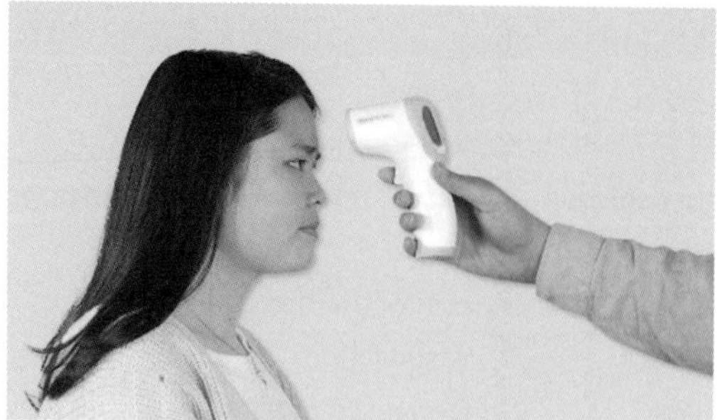

Fig. 5: Digital LED infrared thermometer for forehead temperature monitoring.

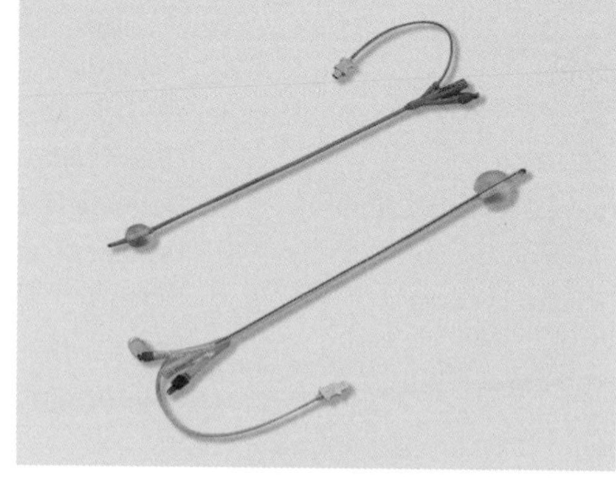

Fig. 7: Urinary bladder temperature monitoring catheter.

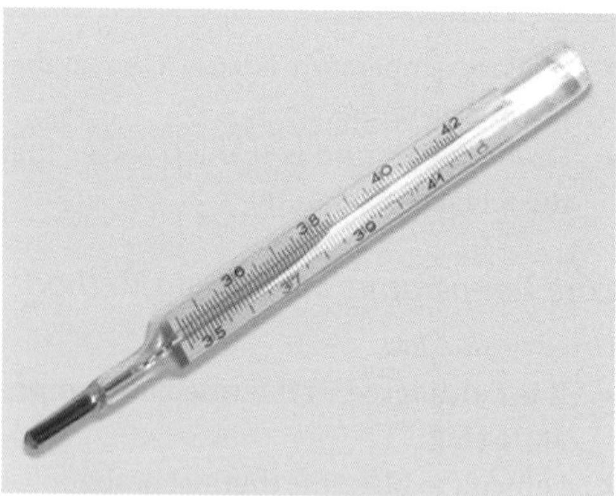

Fig. 6: Universal mercury thermometer.

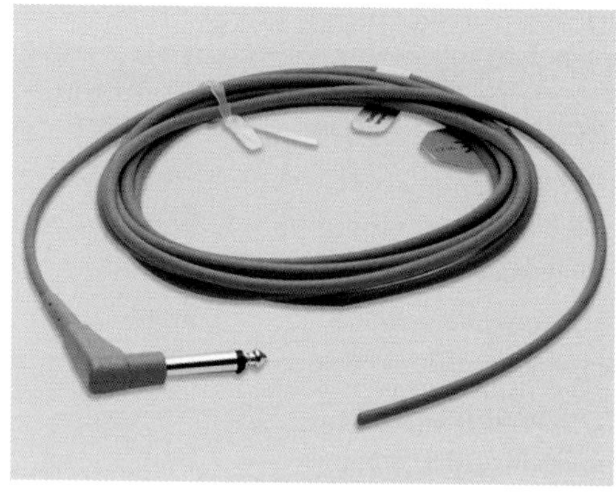

Fig. 8: Rectal and esophageal temperature probe.

Nasopharyngeal temperature:

- Accurate if placed adjacent to nasopharyngeal mucosa
- It is altered by respiratory gases
- Reliable due to close to the ICA
- Risk chances of epistaxis

Esophageal temperature:

- It is positioned 24 cm below larynx in lower third of esophagus behind the heart.
- Position avoids measuring temperature of tracheal gases.
- Reliable even during rapid temperature changes
- Most acceptable method of core body temperature monitoring in ICU and OT setup.

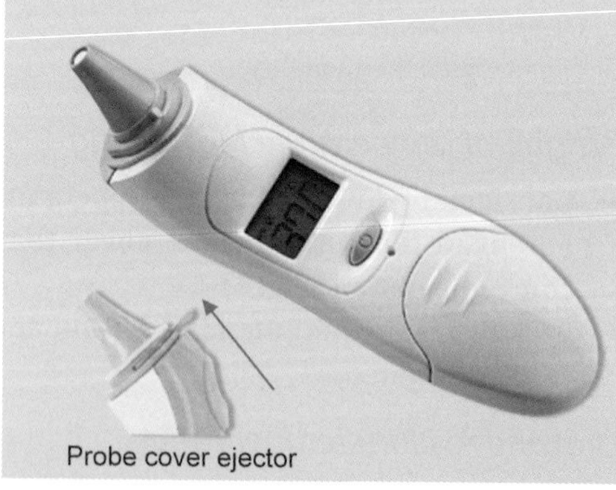

Fig. 9: Tympanic membrane temperature probe.

Tracheal temperature:

- Thermistor is placed within anterior surface of specially designed tracheal tube.

- Inaccurate if there is any fresh gas flow occurs.

Pulmonary arterial temperature:

- Gold standard for core temperature monitoring **(Fig. 10)**
- Approximates jugular bulb temperature

The blood temperature is measured by a *thermistor* at the catheter tip, which lies within the pulmonary artery.

Key Notes

- Gold standard site for core temperature monitoring—pulmonary artery
- Most accurate for brain temperature monitoring—tympanic membrane
- Best for brain temperature monitoring—nasopharynx
- Best site and most commonly used for core body temperature—lower end of the esophagus

CAPNOGRAPHY

Introduction

The first infrared CO_2 measuring and recording apparatus by Luft in 1943, capnography has evolved an essential component in ICU during intubation, on ventilation, and CPR. Capnography helps to identify situations that causes hypoxia and correction.

Principle

End-tidal CO_2 ($EtCO_2$) monitoring is projected as a number and a graph. The number is called capnometry, which is the partial pressure of CO_2 showed at the end of exhalation, ranging between 35 and 45 mm Hg.

The waveform is called capnograph and shows how much CO_2 is present at each phase of the respiratory cycle.

Phases of End-tidal Carbon Dioxide (Fig. 11)

- *Phase I:* Start of exhalation, CO_2 concentration is initially zero
- *Phase II:* CO_2 increases rapidly as alveolar gas exits the airway.
- *Phase III:* CO_2 concentration is relatively constant (reflects the concentration of CO_2 in the alveolar gas). This phase ends with a value of maximum CO_2 concentration
- *Phase IV:* Start of inhalation, CO_2 decreases to zero as atmospheric air enters the airway

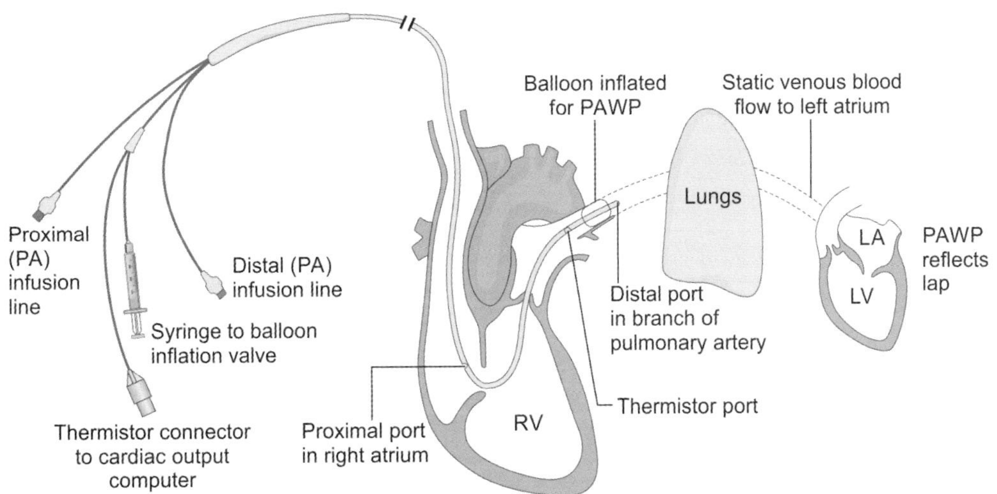

Fig. 10: Pulmonary arterial catheter.

Features

A normal capnogram always has the following features ***(Fig. 12)****:*

- The waveform shape always starts at zero and returns to zero.
- A maximum CO_2 is reached with each breath, corresponding to $EtCO_2$.
- The amplitude of the waveform depends on $EtCO_2$ concentration.
- The width of the waveform depends on expiratory time.
- There is a similar shape for subjects with normal lung function.
- The waveform has four phases.

Why End-tidal CO_2 is Important?

End-tidal CO_2 monitoring is becoming more common in critical care, during sedation practice, in ambulatory settings and in postoperative recovery units.

Several guidelines have supported the use of capnography outside the theater environment:

- Waveform capnography must be used to confirm and continually monitor tracheal tube placement.
- Used to monitor the quality of CPR and to provide an early indication of return of spontaneous circulation (ROSC).
- During moderate or deep sedation, the adequacy of ventilation shall be evaluated by continual observation of qualitative clinical signs.
- Identify patient's airway patency, breathing adequacy, and circulatory status.
- Professionals are able to identify potential breathing complications (such as airway obstruction, hyperventilation, hypoventilation, or apnea) and respond accordingly with a change in clinical management.

BLOOD GLUCOSE MONITORING

Introduction

Blood glucose monitoring helps to identify the fluctuation of blood glucose levels that occur

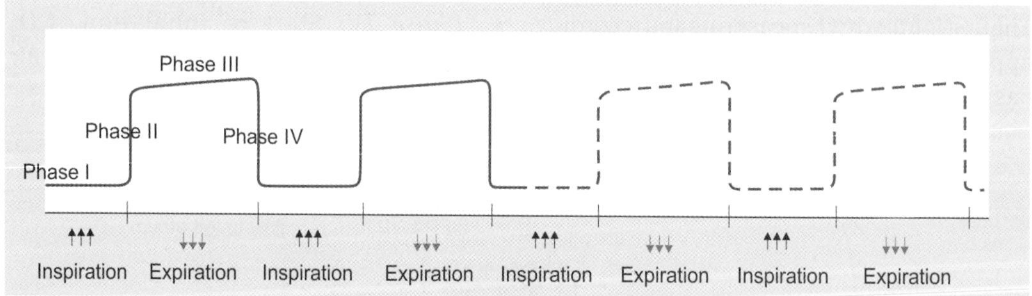

Fig. 11: Capnography waveform.

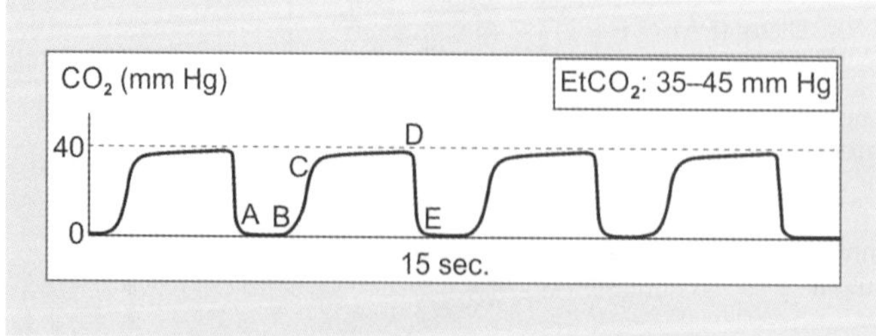

Fig. 12: Normal waveform capnography.

in response to diet, exercise, medications, and pathological processes, such as diabetes mellitus. Unusually high or low blood glucose levels can potentially lead to life-threatening conditions **(Figs. 13 and 14)**. Monitoring is easy and user friendly, it can be easily conducted at home.

Features

Capillary Blood Glucose Test

The blood drop sample is usually collected from a fingertip prick, and can also be drawn from the earlobe, heel, forearm, and palm. Using alternate sites may be less painful for the patient but may need a deeper lancet. Check with the glucometer manufacturer to determine if the machine may be used for alternate site testing **(Fig. 15)**.

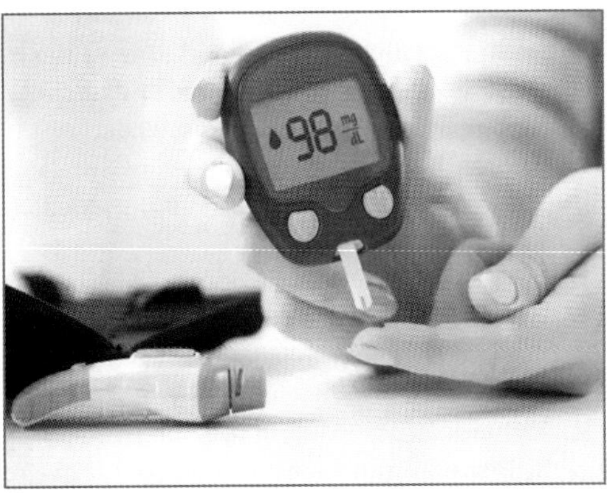

Fig. 13: A glucometer.

Equipment

- Lancet to prick the skin
- Glucometer
- The test strips

Modern "smart" machines require a very small sample of blood (from 0.3 to 1 μL).

Advantages

Advantages are small blood sample, range of alternate testing sites, short testing time, prominent display on glucometer, and less painful than venipuncture.

Disadvantages

Manufacturers often provide low-cost or subsidized glucometers.

The test strips are expensive, time-limited with short expiry dates, and are affected by a range of variables, including temperature, humidity, size, and quality of blood samples.

The clinical presentation of the patient will affect the accuracy of the test result. The reliability of results may vary with the range of hypoglycemia, anemia, altered hematocrit, hypotension, or critically ill patients. The fingers should not be squeezed to get an adequate sample.

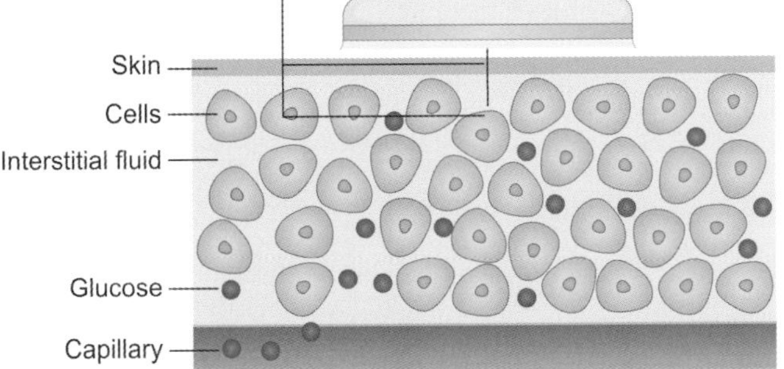

Fig. 14: Glucose in the interstitial space.

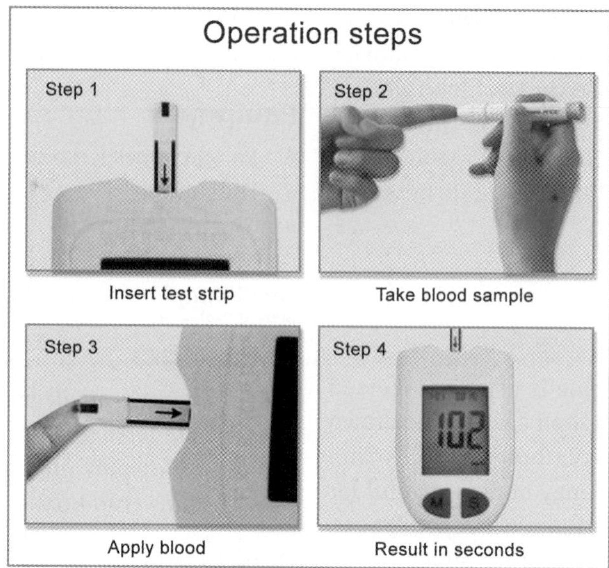

Fig. 15: Steps in the glucometry.

FURTHER READING

1. ALS guideline 2015.
2. Association of Anaesthetists. (2021). Recommendations for standards of monitoring during anaesthesia and recovery 2021. Available from https://anaesthetists.org/Home/Resources-publications/Guidelines/Recommendations-for-standards-of-monitoring-during-anaesthesia-and-recovery-2021. [Last accessed February, 2025]
3. DiLorenzo AN, Schell RM. Morgan & Mikhail's Clinical Anaesthesiology, 5th edition. New York: McGraw-Hill Education; 2014.
4. House of Delegates of ASA 2011.
5. Irwin RS, Lilly CM. Irwin and Rippe's Intensive Care Medicine, 9th edition. Philadelphia: Lippincott Williams & Wilkins; 2023.
6. Jothinath K. Anaesthesia Review for DNB Students. New Delhi: Jaypee Brothers Medical Publisher; 2017.
7. Miller RD, Cohen NH, Eriksson LI, Fleisher LA, Wiener-Kronish JP, Young WL. Miller's Anesthesia, 8th edition. Philadelphia: Elsevier; 2015.
8. NEJM NICE SUGAR Guideline.
9. Richardson M, Moulton K, Rabb D, Kindopp S, Pishe T, Yan C, et al. Capnography for Monitoring End-Tidal CO2 in Hospital and Pre-hospital Settings: A Health Technology Assessment. Ottawa (ON): Canadian Agency for Drugs and Technologies in Health; 2016.

CHAPTER

6 Electrocardiogram and Arrhythmias

Shrikant Suhas Sahasrabudhe, Yogesh Lakkas

INTRODUCTION

Electrocardiogram or ECG is the graphical recording of the electrical activity of the heart. An ECG has several wires with electrodes, which are connected to the limbs and the chest of the patient. **Figure 1** shows the various lead positions.

An ECG tracing is given in **Figure 2**.

ARRHYTHMIA

Arrhythmia is abnormal rhythm of heart. Electric impulse is generated in sinoatrial (SA) node and through atrioventricular (AV) node it travels to right and left bundle of His eventually terminating in Purkinje fibers. Any deviation from this sequence of the pathway will culminate into arrhythmias. As we all know, interpretation of ECG and arrhythmias is vital for not only the doctors but also nurses working in intensive care unit (ICU). Knowledge regarding ECGs will not only help an ICU nurse in picking up the abnormalities early but it will translate it in appropriate and timely management of arrhythmia preventing

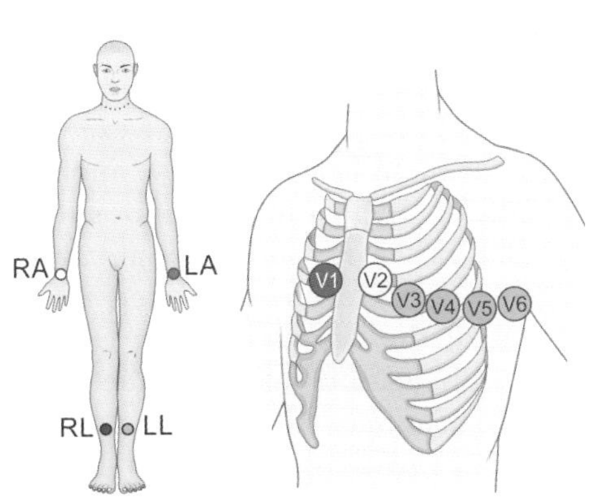

Fig. 1: Various lead positions.

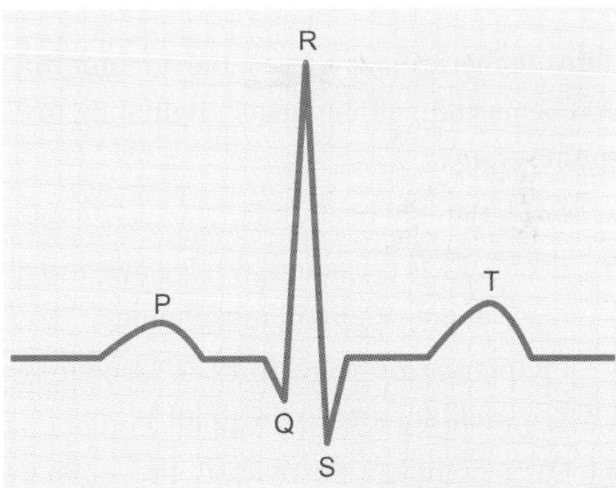

Fig. 2: Electrocardiogram (ECG) tracing.

Note: The P wave is the atrial depolarization, QRS is the ventricular depolarization, and the T wave is the ventricular repolarization. The distance from the beginning of the P wave to the beginning of the QRS is the PR interval. The duration of the QRS complex is from the beginning of the Q or an R if there is no Q, to the end of the S. The duration from the beginning of the QRS to the end of the T is the QT interval. From the end of the QRS to the beginning of the T wave is the ST segment.

catastrophe. It is imperative that any nurse working in an intensive care setting should be conversant with the common arrhythmias.

Broadly arrhythmias are divided into tachyarrhythmias (heart rate >100 beats/min) and bradyarrhythmia (heart rate <60 beats/min). Normal rhythm is called as sinus rhythm. The initial step toward approaching for arrhythmias is to get a 12-lead ECG.

Let us look at the arrhythmias one by one.

Sinus Tachycardia

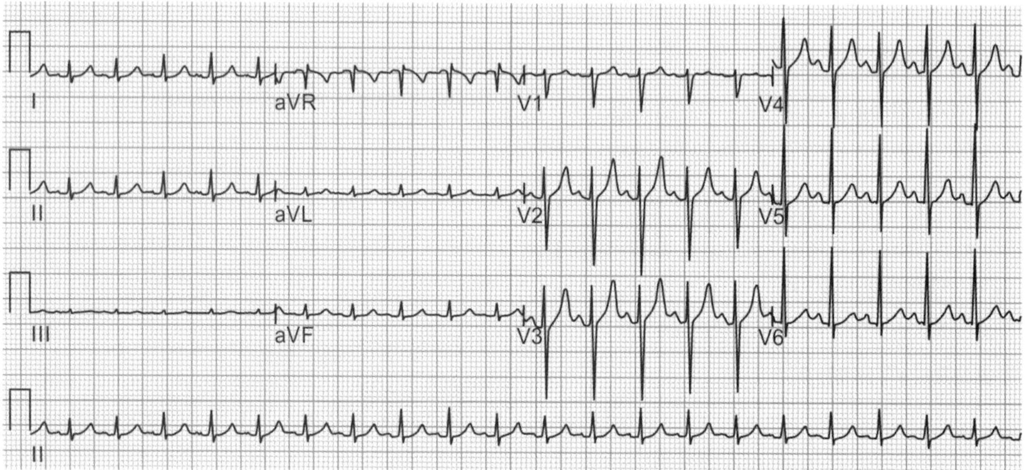

Sinus tachycardia is a heart rate greater than 100 beats/min, all the beats originating from the *sinus node.*

- *Rate:* 100–180 beats/min
- Each QRS is preceded by a P wave and all P waves are similar in morphology.
- PR interval is normal (0.12–0.2 seconds or 3–5 small squares in the graph)
- QRS complex (provided there is no underlying bundle block pattern) is narrow and normal (<0.10 seconds or <2.5 small squares)
- Rhythm is regular.

Causes of sinus tachycardia are exercise, anxiety, fever, infection, drugs, anemia, heart failure, hypovolemia, and shock. Sinus tachycardia is often asymptomatic. Management, however, is directed at the treatment of the primary cause. Carotid sinus pressure (carotid massage) transiently reduces the heart rate. A beta blocker may be used to reduce heart rate.

Sinus Bradycardia

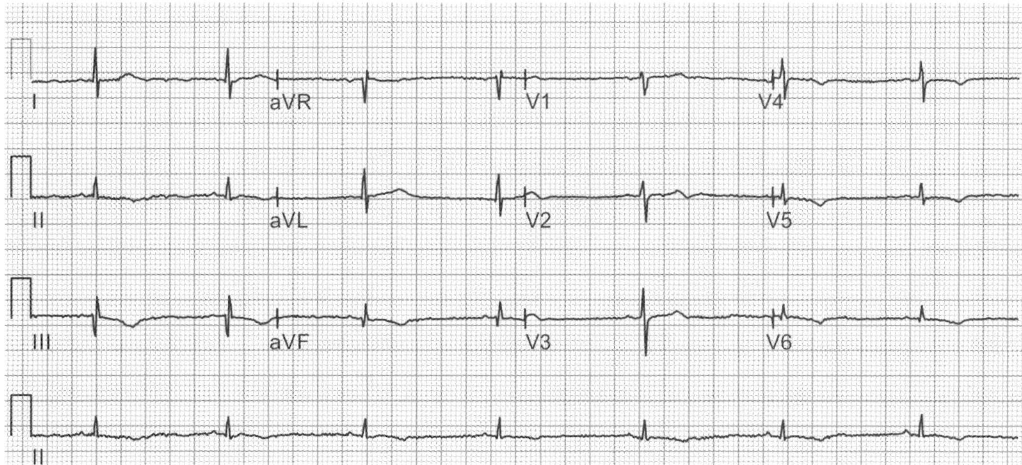

Sinus bradycardia is a heart rate of <60 beats/min and originates from the sinus node (as the term "sinus" refers to the SA node). It has the following characteristics:

- Rate is <60 beats/min.
- P waves precede each QRS complex.
- PR interval is normal.
- QRS complex is normal (provided there is no underlying bundle branch block).
- Rhythm is regular.

Causes may include drugs like beta blockers, vagal stimulation, hypothyroidism, hypothermia, or sinus node involvement in myocardial infarction (MI). This arrhythmia may be normal in athletes. It is often asymptomatic but manifestations may include syncope, fatigue, and dizziness. Management includes treating the underlying cause. Anticholinergic drugs like atropine sulfate or sympathomimetics like dopamine may be used for temporary relief. Symptomatic and significant sinus bradycardia may require temporary or permanent pacemaker.

Atrioventricular Blocks

Atrioventricular blocks are of three types mainly, first degree, second degree, and third degree or complete heart block.

- First degree block usually does not cause any drop in heart rate. By definition, the PR interval is >2.0 seconds (>5 small squares)
- Second degree AV block may be of two types. First is Mobitz type 1 (Wenckebach phenomenon), where the PR interval gradually is prolonged in the consecutive beats and then one P is not conducted and there is no QRS after that, a second P wave comes after this nonconducted P, which is followed by a QRS. In Mobitz type 2, every 2 or 3 P waves are followed by a single QRS (2:1 or 3:1 AV block).
- *Third degree or complete AV block:* The P wave beats at its normal rate; however its impulse is not conducted across the AV node. A rhythm is generated from the AV node (junctional escape which has a usual QRS duration) or from the ventricles (ventricular escape, wide QRS). The P waves and the QRS complexes do not have any relationship to each other and are completely dissociated.

Atrial Flutter

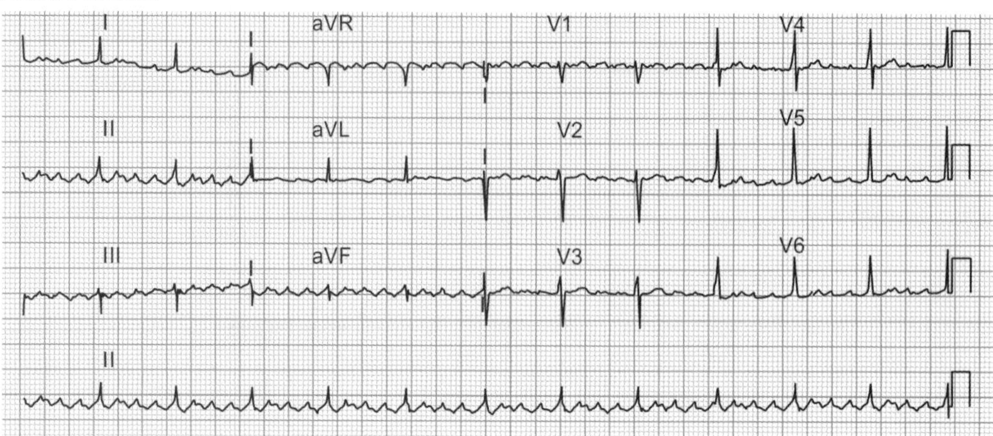

Atrial flutter is an abnormal rhythm that occurs in the atria of the heart. Atrial flutter has an atrial rhythm that is regular but high atrial rate of 250–400 beats/min. On the ECG, this shows as a sawtooth appearance. QRS complexes are uniform in shape and regular in rate, the rate is less than the atrial rate.

- Regular atrial rhythm
- *Abnormal atrial rate*: 250–400 beats/min
- Sawtooth P wave configuration
- QRS complexes uniform in shape and regular in rate
- The QRS complexes are generated for every second or third P wave. This results in an effective heart rate of 150 or 100 beats/min (atrial flutter with 2:1 or 3:1 block).

The causes includes heart failure, tricuspid valve or mitral valve diseases, pulmonary embolism, cor pulmonale, inferior wall MI, myocarditis, and digoxin toxicity.

Atrial Fibrillation

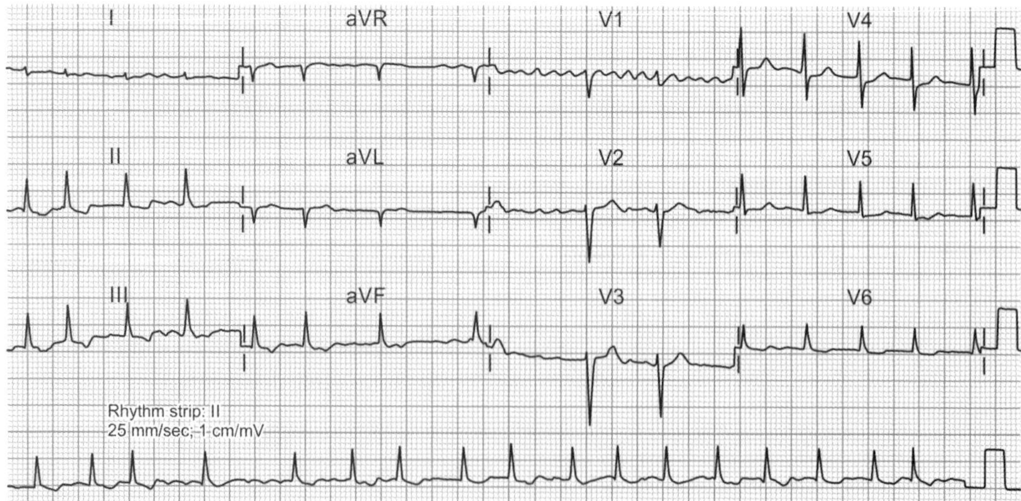

Atrial fibrillation is disorganized and uncoordinated twitching of atrial musculature caused by overly rapid production of atrial impulses. It is the most common tachyarrhythmia among others. This arrhythmia has the following characteristics:

- *Atrial rate*: 350–600 beats/min
- *Ventricular rate:* 120–200 beats/min
- P wave is irregular, fast; sometimes it may show a slightly undulating baseline.
- PR interval is not measurable.
- QRS complex is normal (unless the patient had inherent bundle branch blocks).
- Rhythm is irregular and usually rapid unless controlled.

Causes include atherosclerosis, heart failure, congenital heart disease, chronic obstructive pulmonary disease, and thyrotoxicosis. Atrial fibrillation may be asymptomatic but clinical manifestation may include palpitations, dyspnea, and pulmonary edema. The nursing goal is toward administration of prescribed treatment to decrease ventricular response, decrease atrial irritability, and eliminate the cause. Atrial fibrillation in the long run may cause arterial embolization.

Supraventricular Tachycardia

Supraventricular tachycardia (SVT) is characterized by narrow complex, regular tachycardia. Classically, it comes in paroxysms and is termed as paroxysmal SVT. It is further discussed in detail in the **Table 1**. It can sometimes be aborted by carotid massage.

TABLE 1: Most common arrythmias.

Arrhythmias	*Description*	*Causes*	*Treatment*
Sinus tachycardia	• Rhythm is regular • Rate >100 beats/min • Normal P wave preceding each QRS complex	• Normal physiologic response to fever, exercise, sepsis anxiety, dehydration, or pain • May accompany shock, left-sided heart failure, cardiac tamponade, hyperthyroidism, and anemia • Atropine, epinephrine, quinidine, caffeine, nicotine, and alcohol use	• Correction of underlying cause • Beta-adrenergic blockers, calcium channel blockers, ivabradine for symptomatic patients
Sinus bradycardia	• Regular atrial and ventricular rhythms • Rate <60 beats/min • Normal P wave preceding each QRS complex	• Normal in a well-conditioned heart (e.g., athletes) • Increased intracranial pressure; increased vagal tone due to straining during defecation, vomiting, intubation, mechanical ventilation; medicines like beta blockers	• Follow ACLS protocol for administration of atropine for symptoms of low cardiac output, dizziness, weakness, altered LOC, or low blood pressure • Pacemaker

Contd...

Contd...

Arrhythmias	*Description*	*Causes*	*Treatment*
Paroxysmal supra-ventricular tachycardia	• Rhythm is regular • Heart rate >160 beats/min; rarely exceeds 250 beats/min • P waves regular but aberrant; difficult to differentiate from preceding T wave • P wave may be seen before each QRS complex • Sudden onset and termination of arrhythmia • When a normal P wave is present, it is called paroxysmal atrial tachycardia; when a normal P wave is not present, it is called paroxysmal junctional tachycardia	• Physical exertion, emotion, stimulants, rheumatic heart diseases • Intrinsic abnormality of AV conduction system accessory pathways • Digoxin toxicity • Use of caffeine, marijuana, or central nervous system stimulants	• If the patient is in hypotension, electrical cardioversion is the treatment • If patient is stable, vagal stimulation, or Valsalva's maneuver, carotid sinus massage • Adenosine by rapid IV bolus injection to rapidly convert arrhythmia • If patient has normal ejection fraction, consider calcium channel blockers, beta-adrenergic blocks or amiodarone for prevention on recurrence • If patient has an ejection fraction <40%, consider amiodarone
Atrial flutter	• Atrial rhythm regular, rate 250–400 beats/min • Ventricular rhythm is regular and rate depends on the degree of AV block • Sawtooth shape P wave configuration • QRS complexes uniform in shape	• Heart failure, tricuspid or mitral valve disease, pulmonary embolism, cor pulmonale, inferior wall MI, myocarditis • Digoxin toxicity	• If patient is unstable with ventricular rate >150 beats/min, consider electrical cardioversion • If patient is stable, drug therapy may include calcium channel blockers, beta-adrenergic blocks, or antiarrhythmics • Anticoagulation therapy may be necessary
Atrial fibrillation	• Atrial rhythm grossly irregular rate >300–600 beats/min • Ventricular rhythm grossly irregular, rate 160–180 beats/min • PR interval indiscernible • No P waves, or P waves that appear as erratic, irregular baseline fibrillatory waves	Heart failure, COPD, thyrotoxicosis, constrictive pericarditis, ischemic heart disease, sepsis, pulmonary embolus, rheumatic heart disease, hypertension, mitral stenosis, atrial irritation, complication of coronary bypass or valve replacement surgery; it is one of the most common arrhythmias in the ICU	• If patient is hypotensive with ventricular rate >150 beats/min, prepare for immediate cardioversion • If stable, drug therapy may include calcium channel blockers, beta-adrenergic blockers, digoxin (for only rate control), procainamide, quinidine, ibutilide, or amiodarone (for conversion to sinus rhythm)

Contd...

Contd...

Arrhythmias	***Description***	***Causes***	***Treatment***
			• Anticoagulation therapy to prevent emboli • Dual-chamber atrial pacing, implantable atrial pacemaker, or surgical maze procedure may also be used • The approach can be correction of rhythm to sinus or just a rate control (usually below 110 beats/min) in the chronic atrial fibrillation
First-degree AV block	• Atrial and ventricular rhythms regular • PR interval >0.20 second • P wave preceding each QRS complex • QRS complex normal	• Inferior wall MI or ischemia or infarction, hypothyroidism, hypokalemia, hyperkalemia • Digoxin toxicity • Use of quinidine, procainamide, beta-adrenergic blockers, calcium	Cautious use of digoxin, calcium channel blockers, and beta-adrenergic blockers (stop if PR >0.24 seconds)
Second-degree AV block Mobitz 1 (Wenckebach) Mobitz type 2	• Atrial rhythm regular • Ventricular rhythm irregular • Atrial rate exceeds ventricular rate • PR interval progressively, but only slightly, longer with each cycle until QRS complex disappears • PR interval shorter after dropped beat • In Mobitz type 2, it is 2:1 or 3:1 blocks, i.e., every send of third P wave is conducted so there is a QRS only after every 2 or 3 P waves; PR is constant in the conducted beats	• Severe coronary artery disease, anterior wall MI, acute myocarditis • Digoxin toxicity • AV node disease	• Atropine, epinephrine, and dopamine for symptomatic bradycardia • Temporary or permanent pacemaker for symptomatic bradycardia • Discontinuation of digoxin if appropriate

Contd...

Contd...

Arrhythmias	***Description***	***Causes***	***Treatment***
Third-degree AV block (complex heart block)	• Atrial rhythm regular • Ventricular rhythm regular and rate slower than atrial rate • No relation between P waves and QRS complexes • No constant PR interval • QRS interval normal (nodal pacemaker) or wide and bizarre (ventricular pacemaker)	Inferior or anterior wall MI, congenital abnormality, rheumatic fever	• Atropine, epinephrine, and dopamine for symptomatic bradycardia • Temporary or permanent pacemaker for symptomatic bradycardia
Premature ventricular contraction (PVC)	• Atrial rhythm regular • Ventricular rhythm irregular • QRS complex premature, usually followed by a complete compensatory pause • QRS complex wide and distorted, usually >0.14 second • Premature QRS complexes occurring singly, in pairs, or in threes; alternating with normal beats; focus from one or more sites • Ominous when clustered, multifocal, with R wave on T pattern	• Heart failure; old or acute myocardial ischemia, infarction, or contusion • Myocardial irritation by ventricular catheters such as a pacemaker • Hypercapnia, hypokalemia, hypocalcemia • Drug toxicity by cardiac glycosides, aminophylline, tricyclic antidepressants, beta-adrenergic • Caffeine, tobacco, or alcohol use • Psychological stress, anxiety, pain	• If warranted, procainamide, lidocaine, or amiodarone IV • Treatment of underlying cause • Discontinuation of drug causing toxicity • Potassium chloride IV if PVC induced by hypokalemia • Magnesium sulfate IV if PVC induced by hypomagnesemia
Ventricular tachycardia	• Ventricular rate 140–220 beats/min, regular • QRS complexes wide, bizarre, and independent of P waves • P waves no discernible • May start and stop suddenly	• Myocardial ischemia, infarction, or aneurysm • Coronary artery disease • Rheumatic heart disease • Mitral valve prolapse, heart failure, cardiomyopathy	• If pulseless—initiate CPR; follow ACLS protocol for defibrillation • If with pulse—if hemodynamically stable, follow ACLS protocol for administration of amiodarone; if ineffective initiate synchronized cardioversion

Contd...

Contd...

Arrhythmias	***Description***	***Causes***	***Treatment***
		• Ventricular catheters • Hypokalemia, hypercalcemia • Pulmonary embolism • Digoxin, procainamide, epinephrine, quinidine toxicity, anxiety	
Ventricular fibrillation	• Ventricular rhythm and rate are rapid and chaotic • QRS complexes wide and irregular, no visible P waves	• Myocardial ischemia or infarction, R-on-T phenomenon, untreated ventricular tachycardia • Hypokalemia, hyperkalemia, hypercalcemia, alkalosis, electric shock, hypothermia • Digoxin, epinephrine, or quinidine toxicity	Ventricular fibrillations are always pulseless—start CPR, follow ACLS protocol for defibrillation, ET intubation, and administration of epinephrine or vasopressin, lidocaine, or amiodarone; if ineffective, consider magnesium sulfate
Asystole	• No atrial or ventricular rate or rhythm • No discernible P waves, QRS complexes, or T waves	• Myocardial ischemia or infarction, aortic valve disease, heart failure, hypoxemia, hypokalemia, severe acidosis, electric shock, ventricular arrhythmias, AV block, pulmonary embolism, heart rupture, cardiac tamponade, hyperkalemia, electromechanical dissociation • Cocaine overdose	Start CPR

(ACLS: Advanced Cardiac Life Support; AV: atrioventricular; COPD: chronic obstructive pulmonary disease; CPR: cardiopulmonary resuscitation; ET: endotracheal; ICU: intensive care unit; IV: intravenous; LOC: level of consciousness; MI: myocardial infarction)

Premature Ventricular Contractions

Early or premature ventricular contractions (PVCs) are caused by increased automaticity of ventricular muscle cells. PVCs usually are not considered harmful per se. They may be of concern if more than six occur in 1 minute, if they occur in pairs or triplets, if they are multifocal, or if they occur or near a T wave (R on T phenomenon).

- Atrial rhythm is regular.
- A wide QRS complex coming prematurely, usually followed by a complete

compensatory pause (the distance between two sinus R waves with a PVC in between is same as the distance between two R waves with a sinus beat in between)

- QRS complex is wide and distorted, usually >0.12 second.
- Premature QRS complexes occurring singly, in pairs, or in threes; a sinus beat always followed by a PVC more than a few cycles is called a ventricular bigeminy. Two sinus beats always followed by a PVC is a ventricular trigeminy. Two consecutive PVCs is a couplet, three consecutive ones a triplet, and more than three consecutively is a ventricular tachycardia (VT). if it is spontaneously terminated, it is called a nonsustained VT (NSVT).

Clinical manifestations include palpitations, weakness, and lightheadedness but it is most of the time asymptomatic. Management includes assessment of the cause and treat as indicated. Treatment is indicated if the client has underlying disease because PVCs may precipitate VT or fibrillation. Assess for life-threatening PVCs. Administer antiarrhythmic medication as prescribed.

Ventricular Tachycardia

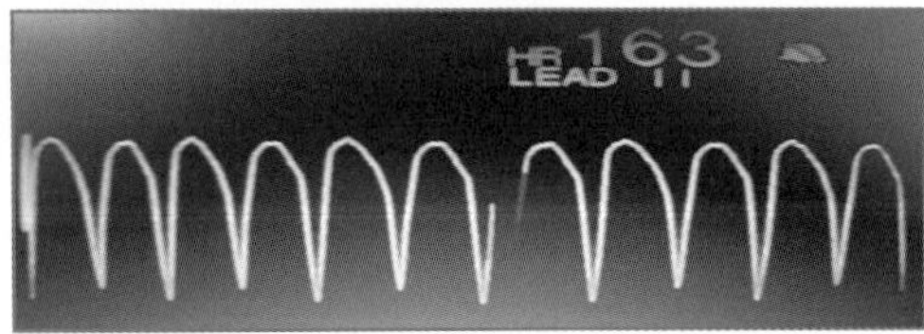

Ventricular tachycardia is three or more consecutive PVCs. It is a medical emergency because cardiac output (CO) cannot be maintained because of decreased diastolic filling (preload) and the patient may become pulseless.

- Rate is 120–250 beats/min.
- P waves are dissociated from the QRS complexes (variable PR intervals; this is the most definitive diagnostic point for VT); sometimes the P wave may be blurred and masked by rapidly occurring QRS complexes.
- QRS complex is wide, T wave is in the opposite direction.
- Rhythm is usually regular.
- May start and stop suddenly
- Ventricular tachycardia may occur with or without a palpable pulse.

Clinical manifestations of VT include lightheadedness, weakness, dyspnea, and unconsciousness. Causes include MI, aneurysm, coronary artery disease (CAD), rheumatic heart diseases, mitral valve prolapse, hypokalemia, hyperkalemia, and pulmonary embolism. Anxiety may also cause VT.

Pulseless Ventricular Tachycardia

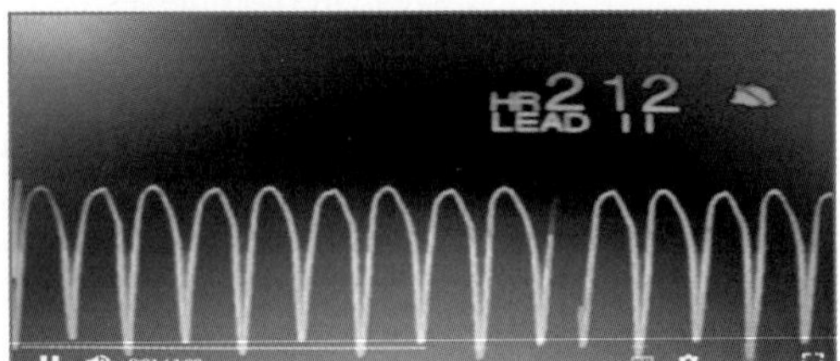

Management for pulseless VT: Initiate cardiopulmonary resuscitation (CPR); follow Advanced Cardiovascular Life Support (ACLS) protocol for defibrillation, ET intubation, and administration of epinephrine.

Ventricular Tachycardia with Pulse

Management with pulse VT: If hemodynamically stable, follow ACLS protocol for administration of amiodarone; if ineffective, initiate synchronized cardioversion. Correction of electrolyte abnormalities remains important (especially hypokalemia).

Ventricular Fibrillation

Ventricular fibrillation is rapid, ineffective quivering of ventricles that may be rapidly fatal.

- Rate is *rapid and uncoordinated, with ineffective contractions.*
- Rhythm is chaotic.
- QRS complexes may be wide, bizarre, and irregular. Sometimes there may just some undulations of the baseline.
- P wave is not seen.

Cause of ventricular fibrillation is most commonly myocardial ischemia or infarction. It may result from untreated ventricular tachycardia, electrolyte imbalances, digoxin or quinidine toxicity, or hypothermia. Clinical manifestation is like cardiac arrest, possible Stokes–Adam attacks and sudden death.

Start CPR if pulseless. Follow ACLS protocol for defibrillation, endotracheal (ET) intubation, and administration of epinephrine.

CONCLUSION

Always remember, do not get afraid or intimidated by abnormalities in ECG. It is just an electrical manifestation of what goes in the heart. In case of any arrhythmia on monitor, follow one *golden rule* of getting a 12-lead ECG immediately when the patient is conscious and pulse is felt. Interpret the ECG alone if possible and take help of the doctors to go ahead for the timely treatment as per the **Table 1**. If monitor shows ventricular fibrillation/ventricular tachycardia, then of course DO NOT WASTE TIME IN CHECKING PULSE and go ahead with defibrillation as soon as possible. At the same time, when monitor shows ventricular tachycardia, remember to check pulse before proceeding for the definitive treatment as patient can still have pulse.

FURTHER READING

1. Allen SM, Abrich VA, Bibby PS, Fishman D, Shen WK, Sorajja D. Prevalence and Prognostic Significance of Nonsustained Ventricular Tachycardia in Patients With a Left Ventricular Ejection Fraction from 35% to 50. Am J Cardiol. 2018;121(3):330-5.
2. Desai DS, Hajouli S. Arrhythmias. In: StatPearls [Internet]. Treasure Island (FL): StatPearls Publishing; 2025.
3. Kaplan J, Lala V. Paroxysmal Atrial Tachycardia. In: StatPearls [Internet]. Treasure Island (FL): StatPearls Publishing; 2025.
4. Kerola T, Eranti A, Aro AL, Haukilahti MA, Holkeri A, Junttila MJ, et al. Risk Factors Associated With Atrioventricular Block. JAMA Netw Open. 2019;2(5):e194176.
5. Lakshminarayan K, Anderson DC, Herzog CA, Qureshi AI. Clinical epidemiology of atrial fibrillation and related cerebrovascular events in the United States. Neurologist. 2008;14(3):143-50.
6. Leonelli FM, De Ponti R, Bagliani G. Challenges in Bradicardias Interpretation. Card Electrophysiol Clin. 2019;11(2):261-81.
7. Ziccardi MR, Goyal A, Maani CV. Atrial Flutter. In: StatPearls [Internet]. Treasure Island (FL): StatPearls Publishing; 2025.

CHAPTER 7

Arterial Blood Gas Analysis and Electrolyte Imbalances

Deven Juneja, Prashant Nasa

INTRODUCTION

Arterial blood gas (ABG) analysis and recognition of electrolyte imbalances form an integral component of management of critically ill patients. ABG is a point-of-care test, which identify life-threatening disturbances including, hypoxemia, hypercapnia, acidosis, and alkalosis. The presence of multiple comorbidities, lack of proper nutrition, multiorgan involvement, and use of some specific medicines may predispose patients to several electrolyte imbalances. Certain electrolyte imbalances such as hypo-/hypernatremia, hypo-/hyperkalemia, and hypo/hypercalcemia are commonly encountered in these patients. Prompt recognition of these disorders may aid in early institution of corrective measures and improving patient outcomes.

ARTERIAL BLOOD GAS ANALYSIS

Arterial blood samples are used to measure the oxygen, carbon dioxide, bicarbonate, and the pH patient.

Collection of the sample: ABGs are collected by puncturing an artery and collecting the sample in a heparinized syringe. Usual sites of arterial puncture are radial, femoral, and brachial arteries. Of these, radial is the preferred site as it is superficial, is not an end artery (hence less likely to cause any ischemic injury if damaged) and does not have many important structures in the vicinity, which can be injured during the sample collection. The disadvantage of the radial artery is that it is a small artery, and needs expertise to be punctured.

The method of collection: Preferably, the Allen test must be performed to confirm the patency of the ulnar artery before puncturing the radial artery. The syringe should be 2 mL or 5mL one, and the needle should be of 20–25 gauge. A narrow gauge needle causes less pain during puncturing but may cause more hemolysis. Local anesthesia may be used to minimize pain. The heparin should be drawn in the syringe and the fully expelled, with only a small amount remaining in the dead space of the syringe. Excess heparin can falsely increase the acidity of the sample. The collector should wash or disinfect his or her hands. The skin should be disinfected by 70% alcohol solution. Usually, about 2 mL of blood is drawn. The artery is palpated and then with the fingers of one hand palpating the artery the collector holds the syringe in the other hand and punctures at 45º angle **(Fig. 1)**. Due to high pressure in the arteries the syringe should fill itself, and the plunger need not be pulled nor vacuum syringes used for normal blood sampling be used. Unless the test is done immediately in a point-of-care analyzer. The syringe should be made air free, capped and transported in a pack or container filled with crushed ice to the laboratory. The usual errors and complications of an ABG testing are:

- Multiple punctures causing local hematoma or setting off a local arterial spasm, which may make further punctures difficult
- Inadvertent venipuncture and collection of a venous sample
- Local hematoma or bleeding
- Injury to the adjacent structure like nerves
- Local infection
- Excess heparin causing an erroneous acidosis in the analysis
- Change in the oxygen content of the sample unless tested immediately or transported in a syringe free of air and in crushed ice

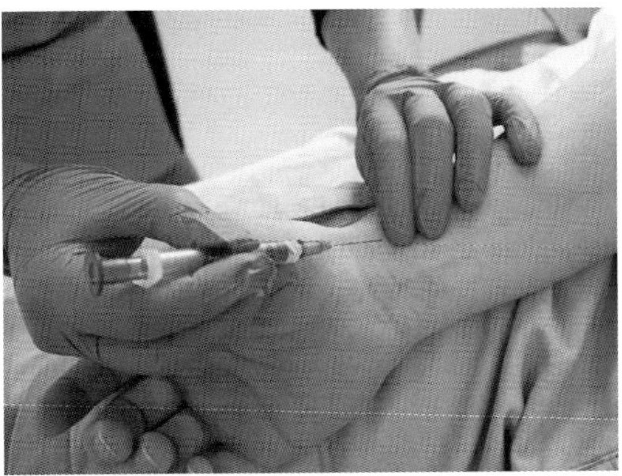

Fig. 1: Site of radial artery puncture.

The different parameters reported in the blood gas analysis report and their normal ranges are provided in **Table 1**.

Several approaches have been described for the analysis of ABG. The commonly applied Boston compensation (6-step) approach is described here.

Step 1

This step involves testing for the validity of the ABG by using the modified Henderson-Hasselbalch equation:

$$[H^+] = 24 \times PaCO_2/HCO_3^-$$

Where $[H^+]$ is the hydrogen ion concentration, $PaCO_2$ is the partial pressure of arterial carbon dioxide and HCO_3^- is the serum bicarbonate levels. The ABG is said to be invalid, if there is any inconsistency in the pH and the $[H^+]$.

Step 2

It involves identifying the presence of alkalemia (pH >7.45) or acidemia (pH <7.35). Whichever is present, it is generally the

TABLE 1: Normal arterial blood gas and electrolyte values.

Variable	*Normal range*	*Basic abnormalities*
pH	7.35–7.45	pH >7.45: Alkalemia pH <7.35: Acidemia
Partial pressure of carbon dioxide (pCO_2)	35–45 mm Hg	pCO_2 >45 mm Hg: Hypercapnia pCO_2 <45 mm Hg: Hypocapnia
Partial pressure of arterial oxygen (PaO_2)	75–100 mm Hg	PaO_2 <75 mm Hg: Hypoxemia
Bicarbonate (HCO_3)	22–29 mEq/L	HCO_3 >30 mEq/L: Alkalosis HCO_3 <22 mEq/L: Acidosis
Anion gap	4–12 mEq/L	Anion gap >12 mEq/L: Acidosis
Serum sodium	135–145 mEq/L	Sodium >145 mEq/L: Hypernatremia Sodium <135 mEq/L: Hyponatremia
Serum potassium	3.5–5 mEq/L	Potassium >5 mEq/L: Hyperkalemia Potassium <3.5 mEq/L: Hypokalemia
Serum calcium	8.5–10.5 mg/dL	Calcium >10.5 mg/dL: Hypercalcemia Calcium <8.5 mg/dL: Hypocalcemia

primary disorder. However, alkalemia or acidemia may be present even in the presence of normal pH. Hence, in the subsequent steps, we need to check the $PaCO_2$, HCO_3^-, and anion gap (AG).

Step 3

To further determine whether the primary disorder is respiratory or metabolic, we have to check the relationship between the direction in change of pH and pCO_2. In primary respiratory disorder, both will change in opposite directions, while in primary metabolic conditions, both will change in the same direction.

Acidosis—pH ↓ and $PaCO_2$ ↑: Respiratory
Acidosis—pH ↓ and $PaCO_2$ ↓: Metabolic
Alkalosis—pH ↑ and $PaCO_2$ ↓: Respiratory
Alkalosis—pH ↑ and $PaCO_2$ ↑: Respiratory

Step 4

This step involves checking for compensation for the primary disorder. However, it must be remembered that compensation is never complete and pH does not return to normal levels. There are different equations to check for compensation for different primary disorders **(Table 2)**. If the observed values are different from those derived from these equations, multiple acid-base disorders are likely present.

TABLE 2: Equations to check for compensation.

Primary disorder	*Equation to check for compensation*
Metabolic acidosis	$PaCO_2 = (1.5 \times [HCO_3^-]) + 8 \pm 2$
Metabolic alkalosis	$PaCO_2 = 0.7 \times [HCO_3] = 20 \pm 5$
Respiratory acidosis (acute)	$\uparrow\Delta[HCO_3] = 0.1 \times \uparrow\Delta PaCO_2$
Respiratory acidosis (chronic, 3–5 days)	$\uparrow\Delta[HCO_3] = 0.35 \times \uparrow\Delta PaCO_2$
Acute respiratory alkalosis	$\downarrow\Delta[HCO_3] = 0.2 \times \downarrow\Delta PaCO_2$
Chronic respiratory alkalosis	$\downarrow\Delta[HCO_3] = 0.4 \times \downarrow\Delta PaCO_2$

(HCO_3: bicarbonate; $PaCO_2$: partial pressure of arterial carbon dioxide)

Step 5

This step involves calculating the AG by subtracting the serum cations (Na^+, K^+) from the serum anion (Cl^-, HCO_3^-) levels.

$$\text{Anion gap} = (Na^+ + K^+) - (Cl^- + HCO_3^-)$$

The normal range is 4–12 mEq/L. Low AG may be present in patients with severe hypoalbuminemia. The common causes of increased AG metabolic acidosis include diabetic ketoacidosis, lactic acidosis, renal failure, and certain poisonings (methanol, ethanol, salicylates, theophylline, and paracetamol). If poisoning is suspected, it is advisable to calculate the osmolal gap (osmolal gap = measured osmolality - (2[Na^+]- glucose/18 - blood urea nitrogen/2.8).

Step 6

In cases where the AG is increased, the ratio of increase in AG (ΔAG) to decrease in bicarbonate $\Delta[HCO_3^-]$ level must be calculated. If it is in the normal range (1.0–2.0), then it shows that the AG is uncomplicated, otherwise it indicates the presence of another metabolic disorder. If $\Delta AG/\Delta[HCO_3^-]$ <1.0, then it indicates the presence of coexisting non-AG metabolic acidosis and if $\Delta AG/\Delta[HCO_3^-]$ >2.0, it indicates coexisting metabolic alkalosis.

ELECTROLYTES

Hypernatremia

Sodium-based disorders signify an imbalance between water and sodium ions. Serum sodium levels >145 mEq/L is classified as hypernatremia. Based on serum sodium levels, it may be further classified as mild (146–150 mEq/L), moderate (151–155 mEq/L), severe (>155 mEq/L), and extreme (>190 mEq/L). Hypernatremia may also be classified as acute (<48 hours) and chronic (>48 hours), depending on the rapidity of the increase in serum sodium levels. Patients with a gradual increase in serum sodium levels and those with chronic hypernatremia are less likely to have symptoms **(Table 3)**.

Correction of hypernatremia depends on the severity of symptoms, onset of time, and volume status of the patient. Management involves identifying and correcting the cause and treating hypernatremia with free water (oral or intravenous 5% dextrose). The water deficit may be calculated as:

Free water deficit (liters) = 0.6 × body weight (kg) × [(serum sodium/148)–1]

TABLE 3: Symptoms secondary to hypernatremia.

Neurological symptoms	*Symptoms secondary to dehydration*	*Other symptoms*
• Nausea • Vomiting • Lethargy • Focal neurological deficits • Muscle spasms • Myoclonic jerks • Nystagmus • Irritability • Seizures • Abnormal speech • Confusion • Altered sensorium • Coma	• Orthostatic hypotension • Tachycardia • Oliguria • Dry skin/oral mucosa • Intense thirst	• Loss of weight • Generalized weakness • Fever • Labored breathing

Hyponatremia

Hyponatremia, defined as serum sodium levels <135 mEq/L, is arguably the most common electrolyte abnormality in hospitalized patients. Based on the extracellular volume status, *hyponatremia* may be defined as hypovolemic, euvolemic, and hypervolemic **(Table 4)**. Symptoms of hyponatremia depend on serum sodium levels and acuity of development of hyponatremia. Symptoms are primarily neurological, and patients may present with nausea, vomiting, anorexia, lethargy, headache, muscular cramps, confusion, altered mental status, restlessness, agitation, seizures, and coma.

The treatment of hyponatremia also depends on the duration, severity, and patient's volume status. Hypertonic 3% saline may be used for severe symptomatic hyponatremia (serum sodium <120 mEq/L). In the presence of severe symptoms, a bolus 100–150 mL of 3% saline may be given over 10–20 minutes, which may be repeated 2–3 times, checking sodium levels every 20 minutes till symptoms resolve or sodium levels increase by 5 mEq/L. In patients with moderate symptoms and low risk of herniation, continuous infusion of 3% saline at 0.5–2 mL/kg/h. The target correction is 10–12 mEq/L in the first 24 hours, after that <8 mEq/L every 24 hours till sodium levels reach >130 mEq/L. Selective vasopressin receptor antagonists (tolvaptan) may be used in patients with chronic hyponatremia secondary to syndrome of inappropriate antidiuretic hormone (SIADH). Treatment of hypervolemic hyponatremia requires restriction of salt and fluids, and cautious administration of loop diuretics. The management of euvolemic hyponatremia requires fluid restriction to <1 L/day. Underlying etiology should also be promptly recognized and treated.

TABLE 4: Causes of hyponatremia.

Causes of hypovolemic hyponatremia	*Causes of hypervolemic hyponatremia*	*Causes of euvolemic hyponatremia*
• Gastrointestinal fluid loss (diarrhea or vomiting) • The third spacing of fluids (pancreatitis, hypoalbuminemia, and small bowel obstruction) • Diuretics • Osmotic diuresis (glucose and mannitol) • Salt-wasting nephropathies • Cerebral salt-wasting syndrome • Mineralocorticoid deficiency	• Renal causes (acute renal failure, chronic renal failure, and nephrotic syndrome) • Extrarenal causes (congestive heart failure and cirrhosis) • Iatrogenic	• Drugs, like vasopressin analogs (desmopressin, oxytocin), thiazide diuretics, antidepressants (serotonin-reuptake inhibitors), carbamazepine, vincristine, nicotine, antipsychotics, chlorpropamide, cyclophosphamide, and nonsteroidal anti-inflammatory drugs • Syndrome of inappropriate antidiuretic hormone (SIADH) • Addison's disease • Hypothyroidism • Primary polydipsia; or potomania, • Iatrogenic

TABLE 5: Causes of hyperkalemia.

Increased potassium intake	*Intracellular potassium shifts*	*Impaired potassium excretion*
• Food and drinks with high potassium content • Intravenous fluids with high potassium contents (parenteral nutrition and potassium-containing drugs) • Massive blood transfusions	• Cellular injury (rhabdomyolysis and hemolysis) • Metabolic acidosis • Insulin deficiency • Diabetic ketoacidosis • Certain medications [succinylcholine, angiotensin-converting enzyme (ACE) inhibitors, and digoxin] • Tumor lysis syndrome • Hyperkalemic periodic paralysis	• Acute/chronic renal failure • Aldosterone deficiency or insensitivity

Hyperkalemia

Hyperkalemia is generally defined as serum potassium levels above 5–5.5 mEq/L. The causes are enumerated in **Table 5**. The development of symptoms depends on potassium level and the rapidity of its increase. Mild hyperkalemia is generally well tolerated, and symptoms generally develop with serum levels above 6.5 mEq/L and levels above 8 mEq/L may have life-threatening complications.

The clinical signs and symptoms of hyperkalemia may include muscular weakness, flaccid paralysis, or depressed deep tendon reflexes. Electrocardiography (ECG) features secondary to hyperkalemia may include small or absent P wave, prolonged PR interval, augmentation of R wave, widening of

QRS complex, and peaking of T waves. Severe hyperkalemia (serum potassium levels >8 mEq/L) may lead to the development of cardiac arrhythmias, sine wave pattern, and even asystole.

Treatment of hyperkalemia involves stopping exogenous potassium, identifying and correcting the cause followed by a three-pronged approach:

- *Cardiac muscle stabilization:* Calcium therapy should be initiated immediately in patients with signs of cardiac toxicity. Both calcium chloride and calcium gluconate (only through the central line) may be used but not together.
- *Enhance intracellular potassium shift:* Insulin and glucose (50 mL of a 50% dextrose with 10 units of insulin), and high doses of beta-2 adrenergic agents (salbutamol nebulization) may aid in driving potassium intracellularly, thereby reducing serum potassium levels. Sodium bicarbonate may also be used in patients with metabolic acidosis.
- *Increasing potassium excretion:* Loop or thiazide diuretics may be used to increase renal excretion of potassium. Potassium binder like sodium polystyrene sulfonate, either orally or as enema, may increase gastrointestinal potassium excretion. Further, hemodialysis may be required in severe or refractory cases and in patients with renal failure, to reduce serum potassium levels rapidly.
- The drugs being taken by the patient must be checked, and any possible drug which may cause hyperkalemia needs to be stopped. The common drugs causing hyperakalemia are: Angiotensin-converting enzyme inhibitors (ramipril), angiotensin receptor blockers (telmisartan and olmesartan), mineralocorticoid receptor antagonists (aldactone), and nonselective beta blockers (propranolol).
- Diet rich in potassium such as fruits and coconut water should be avoided.

Hypokalemia

Hypokalemia, defined as serum potassium levels <3.5 mEq/L, is a more common disorder than hyperkalemia. Renal, gastrointestinal, and even transdermal loses may lead to hypokalemia **(Table 6)**.

Clinical symptoms depend upon the severity and rapidity of development of hypokalemia. Symptoms generally develop when potassium levels fall below 3 mEq/L. These include muscle weakness, which may also involve respiratory muscles leading to respiratory failure and rarely death. Other symptoms include muscle spasms, rhabdomyolysis, and ileus, leading to abdominal distension, nausea, and vomiting. Other serious symptoms are related to

TABLE 6: Causes of hypokalemia.

Decreased potassium intake	*Transcellular shifts*	*Increased potassium loss*
• Malnutrition • Reduced intake	• Alkalemia • Insulin • Beta-adrenergic stimulation • Aldosterone • Xanthines (caffeine) • Hypokalemic periodic paralysis	• *Renal loss:* Primary hyper-reninism and primary aldosteronism, diuretic therapy, magnesium deficiency, and genetic syndromes • *Gastrointestinal loss:* Severe or chronic diarrhea • *Transdermal loss:* Excessive sweating

involvement of cardiac muscles, which may cause arrhythmias, and characteristic ECG changes including T-wave flattening, followed by depression of ST segment and development of U waves.

Treatment involves oral or intravenous potassium supplementation, along with treatment of underlying cause. Oral potassium chloride (10% solution, 20 mEq/15 mL) is preferred in patients with mild deficiency, but must be administered with feeds to avoid gastritis. Intravenous (20 mEq/ampule) route may be used in severe deficiency (serum potassium <2.5 mEq/L) or when the oral route is unavailable. Intravenous potassium should not be dissolved in dextrose water, when it is used as a replacement. Up to 10 mEq/h may be infused through a large-bore peripheral line (2 ampoules of KCl or 40 mEq dissolved in 1 L given over 6 hours or 8 hours) but for a higher dose, central venous access is required.

Hypercalcemia

The normal serum calcium levels are between 8.5 and 10.5 mg/dL. As around 45% of serum calcium is bound to proteins (mainly albumin), corrected or ionized calcium levels (normal range 4.65–5.25 mg/dL) may provide a better estimate. Corrected calcium accounts for the serum albumin levels and may be calculated as:

Corrected calcium (mg/dL) = measured total Ca (mg/dL) + 0.8 (4.0 – serum albumin [g/dL])

Hypercalcemia is classified based on serum calcium levels as mild (10.5–11.9 mg/dL), moderate (12.0–13.9 mg/dL), and hypercalcemic crisis (14.0–16.0 mg/dL). Causes of hypercalcemia have been enumerated in **Table 7**.

The clinical symptoms associated with hypercalcemia are popularly described using mnemonic "groans, bones, stones, moans, thrones, and psychic overtones" **(Table 8)**. These symptoms usually develop when serum calcium levels are >12 mg/dL. Severe hypercalcemia is also associated with involvement of cardiovascular and neuromuscular systems causing arrhythmias and muscle weakness. Hypercalcemia typically causes bradycardia,

TABLE 7: Causes of hypercalcemia.

Excessive parathyroid hormone	*Malignant*	*Hypervitaminosis D*	*Endocrinal*	*Miscellaneous*
• Parathyroid gland adenoma/ hyperplasia • Familial hypocalciuric hypercalcemia • Multiple endocrine neoplasia syndromes • Familial hypocalciuric hypercalcemia	• Renal carcinomas • Leukemias • Lymphomas • Rhabdo-myosarcoma	• Iatrogenic • Excessive milk intake • Granulomatous diseases (sarcoidosis and tuberculosis) • Systemic fungal infections	• Thyrotoxicosis • Hypoadrenalism • Pheochro-mocytomas	• Hypophosphatasia • Hypervitaminosis A • Acute/chronic renal failure • Thiazide diuretics • Lithium • Milk-alkali syndrome • Subcutaneous fat necrosis • Prolonged immobilization • Williams syndrome • Murk Jansen syndrome

TABLE 8: Clinical features of hypercalcemia.

Groans	*Bones*	*Stones*	*Moans*	*Thrones*	*Psychic overtones*
• Gastrointestinal symptoms (pain, nausea, and vomiting) • Peptic ulcers • Pancreatitis	• Bone pain • Osteoporosis • Osteomalacia • Arthritis • Pathological fractures	Renal stones	• Fatigue • Malaise	• Polyuria • Polydipsia • Constipation	• Lethargy • Confusion • Depression • Memory loss • Encephalopathy

TABLE 9: Causes of hypocalcemia.

Hypoparathyroidism	*High parathyroid hormone levels*	*Miscellaneous*
• *Postsurgical:* Thyroidectomy, parathyroidectomy, or radical neck surgery • Autoimmune • Abnormal parathyroid gland development • *Parathyroid gland destruction:* Granulomatous diseases, hemochromatosis, Wilson disease, amyloidosis, aluminum-containing phosphate binders, or irradiation	• Vitamin D deficiency: Absolute/relative • Chronic kidney disease • Pseudohypoparathyroidism	• Pseudohypocalcemia • Acidosis • Alkalosis • Acute pancreatitis • Sepsis • Severe illness/trauma • Hypomagnesemia/hypermagnesemia • Acute hyperphosphatemia • *Drugs:* Cisplatin, foscarnet, bisphosphonates, and denosumab • Massive blood transfusion • Osteoblastic metastasis • Pregnancy

while ECG may show prolongation of PR interval, shortened QT interval, T-wave flattening, widening of QRS complex, and J-waves at the end of QRS.

Active treatment is indicated in symptomatic patients and in those with serum calcium levels >15 mg/dL. Therapeutic strategies include enhancing elimination, reducing bone absorption and decreasing gastrointestinal absorption, and recognizing and managing the cause of hypercalcemia. Restoring intravascular volume using 0.9% saline is the first therapeutic measure to increase renal excretion (target urine output 200–300 mL/h). In patients with hypercalcemia secondary to malignancies, bisphosphonates (etidronate, pamidronate, and alendronate) are the drugs of choice. Subcutaneous calcitonin may be used, but its effects are mild and short-lasting. Hemodialysis may be required in refractory cases and those with severe hypercalcemia and underlying renal or cardiac failure.

Hypocalcemia

Hypocalcemia is defined as serum calcium levels <8.5 mg/dL or ionized calcium levels <4.65 mg/dL. The common causes of hypocalcemia are given in **Table 9**. The clinical manifestations associated with hypocalcemia are generally neuromuscular and cardiovascular. Patients may present with altered mental status, seizures, neuromuscular weakness, paresthesias

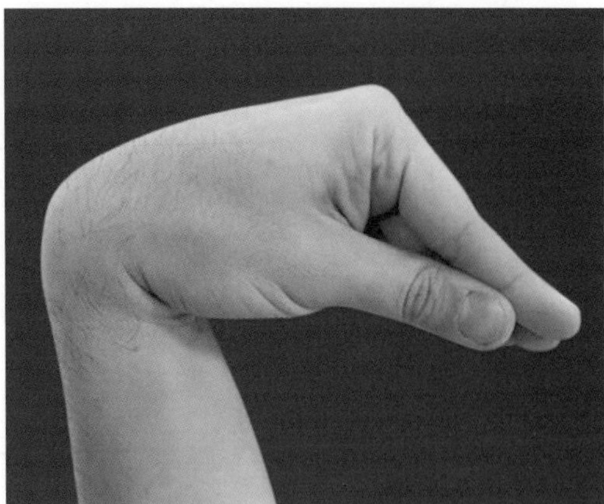

Fig. 2: The flexed wrist and the metacarpophalangeal joint and the extended distal and proximal interphalangeal joint are characteristic of Trousseau Sign (sign of Latent tetany).

(perioral or in the extremities), tetany, and carpopedal spasms. On examination, patient may exhibit a positive Chvostek's sign, Trousseau's sign, and ECG may show prolongation of QTc and rarely, torsades de pointes **(Fig. 2)**.

Hypocalcemia treatment includes identifying and correcting the underlying cause and calcium replacement. Oral calcium supplementation may be done in patients with mild hypocalcemia or with mild symptoms. 1.5–2 g of elemental calcium per day may be given in the form of calcium carbonate (40% elemental calcium) or calcium citrate (21% elemental calcium) in two-three divided doses. Vitamin D supplementation is also generally recommended to increase calcium absorption. Intravenous calcium may be preferred in patients with acute hypocalcemia, and in those with severe symptoms or prolonged QTc. Calcium gluconate (90 mg elemental calcium) 1–2 g or 1 g of calcium chloride (270 mg elemental calcium, only through a central venous catheter) can be transfused over 10–20 minutes. A continuous infusion may be required in patients with persistent hypocalcemia.

CONCLUSION

Acid–base and electrolyte abnormalities are common in hospitalized patients. Certain patients, like those with advanced age, critically ill, underlying renal dysfunction, on parenteral nutrition, and prolonged illness are at higher risk of developing these complications. Multiple electrolyte imbalances may exist in a single patient because of overlapping risk factors and interrelated excretion mechanisms. Hence, other electrolyte abnormalities like hypomagnesemia, hypophosphatemia, and hyperphosphatemia should also be actively sought and ruled out. As most of these are reversible, early identification and correction of these abnormalities and their underlying causative factors may be instrumental in improving clinical outcomes.

FURTHER READING

1. Bove-Fenderson E, Mannstadt M. Hypocalcemic disorders. Best Pract Res Clin Endocrinol Metab. 2018;32(5):639-56.
2. Carrick AI, Costner HB. Rapid Fire: Hypercalcemia. Emerg Med Clin North Am. 2018;36(3):549-55.
3. Castro D, Sharma S. Hypokalemia. (2025). Treasure Island (FL): StatPearls Publishing. Available from https://www.ncbi.nlm.nih.gov/books/NBK482465/. [Last assessed February, 2025].
4. Dépret F, Peacock WF, Liu KD, Rafique Z, Rossignol P, Legrand M. Management of hyperkalemia in the acutely ill patient. Ann Intensive Care. 2019;9:32.
5. Fidkowski C, Helstrom J. Diagnosing metabolic acidosis in the critically ill: bridging the anion gap, Stewart and base excess methods. Can J Anesth. 2009;56:247-56.
6. Fukumoto S, Namba N, Ozono K, Yamauchi M, Sugimoto T, Michigami T, et al. Causes and differential diagnosis of hypocalcemia—recommendation proposed by expert panel supported by ministry of health, labour and welfare, Japan. Endocr J. 2008;55(5):787-94.

7. Goyal A, Anastasopoulou C, Ngu M, Singh S. (2023). Hypocalcemia. Treasure Island (FL): StatPearls Publishing. Available from https://www.ncbi.nlm.nih.gov/books/NBK430912/. [Last assessed February, 2025].
8. Hoorn EJ, Zietse R. Diagnosis and Treatment of Hyponatremia: Compilation of the Guidelines. J Am Soc Nephrol. 2017;28(5):1340-9.
9. Massicotte-Azarniouch D, Canney M, Sood MM, Hundemer GL. Managing Hyperkalemia in the Modern Era: A Case-Based Approach. Kidney Int Rep. 2023;8(7):1290-300.
10. Pepe J, Colangelo L, Biamonte F, Sonato C, Danese VC, Cecchetti V, et al. Diagnosis and management of hypocalcemia. Endocrine. 2020;69(3):485-95.
11. Rondon H, Badireddy M. Hyponatremia. (2023). Treasure Island (FL): StatPearls Publishing. Available from https://www.ncbi.nlm.nih.gov/books/NBK470386/. [Last assessed February, 2025].
12. Rose BD, TW Post (Eds). Clinical Physiology of Acid-Base and Electrolyte Disorders, 5th edition. New York: McGraw Hill Medical Publishing Division; 2001.
13. Sonani B, Naganathan S, Al-Dhahir MA. (2023). Hypernatremia. Treasure Island (FL): StatPearls Publishing. Available from https://www.ncbi.nlm.nih.gov/books/NBK441960/. [Last assessed February, 2025].
14. Sterns RH, Grieff M, Bernstein PL. Treatment of hyperkalemia: something old, something new. Kidney Int. 2016;89(3):546-54.
15. Vanholder R, Van Biesen W, Nagler EV. Treating potassium disturbances: kill the killers but avoid overkill. Acta Clin Belg. 2019;74(4):215-28.
16 Verbalis JG, Goldsmith SR, Greenberg A, Korzelius C, Schrier RW, Sterns RH, et al. Diagnosis, evaluation, and treatment of hyponatremia: expert panel recommendations. Am J Med. 2013;126(10 Suppl 1):S1-42.
17. Walker J. Diagnosis and management of patients with hypercalcaemia. Nurs Older People. 2015;27(4):22-6.
18. Yee J, Frinak S, Mohiuddin N, Uduman J. Fundamentals of Arterial Blood Gas Interpretation. Kidney360. 2022;3(8):1458-66.
19. Yun G, Baek SH, Kim S. Evaluation and management of hypernatremia in adults: clinical perspectives. Korean J Intern Med. 2023;38(3):290-302.

CHAPTER 8

Hemodynamic Monitoring

Saswati Sinha, Amit Das

INTRODUCTION

Patients admitted to the critical care unit are often experiencing life-threatening effects of respiratory failure, kidney failure, heart failure, sepsis, trauma, shock, intracranial hemorrhage, burns, major surgery, myocardial infarction, etc. Each of these conditions can cause hemodynamic instability, multiorgan failure, and death. Hemodynamic monitoring helps to identify the problem and guides resuscitation.

ASSESSMENT

- *Basic assessment:*
    - Heart rate and rhythm
    - Peripheral systolic, diastolic, and mean pressures
    - Capillary refill time (CRT)
    - Lactate
    - Urine output
    - Mentation
- *Advanced:*
    - Echocardiography
    - Central venous pressure (CVP)
    - Invasive and noninvasive arterial blood pressure (ABP) monitoring
    - Pulmonary artery pressure (PA pressure)
    - Cardiac output (CO)

Most of the advance monitoring needs calibration/zeroing, maintenance, and trouble shooting.

Heart Rate and Rhythm

- Heart rate is a component of cardiac output (cardiac output = heart rate × stroke volume)
- A 12-lead electrocardiogram (ECG) allows one to check the cardiac rhythm and pick up other abnormalities if any. ECG may also be monitored in real time.

One needs to note heart rate >100 beats/minute (tachycardia) and heart rate <60 beats/minute (bradycardia). Hypovolemia, shock, myocardial ischemia, and many other acute conditions can be picked up by doing continuous monitoring of heart rate, rhythm, and ST segments. Monitoring of the heart rate and rhythm reveals different types of arrhythmias signifying various clinical conditions, e.g., sinus tachycardia, sinus bradycardia, atrial fibrillation, atrial flutter, complete heart block, etc. some common ECG abnormalities **(Fig. 1)**.

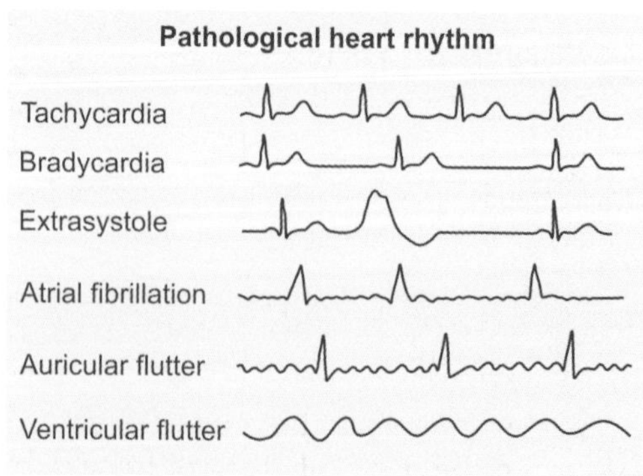

Fig. 1: Different cardiac rhythms.

Peripheral Pulse, Systolic, Diastolic, and Mean Pressures

Pulse remains perhaps the first observed clinical sign in a patient. Although usually checked in the radial area in the wrist, please note a feeble pulse in a collapsed or unstable patient who should be palpated in the carotid artery. No patient can be diagnosed as pulseless without palpating the carotid pulse. Pulse can also be palpated in any artery like the dorsalis pedis, femoral, or brachial arteries. Palpated pulse may or may not match the heart rate shown in the ECG monitor, as ectopic beats may have a lesser stroke volume and may not produce a palpable pulse.

Systolic blood pressure (SBP) is the maximum blood pressure during contraction of the ventricles. Diastolic blood pressure (DBP) is the minimum pressure recorded just prior to the next contraction. Mean arterial blood pressure (MAP) = SBP + (2 × DBP)/3. MAP is an approximation of organ perfusion pressure.

Hypotension is seen in states of decreased vascular resistance (e.g., septic shock, anaphylactic shock, etc.), whereas hypertension is associated with increased vascular resistance (acute renal failure, hypertensive encephalopathy, etc.). Sometimes hypotension may also be present with increased vascular resistance like in cardiogenic shock.

Capillary Refill Time

Capillary refill time is a simple bedside method to check the peripheral perfusion of critically sick patients, who are in shock due to sepsis or hypovolemia, etc.

How to Check for Capillary Refill Time? (Fig. 2)

The performing examiner applies finger pressure to the distal phalanx of fingers or toes until the nail is blanched.

This pressure is maintained for 10 seconds and then released.

If after the release of the pressure the normal color returns by 3 seconds or less, capillary refill is said to be normal.

Lactate

Lactic acid is produced in physiologically normal processes, but its production may be severely elevated in diseased states secondary to poor tissue perfusion. This means there is a profound hemodynamic compromise.

The common causes of lactic acidosis are as follows:

- Shock
- Sepsis
- Metformin
- Heart failure
- Renal failure

The tissues that produce excess lactic acid include skin, red cells, brain tissue, muscle, and gastrointestinal tract. It is metabolized mostly via the liver and kidney.

The higher the level of lactate and longer the time needed for normalization, the greater the mortality.

Patients with lactic acidosis usually present with clinical signs of tissue hypoperfusion, such as severe hypotension, altered mental status, oliguria, tachypnea, or Kussmaul's respiration.

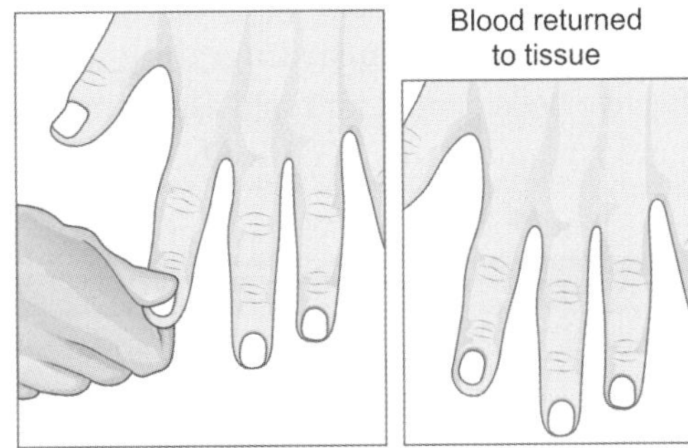

Fig. 2: Checking capillary refill.

Management of lactic acidosis is targeted on the underlying cause.

Urine Output

Monitoring hourly urine output in a critically ill patient is a simple, reliable, and inexpensive tool for hemodynamic assessment.

Passing of large amount of urine may be seen in patients on diuretic infusion, glycosuria, resolving phase of acute tubular necrosis, diabetes insipidus, etc.

Improvement in urine output in a patient after transfusing crystalloid is an indicator of fluid responsiveness.

Decreasing urine output (oliguria) or no urine output (anuria) may also be seen in conditions like acute on chronic kidney disease, acute tubular necrosis, etc. The stages of acute kidney injury are shown in **Table 1**.

Mentation

Critically ill patients may present with altered mental status or drowsiness, attributed to cerebral hypoperfusion as a consequence of hemodynamic instability. MAP should be kept at a higher value apart from treating the underlying cause of hypoperfusion in such patients.

Echocardiography

Transthoracic echocardiography is an effective bedside tool for rapid assessment of hemodynamic status in critically ill patients admitted to intensive care unit with features of hypoperfusion.

The different views that can be obtained on echocardiography are parasternal long axis (PLAX), parasternal short axis (PSAX), apical four-chamber, apical five-chamber, apical long axis, subcostal four-chamber, and suprasternal views.

Echocardiography helps in the management of intravenous (IV) fluid prescription, to rule out regional wall motion abnormalities in myocardial infarction patients, any chamber clots, valvular vegetations, pericardial effusion or tamponade, right ventricular dysfunctions, etc.

Performing bedside echocardiography, however, needs expertise and regular hands-on practice on patients.

Invasive Hemodynamic Monitoring

The measurement of various pressures with cannulas placed inside the vessels is called invasive monitoring. Usually, these are more accurate than noninvasive monitoring and allow real time.

Invasive Arterial Blood Pressure

Indications of invasive arterial pressure monitoring

- Patients in shock after initial resuscitation needing high dose vasopressors
- Significant blood loss and major surgery
- Frequent sampling of blood for laboratory analysis or ventilatory impairment

TABLE 1: Stages of acute kidney injury based on KDIGO.

Stage 1	Increase in serum creatinine ≥0.3 mg/dL (48 hours) or 1.5–1.9 times the baseline (in 7 days)
Stage 2	Serum creatinine 2–2.9 times the baseline
Stage 3	Serum creatinine 3 or more times the baseline; increase in creatinine ≥4 mg/dL; or beginning of renal replacement therapy regardless of a previous Kidney Disease: Improving Global Outcomes (KDIGO) stage

- Patients in whom noninvasive measurement is unreliable, e.g., morbid obesity, large surface area burns, and multiple extremity fractures.
- Cardiac output calculation (stroke volume and fluid responsiveness)
- Insertion of intra-aortic balloon pump (IABP)—femoral artery

Contraindications to insertion of an arterial cannula

- Peripheral or distal arterial insufficiency
- Peripheral arterial vascular diseases
- A lack of collateral circulation due to anatomical anomalies, such as the congenital absence of the ulnar artery. Allen's test is helpful in this matter.
- Infection at the catheter insertion site (less risk with the more peripheral locations)
- Synthetic vascular graft

Relative contraindications

- Coagulopathy
- Post-thrombolysis (for first 24 hours)

Sites of arterial line placement

The most common sites of arterial line placement are as follows:

- Radial artery
- Femoral artery
- Brachial artery (not a preferred site as it does not have adequate collateral supply)

Other sites which may be used include axillary, dorsalis pedis, and ulnar arteries.

Modified Allen's test: The modified Allen's test is used to assess collateral blood flow to the hands. It is done before placing any arterial line in a radial artery. It evaluates the capacity of the ulnar artery to supply blood to the digits when radial artery is occluded **(Fig. 3)**.

Technique:

- Hold the patient's hand high with fist clenched
- Occlude radial and ulnar arteries with both thumbs which allow the blood to drain from the hand
- Release the pressure from the ulnar artery while maintaining the pressure over radial artery
- Record the time for the return of normal color to the fingers
  Normal response time ≤6 seconds
  Abnormal ≥14 seconds

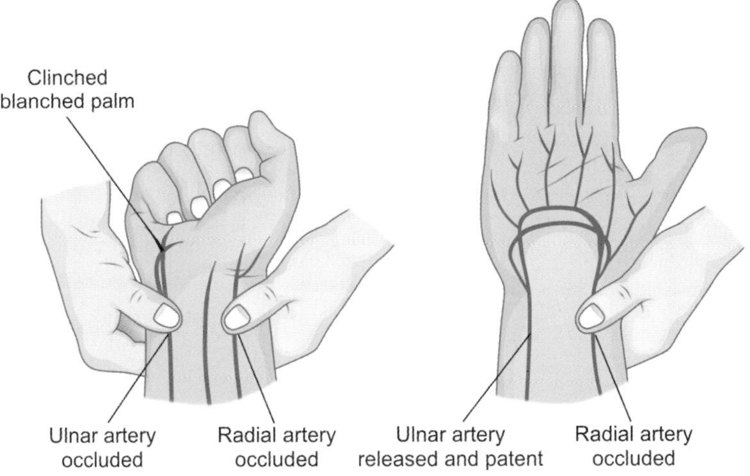

Fig. 3: Allen test for blood flow.

Arterial waveform interpretation **(Fig. 4)**: The arterial waveform results from each left ventricular systole ejecting blood into the aorta and later the run-off of that blood into the peripheral arteries. The several components include:

- Systolic upstroke—systolic ventricular ejection
- Peak systolic pressure—highest pressure
- Systolic decline—rapid decrease in pressure as ventricular contraction
- Dicrotic notch—represents the closure of the aortic valve. The diastole starts after that.
- Diastolic run-off
- End-diastolic pressure—lowest pressure at the end of the diastolic cycle occurs immediately before the next arterial upstroke.

Apart from systolic and diastolic blood pressure, the other useful information which can be derived from the arterial waveform includes:

- Mean arterial pressure (MAP)—area under the curve
- Pulse pressure—(SBP – DBP)
- Pulse pressure variation (PPV)—to assess volume status

SETTING UP THE PRESSURE TRANSDUCING SYSTEM

This consists of a pressure transducing assembly with a flushing system **(Fig. 5)**.

- The accuracy of invasive pressure measurement will be compromised if the proper setup and function of the pressure transducing system is not maintained.
- The pressure transducing assembly consists of coupling system, pressure transducer, amplifier and signal conditioner, analog to digital converter, and microprocessor which converts the signal received from the vein or the artery into a waveform on a bedside monitor.
- The flushing system is set up using a 500-mL sterile saline bag encased in a pressurized system to 300 mm Hg. At this pressure, the catheter will be flushed with 3 mL saline per hour and help keep the catheter patent. The flushing device helps to flush the assembly as required. Before

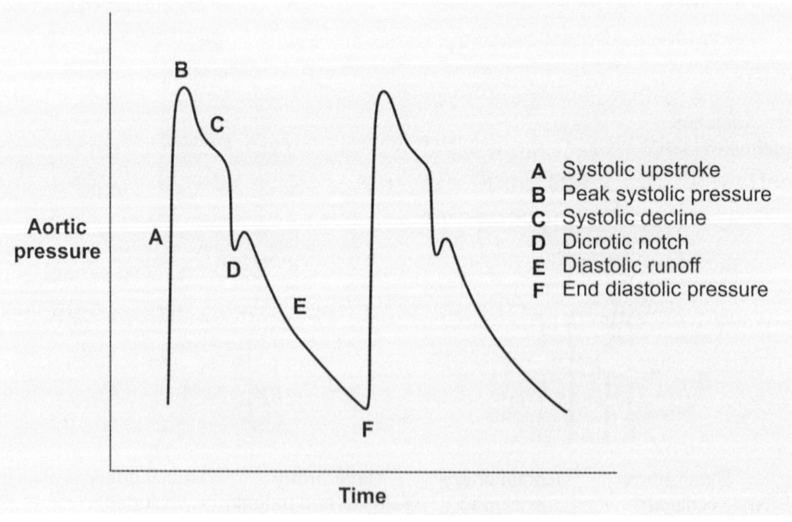

Fig. 4: Arterial waveform interpretation.

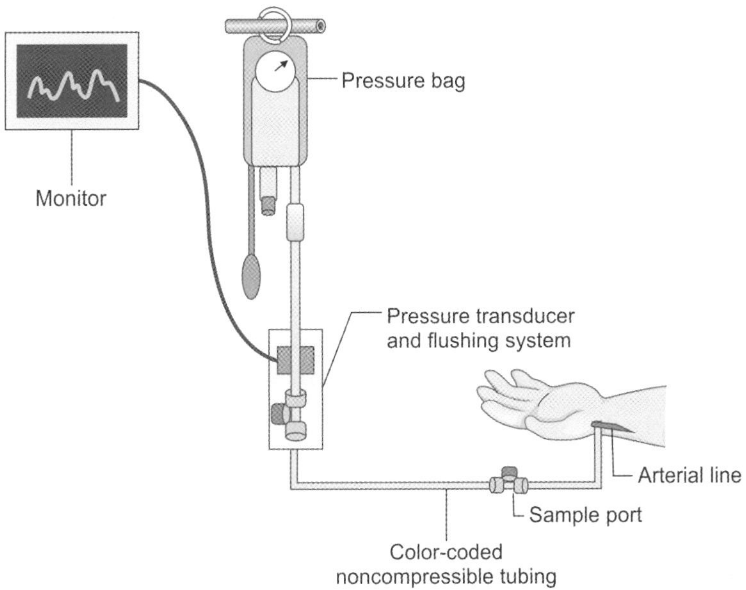

Fig. 5: Setting up the pressure transducing system.

connecting, the system should be flushed and made free of air bubbles.

- Because of concerns of heparin-induced thrombocytopenia, and errors in coagulation tests if the sample for the test is collected from this system, the system is not heparinized.

Zeroing the transducer (static calibration): The air fluid interface of the system must be aligned with the cardiac chamber or the vessel (artery/vein) which is being measured.

- The reference point is usually at the level of the heart. The junction of the fourth intercostal space and the midpoint between the anterior and posterior chest walls or 5 cm behind the sternum (called the phlebostatic axis) **(Fig. 6)**.
- A spirit level should be used to level this point with the stopcock of the pressure transducing system which is used for zeroing.

The stopcock is opened to air, and the recorded pressure (atmospheric pressure) is used by convention as the reference value of 0 mm Hg.

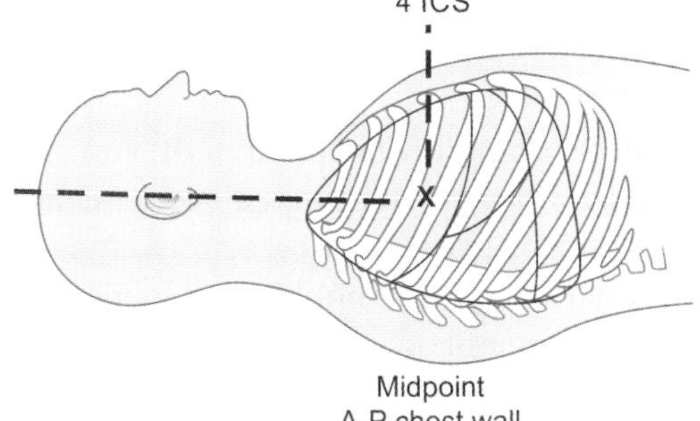

Fig. 6: Phlebostatic axis.

Phlebostatic Axis

- Check if the system is optimally damped **(Figs. 7A to C)**.
- Damping indicates the tendency of an oscillating system to return to its resting state.
- Underdamped waveform is a narrow and peaked tracing which will show a

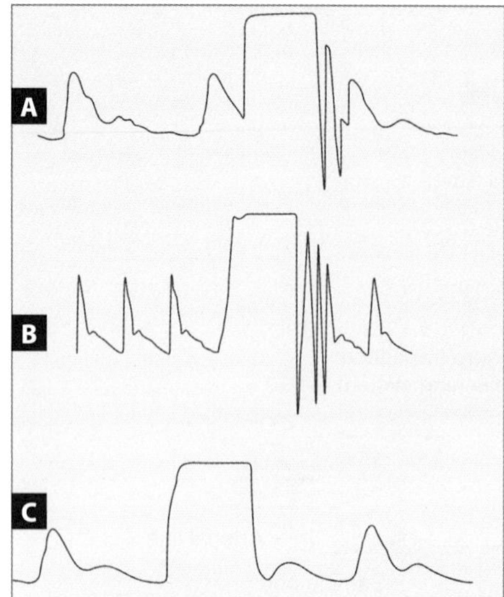

Figs. 7A to C: (A) Optimally damped; (B) Underdamped; and (C) Overdamped.

falsely higher systolic and falsely lower diastolic pressure. This is seen when long tubing is used or with increased vascular resistance.

- Overdamped waveform will show a falsely lower systolic and a falsely higher diastolic pressure. This is commonly seen when there are air bubbles or blood clots, overly compliant tubing, catheter kinks, stopcocks not properly closed, no fluid in flush bag, or low flush bag pressure.
- The MAP will not change with either overdamping or underdamping. Hence, the MAP is usually taken as the standard for ABP monitoring
- Damping can be checked by performing a "square wave test": this is performed by activating the flush device and then quickly releasing it and observing the waveform on the monitor. The waveform sharply rises and "squares off" at the top when the flush is activated, and then, the tracing returns to baseline when it is released. Check the number of oscillations.
    - *Optimally damped:* One or two oscillations before returning to tracing.
    - *Underdamped:* More than two oscillations before returning to tracing.
    - *Overdamped:* Less than one oscillation before returning to tracing.

The square wave test may be done on every shift change or whenever the waveform looks over- or underdamped, when the accuracy of the measurement is doubtful and when intra-arterial pressure is to be used for guiding some intervention.

Central Venous Pressure

Central venous pressure is taken as a direct measurement of the right atrial pressure and vena cava. The tip of the catheter should rest in the lower third of the superior vena cava. The pressure monitoring assembly is attached to the distal port of a multilumen central venous catheter. CVP is used to assess intravascular volume status and right ventricular function.

However, the CVP is influenced not only by the volume status but also by myocardial contractility, afterload, and intrathoracic and intraabdominal pressures. Hence, the CVP can be confusing at times and difficult to interpret.

In order to minimize the effects of respiration, the CVP measurement should be taken at end exhalation when the muscles of respiration are at rest and intrathoracic pressure is stable at its resting level. In mechanically ventilated patients, inspiration is positive and expiration is negative, and end-expiratory values should be read just before the beginning of inspiration. In spontaneously breathing patients, it is the reverse **(Fig. 8)**.

In some patients, "a" and "v" waves are identifiable in CVP tracing. To identify these waves, a parallel ECG tracing should be used.

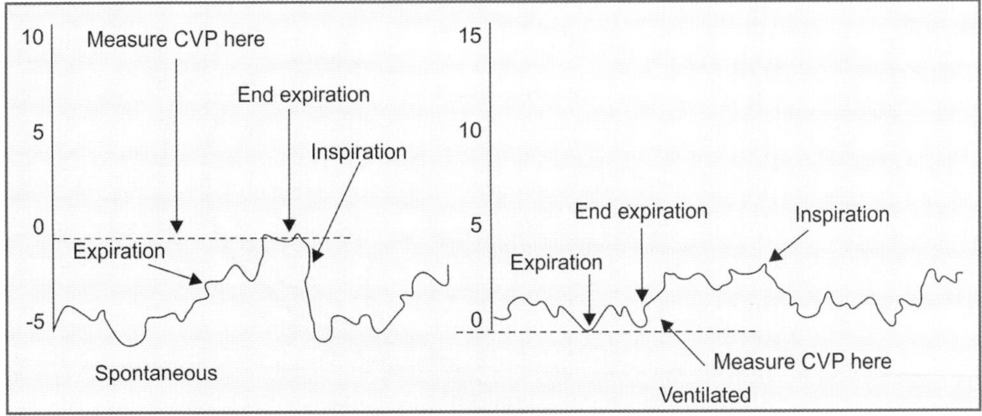

Fig. 8: Central venous pressure (CVP) measurement in spontaneous breathing and mechanical ventilated patient.

The "a" wave is located corresponding to the PR interval and "v" wave to the QT interval. CVP should be measured at the end of "a" wave.

Pulmonary Artery Occlusion Pressure

The pulmonary arterial catheter (PAC) has been regarded as the gold standard for hemodynamic measurements for many years. Lately, the use of PAC has decreased due to availability of other less invasive techniques of measuring CO.

Pulmonary arterial catheter is a percutaneous, nontunneled, multi-lumen, flow-directed, central venous catheter that is inserted through an introducer into a large vein, e.g., internal jugular or femoral vein, and antecubital vein. The balloon is inflated in the right atrium. The catheter is advanced; blood flow directs the balloon through the tricuspid valve into the right ventricle and then through the pulmonary valve into the pulmonary artery **(Fig. 9)**.

Hemodynamic Parameters Measured with PAC

- Pulmonary artery occlusion pressure (PAOP)/wedge pressure
- Pulmonary artery systolic pressure (PASP) and pulmonary artery diastolic pressure (PADP)
- Thermodilution CO
- Mixed venous oxygen saturation

Indications

- Differentiate shock conditions
- Assess intracardiac pressure, valvular abnormalities, congenital heart disease, cardiac shunts, and pre- and postsurgical repair.
- Diagnose and classify pulmonary hypertension

Other methods to assess cardiac output:

- *Pulse contour analysis:* CO—PiCCO, Flotrac
- Lithium dilution CO—LiDCO
- Esophageal Doppler
- Transesophageal echocardiography (TEE)

ASSESSMENT OF FLUID RESPONSIVENESS

Both excess and less fluid therapy may be harmful for a patient. The ability of a patient to increase the CO with fluid infusion is called fluid responsiveness. In patients with

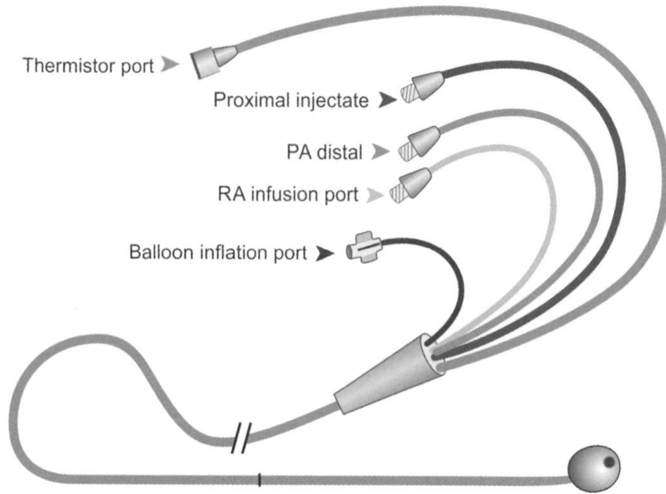

Fig. 9: Pulmonary arterial catheter.

complex shock, it is sometimes difficult to judge if the patient is fluid responsive using basic hemodynamic monitoring parameters. Hence, assessment of fluid responsiveness is important.

A patient who can increase their stroke volume/CO by >10–15% after a fluid bolus is called a fluid responder.

Methods to Assess Fluid Responsiveness

Several methods can be used to assess fluid responsiveness of which most of them require some form of CO monitoring.

- Pulse pressure variation/stroke volume variation (PPV/SVV)
- Inferior vena cava/superior vena cava (IVC/SVC) diameter—variations
- Tidal volume challenge
- End-expiratory occlusion test
- Conventional fluid challenge
- Echocardiography
- Mini-fluid challenge
- Passive leg raising test

Passive Leg Raising Test (Fig. 10)

Technique

- Start always from the 45° semirecumbent position
- Use a direct measurement of CO—not arterial pressure
- Use "real time assessment" of CO
- Raise legs by changing bed position not manually raising legs
- Reassess CO in semirecumbent position before infusing fluid—return to baseline

CONCLUSION

The goal of hemodynamic monitoring is to identify and improve organ function and oxygen delivery to tissues. No single monitoring tool is perfect. The method used needs to be individualized for each patient. Integrating findings from the monitoring and serial reevaluation of the patient's clinical condition is essential to improve outcomes **(Flowchart 1)**.

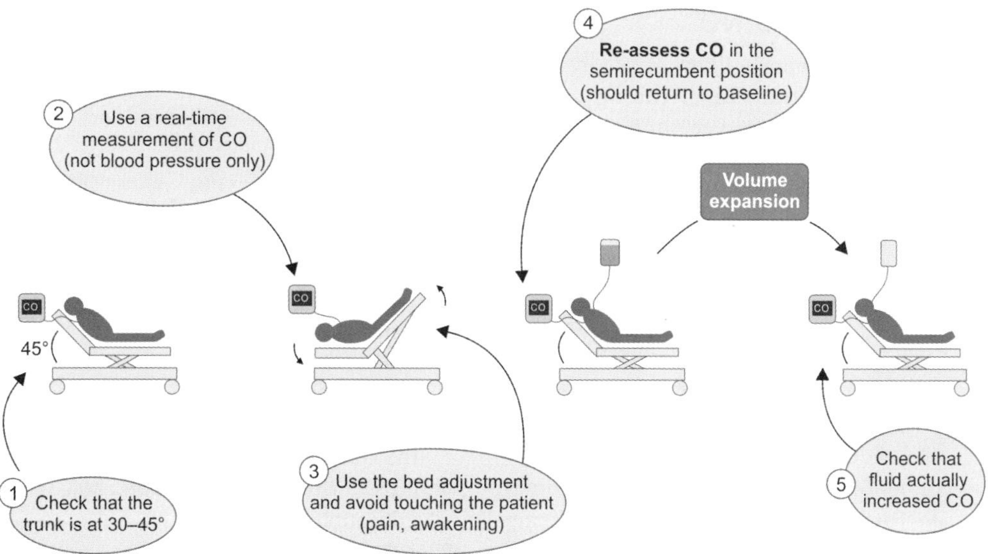

Fig. 10: Passive leg raising technique.

Flowchart 1: Algorithm for hemodynamic monitoring.

Patient in shock
↓
Basic monitoring + Tissue perfusion
↓
Echocardiography
↓
Assess response
↓

- • Rapid improvement • No cardiac dysfunction → Continue basic monitoring + frequent re-assessment
- Continue basic monitoring + add Flotrac (non-calibrated CO)
- High dose vasopressors + No cardiac dysfunction → LV dysfunction → Consider transpulmonary thermodilution
- High dose vasopressors + Cardiac dysfunction → RV dysfunction → Consider PA catheter

(LV: left ventricular; PA: pulmonary arterial; RV: right ventricular)

FURTHER READING

1. Boutros A, Albert S. Effect of the dynamic response of transducer-tubing system on accuracy of direct blood pressure measurement in patients. Crit Care Med. 1983;11(2):124-7.
2. Courtois M, Fattal PG, Kovács SJ Jr, Tiefenbrunn AJ, Ludbrook PA. Anatomically and physiologically based reference level for measurement of intracardiac pressures. Circulation. 1995;92(7):1994-2000.
3. Esper SA, Pinsky MR. Arterial waveform analysis. Best Pract Res Clin Anaesthesiol. 2014;28(4):363-80.
4. Kidney Disease: Improving Global Outcomes (KDIGO) Acute Kidney Injury Work Group KDIGO Clinical Practice Guideline for Acute Kidney Injury. Kidney Int Suppl. 2012;2:1-138.
5. Lara B, Enberg L, Ortega M, Leon P, Kripper C, Aguilera P, et al. Capillary refill time during fluid resuscitation in patients with sepsis-related hyperlactatemia at the emergency department is related to mortality. PLoS One. 2017;12(11):e0188548.
6. Monnet X, Teboul JL. Passive leg raising: five rules, not a drop of fluid! Crit Care. 2015;19(1):18.
7. Pierre L, Pasrija D, Keenaghan M. Arterial Lines. In: StatPearls [Internet]. Treasure Island (FL): StatPearls Publishing; 2024.
8. Weiner R, Ryan E, Yohannes-Tomicich J. Arterial line monitoring and placement. In: Oropello JM, Pastores SM, Kvetan V, (Eds). Critical Care. New York: McGraw-Hill Education; 2016.
9. Zisquit J, Velasquez J, Nedeff N. Allen Test. In: StatPearls [Internet]. Treasure Island (FL): StatPearls Publishing; 2024.

SECTION 3

Organ Support

Section Editor: *Pragyan Kumar Routray*

9. **High-flow Nasal Oxygen and Noninvasive Ventilation**
Manoj K Singh, Rakesh Panchal

10. **Mechanical Ventilation Simplified**
Pragyan Kumar Routray, Dharmajivan Samantaray

11. **Renal Replacement Therapy**
Ranajit Chatterjee, Lalit Gupta

12. **The Role of Nurses in the Care of Extracorporeal Membrane Oxygenation Patients**
Rahul Anil Pandit, Arindam Kar

CHAPTER 9

High-flow Nasal Oxygen and Noninvasive Ventilation

Manoj K Singh, Rakesh Panchal

HIGH-FLOW NASAL CANNULA

INTRODUCTION

Humidified high-flow nasal prong (HFNP), also called high-flow nasal oxygen (HFNO)/ high-flow nasal cannula (HFNC), therapy is a form of noninvasive respiratory support. HFNC therapy is an oxygen supply system capable of delivering up to 100% humidified and heated oxygen at a flow rate of up to 60 L/min. All settings are controlled independently, allowing for greater confidence in the delivery of supplemental oxygen as well as better outcomes when used. In addition to greater control over the delivery of fraction of inspired oxygen (FiO_2), there are several benefits to using a HFNC. At high flows (2 L/kg/min, in children) using appropriate nasal prongs, a positive distending pressure may be achieved. The high flows and humidification improve functional residual capacity and mucociliary clearance of secretions, thereby reducing work of breathing. The high flows may also affect pulmonary and systemic circulation, which is an important consideration when applying HFNP therapy to children with cardiac disease.

MACHINE

Basic components include a *flow generator* providing gas flow rates up to 60 L/min, *an air-oxygen blender* that achieves escalation of FiO_2 from 21% to 100% irrespective of flow rates, and a *humidifier* that saturates the gas mixture at a temperature of 31°–37°C. To minimize condensation, the heated humidified gas is delivered via heated tubings through a wide-bore nasal prong **(Fig. 1)**.

BENEFITS

We can divide the benefits of HFNC into clinical and physiologic as follows:

Clinical benefits:

- Improved patient comfort and compliance with the treatment
- Better patient tolerance due to the warmth and humidity of inspired air
- Ease of use

Physiologic benefits:

- Although technically high FiO_2 may be achieved through devices like Venturi masks or non-rebreathing masks, the oxygen flow through a low-flow system does not match the minute ventilation demand of a patient with severe dyspnea. A patient with high minute ventilation demand connected to a low-flow oxygen delivery draws in atmospheric air by the sides of the mask, which dilutes the oxygen. This is taken care of by the high flow of the HFNO system.
- Reduction of dead space and CO_2 rebreathing compared with low-flow oxygen therapy and noninvasive ventilation (NIV).
- Reduced work of breathing associated with an improvement in respiratory rate,

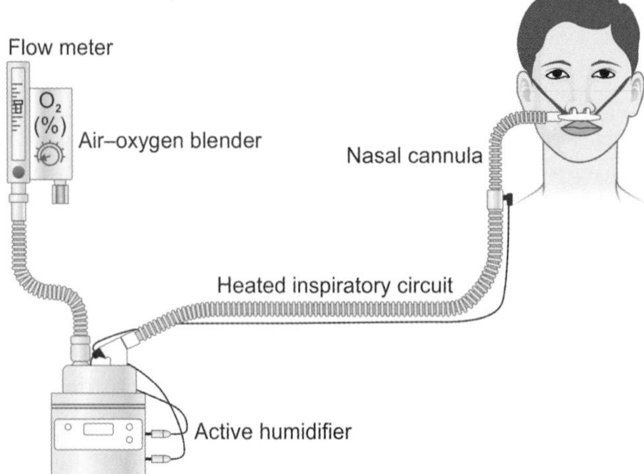

Fig. 1: High-flow nasal cannula setup. An air/oxygen blender, allowing from 0.21 to 1.0 fraction of inspired oxygen (FiO_2), generates up to 60 L/min flow. The gas is heated and humidified through an active heated humidifier and delivered via a single-limb heated inspiratory circuit. The patient breathes the adequately heated and humidified medical gas through nasal cannulas with a large diameter.

as well as a reduction in heart rate with a significant improvement in peripheral oxygen saturation (SpO_2) measurements.

- Generation of positive-end expiratory pressure (PEEP)
- Increase in the tidal volume

INDICATIONS

Patients requiring respiratory support:

- Acute respiratory distress associated with respiratory illness, hypoxemia ($SpO_2 < 90\%$) and/or moderate-to-severe work of breathing
- Respiratory distress in association with nonrespiratory issues, e.g., congestive cardiac failure and fluid overload
- Postoperative respiratory support, e.g., tonsillectomy and adenectomy
- Respiratory support to infants and children with chronic lung disease
- Weaning therapy from mask continuous positive airway pressure (CPAP) or bilevel positive airway pressure (BiPAP)
- Preintubation and postextubation oxygenation

CONTRAINDICATIONS

- Critically ill patients requiring immediate higher level of respiratory support, i.e., NIV or invasive ventilation or decreased level of consciousness
- Upper airway obstruction
- Central apnea
- Blocked nasal passages/choanal atresia
- Trauma/surgery to nasopharynx
- Pneumothorax

SETUP

Follow these steps for setting up HFNC:

- Collect proper equipment, including correct size of nasal prong and tubing length. You may have to choose between small or larger adult sizes depending on the manufacturer.
- Ensure humidification fluid is in place and heating circuit is functioning. A dust filter may be used over the room air intake port.
- Adjust the flow rate first, then titrate FiO_2 to appropriate levels.

- Insert the cannula into the patient's nostrils and secure it to the patient's head with an elastic strap to prevent lateral air loss.
- Monitor the patient's skin surrounding the nostrils under and around HFNC to identify potential skin breakdown or pressure injuries.
- Adjust the head strap to patient's head, carefully avoiding the ears; do not overtighten.
- Secure the head strap clip to the nasal cannula and clip HFNC tubing to the patient's gown to relieve tension.
- Maintain the patient in semi-Fowler's position and consider periodic prone positioning to promote lung expansion.
- Ensure suction equipment is present in the room.
- Monitor the patient for comfort and tolerance.
- Note that although the flow rate and the temperature can be directly controlled by knobs, the oxygen has to be controlled by knobs as well as the flow meter. Every time the flow rate is changed, the FiO_2 may change automatically and will need readjustment.

PATIENT MONITORING AND ASSESSMENT

- The greatest concern for patients on HFNC is the need for emergent intubation if treatment fails, so your early recognition of changes in the patient's condition is essential.
- Track trends in vital signs and look for any increased work of breathing (elevated heart rate, elevated respiratory rate, blood pressure changes, and decreased oxygen saturation levels). Titrate oxygen flow rates according to the patient's respiratory rate and work of breathing for a targeted oxygen saturation no higher than 96% or per facility protocol.
- Monitor the patient for potential respiratory compromise such as declining oxygen saturation (as measured by pulse oximetry), tachypnea, use of accessory muscles, intercostal recession, abdominal distension, secretions in the tubing, and changes in lung sounds.
- ROX index calculated using SPO_2, FiO_2, and respiratory rate may be used to predict HFNC failure and the need for intubation.
- Measure arterial blood gases daily and watch for FiO_2 titrations or changes in patient condition. Interpret and report results to the provider immediately.

The American Heart Association recommends that providers assess patients at 1 hour and 3 hours after HFNC initiation to determine response and whether intubation should be considered. Intubation should not be delayed if the patient is not improving.

NURSING CARE

- Do not feed during the initial 2 hours following commencement of HFNP therapy.
- Once stable, patient should be assessed as to whether they can tolerate oral feeds.
- If oral feeding is not tolerated, commence 2-hourly nasogastric (NG) bolus feeds.
- Oral and nasal care must be performed 4 hourly.
- Check for pressure areas, ensure nasal prongs are in correct position and saturation probe moved regularly.
- Monitor for abdominal distention and aspirate nasogastric tube (NGT) if clinically indicated.
- Cluster cares and minimal handling.

CONCLUSION

High-flow nasal cannula is a more sophisticated oxygen delivery device with added advantage of flow and humidified temperature-regulated oxygen. Nursing excellence in monitoring and safety aspects during the patient care will give patient advantage in overcoming the respiratory crises. The bedside nurse can assist the medical team by monitoring the patient's vital signs and respiratory effort while on high-flow therapy to ensure there is no risk of impending respiratory compromise.

NONINVASIVE VENTILATION: WHAT NURSES SHOULD KNOW?

INTRODUCTION

Noninvasive ventilation has proven to be an effective ventilatory support in many situations. It is viewed as a viable alternative to invasive ventilation and primarily a means of preventing some patients go into full invasive ventilation. Nurses are the ones who are involved in the care, monitoring, and troubleshooting of the patients requiring NIV. Most of the troubleshooting is managed well if a nurse knows the detailed aspects of daily care.

Noninvasive ventilation is a form of mechanical ventilation that uses a ventilator connected to some interfaces like a well-fitting face mask or a helmet in place of an endotracheal tube. This ventilatory mode allows patients' airways to remain free. Then the NIV device supports the patients' breathing effort with an inspiratory positive airway pressure (IPAP), resulting in increased tidal volume and improved ventilation. The expiratory positive airway pressure (EPAP) keeps the smaller airways and the alveoli open. Thus, NIV helps the patients when they are critical and need breathing assistance.

Advantages of a noninvasive interface:

- Flexibility in initiating and removing the device (as no intubation/extubation is needed)
- Allows intermittent application
- Improves patient comfort
- Reduces the need for sedation
- The mouth remains free
- Allows the patient to speak, take food orally, and expectorate
- Avoids the major adverse effects of intubation, like intubation-associated infections, local trauma, etc.

NONINVASIVE VENTILATION CIRCUIT COMPONENTS

- *NIV device:* NIV can be given from some standard ICU ventilators with NIV modes and portable smaller machines, which have inbuilt compressors. Patients coming to emergency and those needing ICU care are managed with flow-driven machines where FiO_2 can be titrated along with tidal volumes and PEEP more efficiently.
  - *ICU ventilator-driven NIV:*
    - *Advantages:*
      - High FiO_2 can be given.
      - It can give high flows and reduce discomfort in tachypneic patients in acute settings.
  - *NIV machines **(Fig. 2)**:*
    - *Advantages:*
      - They are portable.
      - Easy to handle
      - Better compensation for leaks (some newer ICU ventilators may have dedicated NIV modes with leak compensation)
    - *Disadvantages:*
      - Cannot develop pressures >30 cmH_2O
      - Lack O_2 blenders
      - Lack of sophisticated alarm systems, battery backup

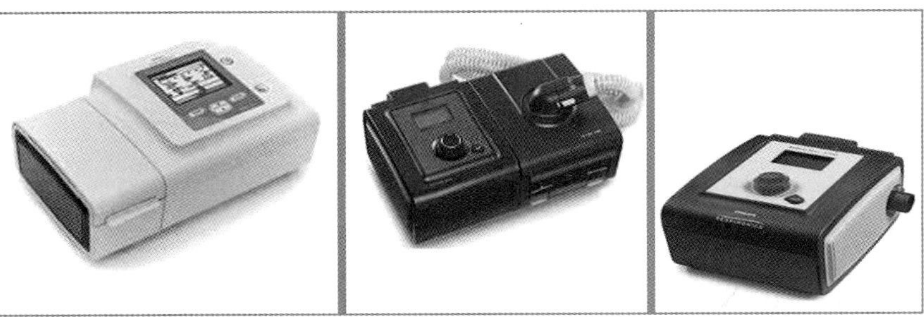

Fig. 2: Various types of noninvasive (NIV) machines available for critical care nurses.

- *NIV modes:*
    - CPAP is delivered using a continuous flow; this acts like a "pneumatic splint" for the upper airway, preventing the airway from narrowing and collapsing. It also maintains a positive pressure during expiration and keeps the alveoli patent and free from edema. It is recommended in obesity-related breathing disorders (sleep apnea), atelectasis, tracheomalacia, and cardiogenic pulmonary edema.
    - BiPAP uses different IPAP and EPAP. This bilevel support reduces the patient's work of breathing. Airway pressure switches from an IPAP to an EPAP synchronizing with patient's own respiratory cycle. Patient's inspiratory effort triggers the switch from EPAP to IPAP. It is recommended in chronic obstructive pulmonary disease (COPD) and mild-to-moderate lung injury.
    - Spontaneous or spontaneous/timed (S/T); spontaneous mode (S) is where the machine augments the patient's spontaneous breaths only. The S/T mode includes a backup rate, which takes over in case the patient initiates less number of breaths.
    - Average volume-assured pressure support (AVAPS) device delivers a constant tidal pressure-volume to patients and uses a specific algorithm that automatically adjusts the pressure to maintain an optimal tidal volume.
    - In addition, AVAPS can be combined with auto-expiratory positive airway pressure (AVAPS-AE) to maintain a patient's upper airway patency.
- *Masks can be of various types* ***(Figs. 3A to F)****:* (1) Nasal mask, (2) oronasal mask, (3) nasal pillows, (4) oral mask, (5) total face mask, and (6) helmet photograph.
- *Tubing:* Specialized tubes are required, which are available compatible only to same company machines. For ICU ventilators, ventilator circuits with one mask attachment device suffice to hook on the patient. The tubes can be single or double. Note in case of a single tube, there is no port for expiration. In this case, there has to be at least one port in the circuit open to atmosphere for the exhaled air to go out.
- *Oxygen supply:* Additional wall oxygen supply is used for small NIV machines, which can be given via nasal prongs or by a separate tube attached on the NIV tube or mask. ICU ventilators have inbuilt oxygen supply with blenders. In case there is no blender, the oxygen delivered depends not only the flow meter of the oxygen supply but also the positive airway pressure set on the NIV. Higher the positive pressure less is the oxygen mixed

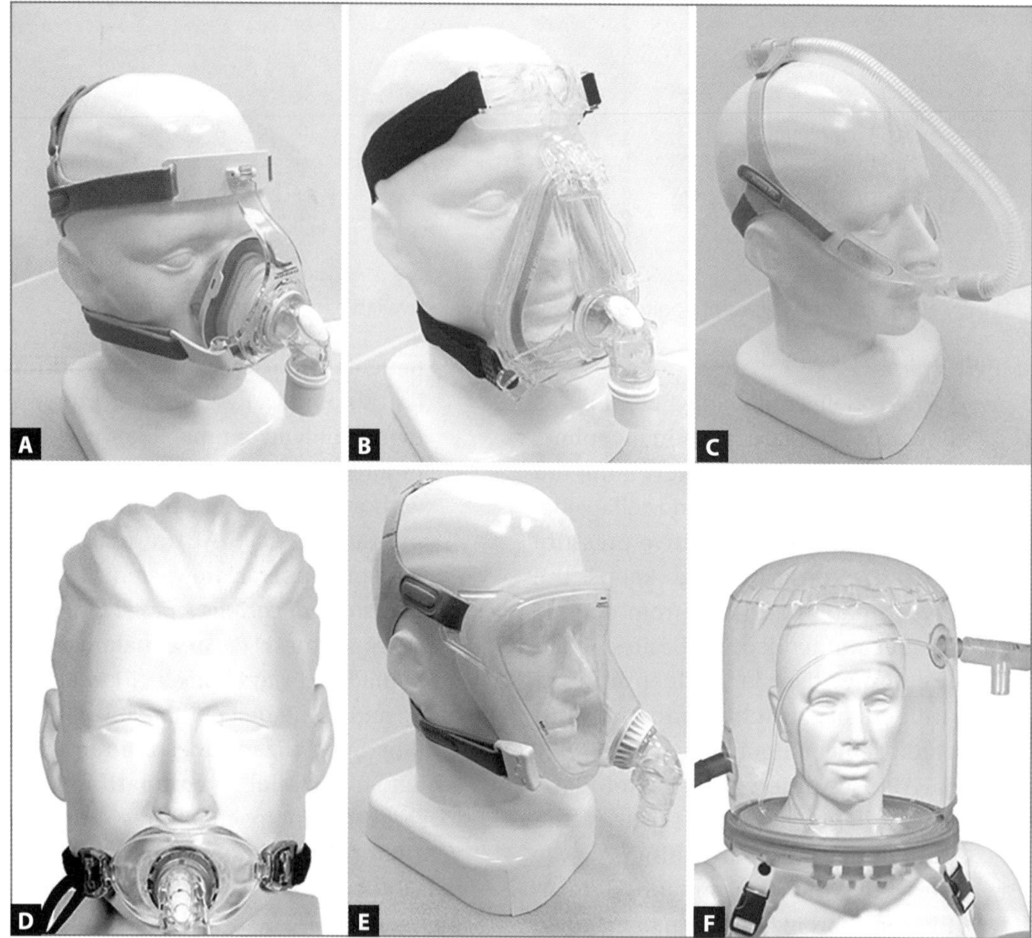

Figs. 3A to F: Various interfaces used for noninvasive ventilation (NIV).

through a side port due to Venturi effect and the oxygen flow needs to be increased accordingly.

- *Power supply:* All NIV machines are power-driven.
- *Humidifier:* It is a key ignored area during NIV. Humidification should be applied to all patients on NIV as inhaling the dry gas will have deleterious consequence on already diseased lung.

ASSESSMENT AND DIAGNOSES

The patient should be assessed for discomfort, consciousness level, chest wall motion, accessory muscle recruitment, synchronization of respiratory effort with the ventilator, respiratory rate, and hemodynamic parameters. Patients receiving NIV should be reviewed regularly to assess their response to treatment and the settings should be changed as needed. The arterial blood gas analysis will be governed by the patient's clinical progress but should be measured in most patients after 1–2 hours of NIV and after 4–6 hours if the earlier sample showed little improvement. If there has been no improvement in partial pressure of arterial carbon dioxide ($PaCO_2$) and pH after this period, despite optimal ventilator settings, NIV should be discontinued and invasive ventilation be considered. Oxygen saturation should be monitored regularly. Breaks from NIV should be made for drugs, physiotherapy, meals, etc. Patients who show benefit from NIV in the first few hours should be continued on NIV till improvement.

INDICATIONS OF NONINVASIVE VENTILATION IN INTENSIVE CARE UNIT

Evidence-based recommendation for the following in the setting of acute respiratory failure (ARF):

- BiPAP for acute or acute-on-chronic respiratory acidosis secondary to COPD exacerbation where pH ≤7.35 and partial pressure of carbon dioxide (pCO_2) is >48 mm Hg
- BiPAP is the prevention of endotracheal intubation and mechanical ventilation in a patient who has refused invasive ventilation.
- BiPAP or CPAP for cardiogenic pulmonary edema

Conditional recommendation for the following in the setting of ARF:

- Early NIV for immunocompromised patients with ARF
- In select patients with mild acute respiratory distress syndrome (ARDS)
- In select patients with asthma
- Obesity hypoventilation
- Postoperative ARF
- As palliation to patients with respiratory failure in the setting of terminal cancer or other terminal conditions or advance neuromuscular disorders
- Chest trauma patients with compromised respiration
- Prevention of postextubation respiratory failure in high-risk patients

In addition, noninvasive positive-pressure ventilation (NPPV) has been effective in treating various chronic respiratory diseases. These diseases include chronic stable COPD with hypercapnia, obesity hypoventilation syndrome, obstructive sleep apnea, respiratory failure secondary to neuromuscular disease, and restrictive thoracic disorders.

CONTRAINDICATIONS

Absolute contraindications:

- Facial trauma/burns
- Fixed upper airway obstruction
- Active vomiting
- Respiratory or cardiac arrest

Relative contraindications:

- A recent facial, upper airway, or upper gastrointestinal (GI) tract surgery
- Patient is unable to protect the airway
- Life-threatening hypoxemia
- Hemodynamic instability (hypotension, shock, pulmonary edema, and serious arrhythmias)
- Altered mental status/agitation, requiring deep sedation
- Bowel obstruction
- Profuse respiratory secretions
- Undrained pneumothorax
- Serious comorbidity
- Uncooperative patients

SETTING UP NONINVASIVE VENTILATION

The equipment required for NIV should be adapted depending on the type of NIV device and its accompanying consumables. Before use, it is essential to prepare the equipment, including:

- Noninvasive ventilator device
- Tubing (single- or dual-limb, depending on the device)

- Face mask (sizing gauge if needed)
- Oxygen port if the NIV does not have an oxygen blender
- Exhalation port for CO_2 clearance if this is not built into the face mask
- Bacterial and viral filter

Intensive care unit patients need oronasal or full-face mask or helmets.

Many acute hospital wards have guidelines for initial NIV settings. These often start on a spontaneous timed mode with conservative pressures such as IPAP 10–12 cmH_2O and EPAP 4–5 cmH_2O. Starting NIV at these pressures allows the patient to get used to the treatment. The initial settings vary as per different patient groups. Patients with neuromuscular weakness or chest trauma will need lower opening IPAP (10–12 cmH_2O) than a COPD patient (15–20 cmH_2O). Obese patients may require even higher pressures. Initial settings and any changes should be documented on a standardized proforma.

MONITORING DURING NONINVASIVE VENTILATION

- *Clinical parameters:*
  - Whether the patient is comfortable or not
  - Is the interface well tolerated
  - Respiratory rate
  - Whether the patient is still dyspneic and whether the accessory muscles of respiration are working
  - Consciousness
  - Ability to protect the upper airways and presence of an effective cough reflex
  - Gastric distention
  - Disease severity scores (APACHE II)
  - Sedation–delirium scores
  - Monitoring of side effects
- *Physiological parameters:*
  - Oxygen saturation
  - Arterial blood gas analysis [pH, $PaCO_2$, partial pressure of arterial oxygen (PaO_2)]
- *Ventilatory parameters:*
  - Respiratory frequency
  - Tidal volume
  - Leaks
  - Waveforms (flow-time, pressure-time, capnography)
  - Intrinsic PEEP
  - Patient–ventilator interaction
- *Cardiac parameters:*
  - Blood pressure
  - Electrocardiogram (ECG)
  - Echocardiography
- *Others:*
  - Radiological evaluation (chest radiography, computed tomography)
  - Lung and diaphragm ultrasonography

Complications of NIV which need to be monitored by bedside nurse:

- *Pressure sores:* Rash, abrasions, necrosis on the nasal bridge, and on the cheeks
- Nasal congestion/dryness
- Eye dryness/irritation
- Aspiration pneumonia
- Air leaks may offset the trigger.
- Pneumothorax, leading to sudden patient worsening
- Claustrophobia
- Rapid deterioration, although not a complication, should be a red flag warning sign.

Predictors of success of NIV:

- Strong and well-trained nursing team
- Ability of the patient to cooperate; patient's alertness
- Ability to synchronize breathing with noninvasive ventilator
- Less air leakage; intact dentition
- Hypercarbia is not too severe

- Acidemia, but not too severe (pH between >7.1)
- Improvements in gas exchange, heart and respiratory rates within first 2 hours.
- HACOR score (Heart rate, Acidosis, Consciousness, Oxygenation, and Respiratory rate) may be used to predict NIV failure.

KEY POINTS

- In respiratory failure, if a patient needs breathing assistance over and above oxygen, it can be given via NIV.
- NIV delivers positive pressure to a patient's airway and lungs via a face mask and avoids intubation.
- The equipment should be adapted depending on the patient, device used, and mode of treatment.
- Patients receiving treatment require regular monitoring for a number of complications.
- Therapy duration varies and patients need to be weaned off the treatment if they show signs of improvement.

CHAPTER 10

Mechanical Ventilation Simplified

Pragyan Kumar Routray, Dharmajivan Samantaray

INTRODUCTION

Mechanical ventilation is pumping of gas into patient's lungs and allowing it to flow out passively. A ventilator is a machine which delivers air into the patient's lung. The parameters which can be controlled by the operator are volume, pressure, flow, cycle, time, etc.

Indications of mechanical ventilation: The various indications of mechanical ventilation are summarized in **Table 1**.

Contraindications: There are no absolute contraindications.

PHYSICS OF MECHANICAL VENTILATORS

A mechanical ventilator either fully or partially supports a patient's work of breathing. The design of a mechanical ventilator can be classified according to (1) input power, (2) source of pressurized gas, (3) drive mechanism, or (4) control circuit.

The various components of the design of a mechanical ventilation are shown in **Table 2**.

The various physiological aspects of the respiratory system when connected to a ventilator are as follows:

Airway resistance: This is the obstruction to flow of the air in the circuit and airways; normally, it is 0.5–2.5 $cmH_2O/L/s$. It is affected by two main factors: Velocity of the gas flowing through it and the length and the radius of the airway. A longer airway tube increases the resistance. Airway resistance can also be calculated in the following way:

Change in pressure/change in volume or (peak pressure – plateau pressure)/flow.

TABLE 1: Indications of ventilation.

Indication	*Definition*	*Possible etiologies*
Inadequate oxygenation	Hypoxemia	• Pneumonia • Heart failure • ARDS
Inadequate ventilation	Hypercapnia	Obstructive airway diseases
Increased work of breathing	Normal oxygen and carbon dioxide but severe dyspnea compromising hemodynamics or causing extreme fatigue	• Severe metabolic acidosis • Hepatic encephalopathy
Poor sensorium and inability to protect airway		• Following head trauma • CVA • Intoxication • Postictal state

(ARDS: acute respiratory distress syndrome; CVA: cerebrovascular accident)

TABLE 2: Various components of the design of a mechanical ventilation.

Various sources of input power	Air and oxygen supply	*Drive mechanism* (converts the electrical power to the power driving the air)	*Ventilator circuit:* The tubes going out and coming into the ventilator
Pneumatic: Compressed gases are used as the source of power	From the hospitals centralized supply through a manifold	Bellow driven	Open circuit
Electrical: AC or DC power	Oxygen from cylinders and pressurized air from built-in compressors/ pistons in the ventilator	Piston driven	Closed circuit
Combined		Pneumatic circuits	

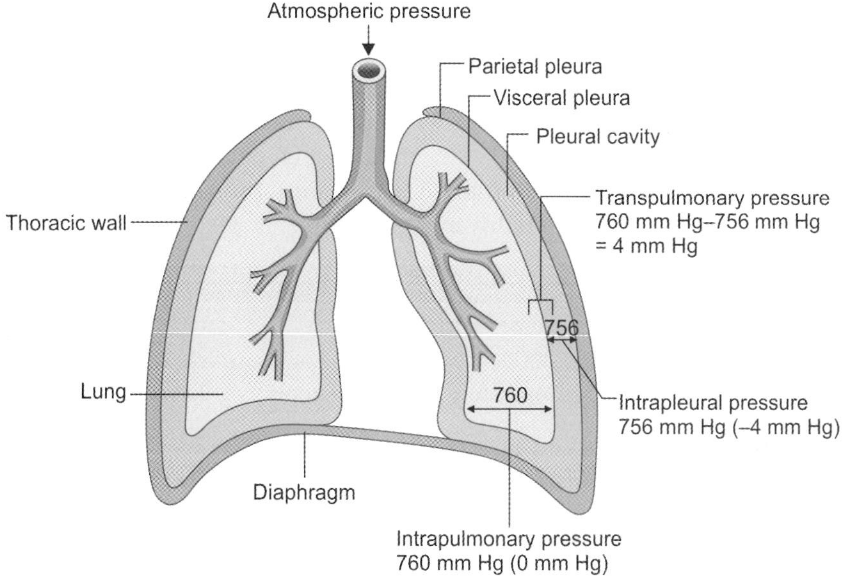

Fig. 1: Factors determining compliance of the respiratory system.

Compliance: Lung compliance is the measure of distensibility of the lungs—it is the change in volume per unit change in transpulmonary pressure (which in turn is the difference between the pressure in the pleural space and the pressure in the alveoli) **(Fig. 1)** and is calculated in the following way:

$$C = \Delta V/\Delta P$$

where C is compliance, ΔV is change in volume, and ΔP is the change in transpulmonary pressure.

Low compliance means that the lungs are stiff or noncompliant, making lung expansion difficult and increasing the work of breathing [e.g., acute respiratory distress syndrome (ARDS)].

High compliance occurs when there is an incomplete exhalation and air trapping, due to a lack of elastic recoil in the lung (a typical example is emphysema).

For a normal lung at its functional residual capacity, compliance is 200 mL/cmH_2O.

The total compliance of the respiratory system includes both lung compliance and thoracic cage compliance.

Compliance can be divided into static and dynamic compliance.

Static compliance is measured by stopping the airflow in the circuit. It relates to the elastic resistance of the lung and the chest wall only.

Dynamic compliance is measured with the air flowing. It includes both airway resistance and the elastic resistance of the lung and the chest wall. As the airway resistance is included, it is therefore always lower than static compliance.

The common abnormalities in the compliance are summarized in **Table 3**.

MECHANICS OF VENTILATION

Nowadays, most of the ventilators are positive-pressure ventilators. The air is driven into the lung by a positive pressure. This is called the driving pressure which is in turn equal to the airway pressure (generated by the ventilator) - alveolar pressure.

The lung and the ventilator can be seen as a unit, as shown in **Figure 2**. They can be thought of as a tube (representing the ventilator tubing, the endotracheal tube, and the airways) with a balloon at one end (representing the alveoli).

Pressure when measured at point B represents the alveolar pressure. Pressure at point A is equivalent to the airway pressure which is actually measured by the ventilator. This pressure at point A is a product of flow and resistance added to the pressure at point B (i.e., the alveolar pressure). If the flow is stopped in the airway by the inspiratory hold switch or manually, it makes the flow zero; hence, the product of flow and airway resistance is also zero. So the pressure

TABLE 3: Common abnormalities of compliance.

Conditions increasing static compliance	*Conditions decreasing static compliance*	*Conditions decreasing dynamic compliance*
• Flail chest • Sternotomy • Emphysema	• Acute respiratory distress syndrome • Consolidation • Distended abdomen • Pleural effusion • Obesity • Pneumothorax • Atelectasis	• Airway obstruction • Kinked endotracheal tube • Bronchospasm

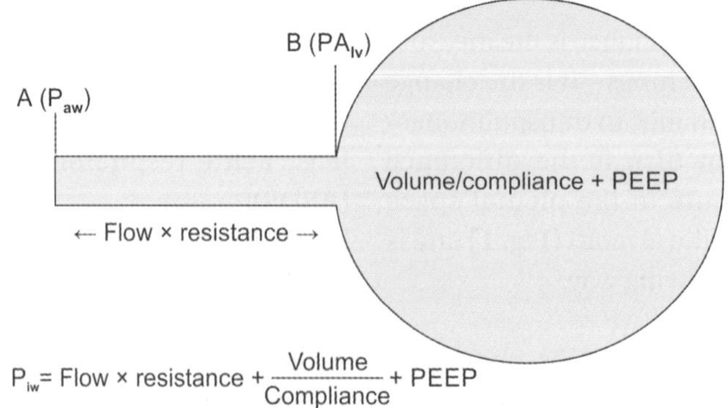

Fig. 2: Lung–ventilator unit.

measured at point A will be the same as that of point B, which will be the alveolar pressure. This is also called the plateau pressure or the occlusion pressure **(Fig. 3)**.

HOW TO START VENTILATION?

Although the ventilator may deliver various modes of ventilation, these various modes can be understood by three underlying parameters **(Fig. 4)**:

1. Trigger (this initiates a respiratory cycle)
2. Limit (there can be a limit to the volume delivered or pressure generated)

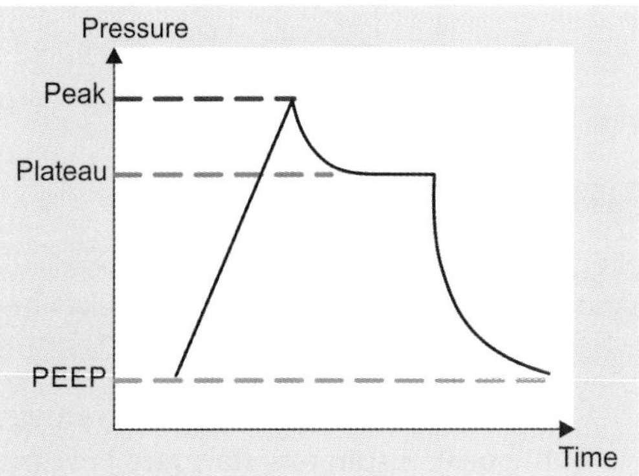

Fig. 3: Peak and plateau pressures. (PEEP: positive end-expiratory pressure)

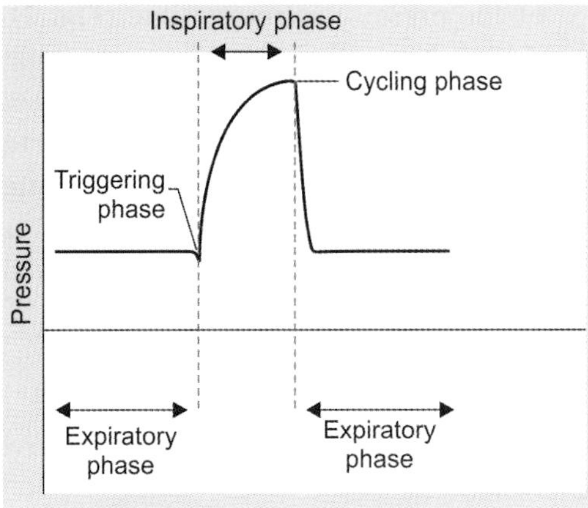

Fig. 4: Ventilatory breaths showing trigger, limit, and cycling.

3. Cycle (what ends the inspiration and starts the expiration)

Triggers

A trigger is the cue that initiates each breath cycle. The following parameters can act as triggers:

- *Time:* There is a set breathing rate. The ventilator will time the breaths accordingly. It the rate set at 20 per minute. The ventilator will be triggered automatically at every 3 seconds. It is to be noted that nowadays, most ventilators are assist controlled. So if the patient breaths spontaneously, the ventilator will synchronize and deliver with each effort of the patient.
- *Pressure:* A breath in its expiratory phase drops its pressure. When the pressure drops below a certain level, a new breath is initiated **(Fig. 5)**.
- *Flow:* A spontaneous breath effort causes a gradual drop in the expiratory flow. When this flow drops down below a certain level, the ventilator detects that at the end of the expiration and then an inspiratory flow of gas starts **(Fig. 6)**.
- *Neural assist:* In neural-adjusted ventilatory assist (NAVA), the ventilator detects the diaphragmatic effort for an inspiration and is triggered by that.

Limits

A *limit* is the mechanism that determines how the breath is delivered. It can be one of the following:

- *Flow limited:* Over a preset time, a preset flow is maintained. This delivers a tidal volume.
- *Pressure limited:* Over a preset inspiratory time, a preset pressure is delivered. The volume delivered varies with patient

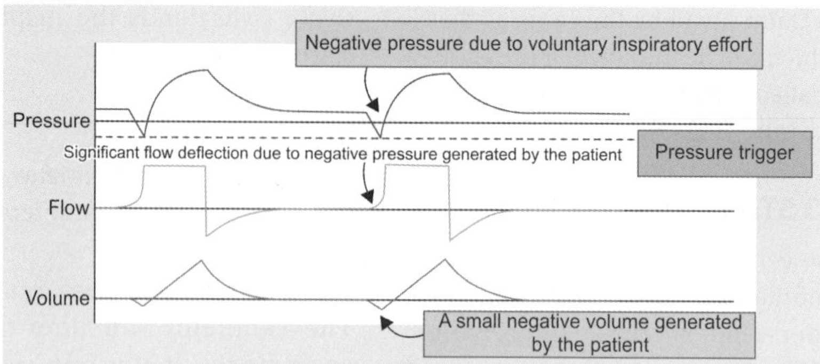

Fig. 5: Pressure trigger set to initiate breath.

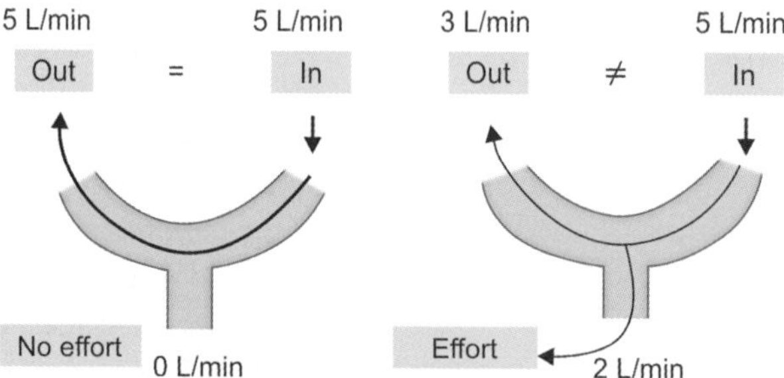

Fig. 6: In flow triggering, a change in the flow of gas during an inspiratory effort is sensed by the ventilator and breath initiated. A ventilator can be also be falsely triggered by many factors: (1) Water accumulating in the expiratory limb of the breathing circuit or (2) a high cardiac output state.

characteristics such as lung compliance or airway obstruction.

Cycling

Cycling is the factor that governs the changeover from inspiration to expiration. Inspiration ends on attaining a preset parameter. This preset parameter can be one of the following:

- *Volume:* The inspiration ends after a preset volume is delivered.
- *Time:* The inspiration ends after the inspiratory time. This can be set directly as the inspiratory time or indirectly as the inspiration:expiration (I:E) ratio.
- *Flow:* During a pressure-supported breath, inspiratory flow declines after reaching a peak inspiratory flow rate. Once this flow declines to a preset expiratory flow rate (this is usually described as a percentage of the peak inspiratory flow rate,) cycling occurs due to expiration.
- *Pressure:* Inspiration ends after a preset pressure is reached and maintained for the preset inspiratory time **(Fig. 7)**. This reduces the risk of barotrauma. If the airway pressure exceeds the set maximum, the ventilator will cycle to expiration, regardless of the tidal volume being delivered. Thus, high airway or alveolar pressures may lead to less tidal volumes being delivered.

TYPES OF VENTILATOR BREATH

Ventilator-delivered breaths can be controlled or assisted.

- *Controlled breath:* Initiated by the ventilator. The preset parameters may be

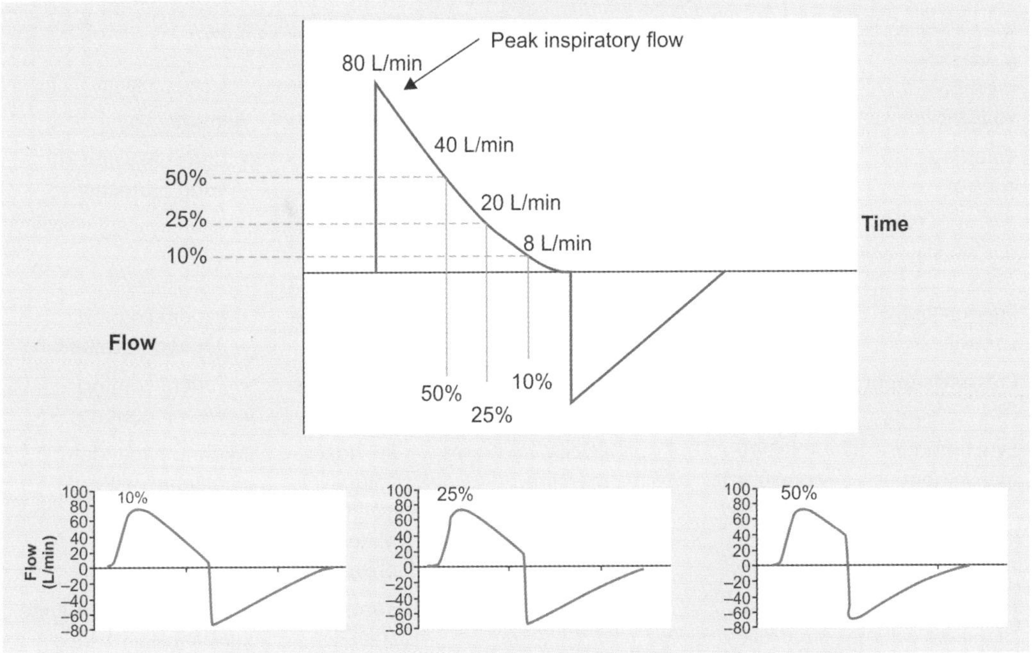

Fig. 7: Flow cycling at 10%, 20%, and 50% expiration trigger sensitivity (ETS).

- Volume
- Pressure

- *Assisted breath:* Initiated by the patient and assisted by the ventilator

Note that all the ventilators nowadays are set as assist control, which means that the patient's efforts are assisted. It is only if the patient takes less number of breaths than the set rate in the ventilator or the patient is sedated and paralyzed that the control mode sets in.

Volume-controlled breaths are delivered by a constant flow. The flow tries to deliver a preset volume. The pressure may vary as per the lung compliance and the airway resistance. These breaths can be mandatory or assisted depending on the patient's effort.

Preset pressure breaths use an inspiratory flow, which is high initially and then decreases over the course of inspiration. The resultant tidal volume varies and will depend upon inspiratory time plus the resistance and compliance of the patient's respiratory system.

MODES OF VENTILATION

Different modes of ventilation are described in **Table 4**. We describe the three most common conventional modes of ventilation. The graphics of the different modes of ventilation are shown in **Figures 8 to 10**.

1. Continuous mandatory ventilation (CMV) [also may be called intermittent positive pressure ventilation (IPPV)]
2. Synchronous intermittent mandatory ventilation (SIMV)
3. Pressure-support ventilation

Continuous Mandatory Ventilation

Nowadays, all ventilators have assist control modes. That is to say that the patient's own efforts trigger the ventilator to deliver

TABLE 4: Different modes of ventilation.

Modes of mechanical ventilation	***Types of breaths***	***Independent variable***	***Dependent variables***	***Remark***
Volume assist/ control	Assisted/ controlled	Preset tidal volume	Peak inspiratory pressure (PIP) and plateau pressures	• Control TV and MV • Lung protective
Pressure assist/ control	Assisted/ controlled	Preset pressure	Tidal volume	• Patient comfort • Avoid barotrauma
Pressure support (PS)	Supported	Preset pressure	Tidal volume	• Patient comfort • Weaning mode
Synchronous intermittent mandatory ventilation (SIMV) PS	Assisted/ controlled/ supported	• PC-SIMV = Preset pressure • VC-SIMV = Preset tidal volume	• PC-Tidal volume • VC-PIP and plateau pressures	Minimum mandatory ventilation with pressure support
Pressure regulated volume control (PRVC)	Assisted/ controlled	Preset	PIP and plateau pressures	Advance mode, volume guarantee with little change in pressure

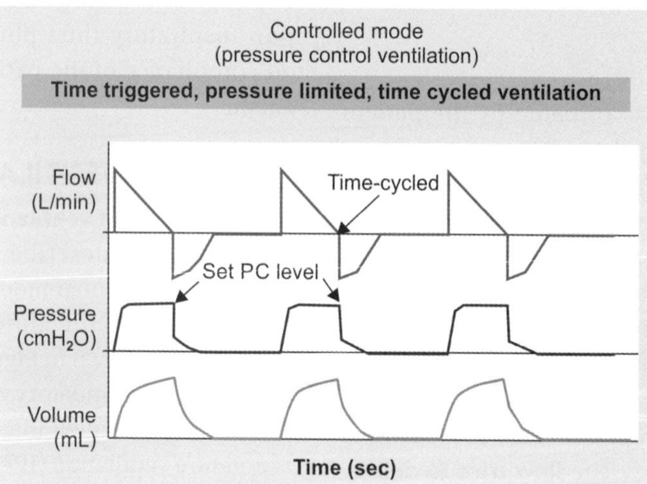

Fig. 8: *Basic types of breath:* Comparison on pressure, flow, and volume time scalars.

a certain volume or certain pressure. Moreover, the mode also has a backup rate. If the patient takes breath at a rate less than the backup rate or is sedated and/or paralyzed, the ventilator delivers the breath by itself.

Volume Control

In volume control (VC) mode, the ventilator delivers a preset volume of air with each breath. The mode is time triggered, which depends on the set frequency. When the patient is making spontaneous efforts, the

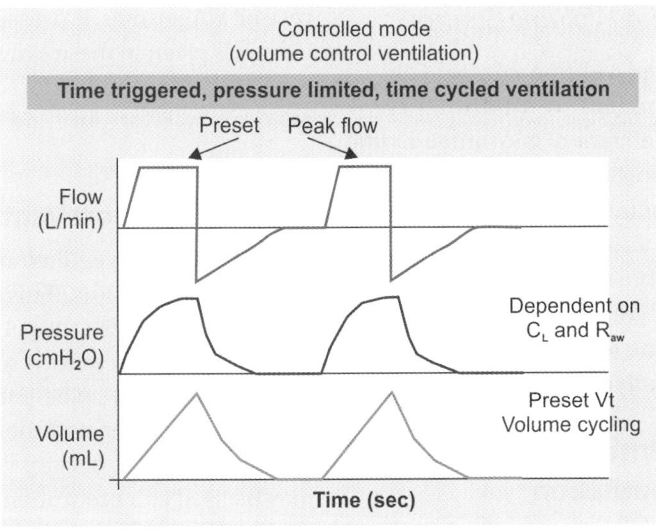

Fig. 9: Control mode–Pressure control ventilation.

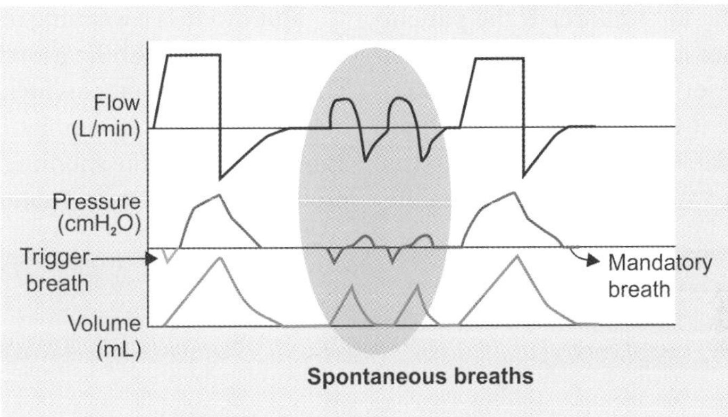

Fig. 10: SIMV, volume control mode.

trigger is the patient's own efforts detected by the ventilator. The user sets the tidal volume, respiratory rate, inspiration:expiration ratio, and positive end expiratory pressure (PEEP).

Volume-control ventilation tries to maintain a constant minute ventilation, but it is subject to lung compliance, airway resistance, etc. Usually there is a set pressure limit above which the ventilator does not allow the airway pressure to rise. This prevents lung trauma due to high pressure (barotrauma).

Pressure Control

In pressure control mode, the trigger is time. In this mode, the ventilator delivers a set inspiratory pressure over a set inspiratory time at a set rate. The peak pressure is controlled; hence, there is a lesser chance of barotrauma or exceeding and pressure limits like plateau pressure limit in patients with ARDS. This mode may also compensate for leaks.

Pressure-regulated Volume Control

Pressure-regulated volume control (PRVC) is a hybrid mode of ventilation. Here, the ventilator delivers a guaranteed tidal volume with a pressure-control waveform. This is done by combination of alteration in inspiratory time and peak flow in response to the breath-by-breath changes in airway or compliance characteristics.

It combines the advantages of the above two modes of breath delivery.

Synchronous Intermittent Mandatory Ventilation

In SIMV, the ventilator delivers a prefixed number of assisted breaths (either volume control or pressure control) synchronizing them with the patient's efforts. If the patient takes less number of breaths than the preset breaths, the preset breaths act as a backup rate. If the patient takes more breaths than the preset number, the ventilator only assists up to the preset value; it does not assist the rest or sometimes a pressure support (see below) is given to these extra breaths.

This mode can allow for some spontaneous respiratory effort and aid weaning from a ventilator.

Pressure-support Ventilation

Pressure-support ventilation is a spontaneous mode of ventilation. This means that the ventilator only assists the patient's own efforts. The inspiratory pressure is set which supports the patient's effort. The patient decides the number of breaths and the inspiratory time for each breath. A backup ventilation setting may be used as a precaution in case of apnea.

The tidal volume will be decided by the pressure support, the inspiratory time of each breath, and the patient's lung physiology.

This mode is a weaning mode and is used only after the stabilization of the patient. The basic parameters which have to be set in various modes of ventilation are shown in **Table 5**. The trouble shooting of the common problems are shown in **Table 6**.

TABLE 5: Mechanical ventilation settings.

Parameters	*Volume preset assist control*	*Pressure preset assist control*	*Pressure support*	*SIMV and PS*
FiO_2	√	√	√	√
Respiratory rate	√	√		√
Tidal volume	√			√
Inspiratory pressure		√	√	√
Inspiratory flow	√			√
I:E ratio	√	√		√
Inspiratory pause	√			√
SIMV period				±
PEEP	√	√	√	√
Trigger	√	√	√	√

(I:E: inspiration:expiration; PEEP: positive end-expiratory pressure; SIMV: synchronous intermittent mandatory ventilation)

TABLE 6: Troubleshooting of common alarms.

Alarms	*Definitions*	*Potential cause*
High pressure	Pressure required to ventilate exceeds the preset pressure	Pneumothorax, secretion, mucous plug, decrease compliance, bronchospasm
Low pressure	Resistance to inspiratory flow is less than preset pressure	Disconnected from ventilator, break in circuit
Low expiratory tidal volume	Exhaled tidal volume drops below preset volume	Leaks in system, increased airway resistance, decrease compliance
Rate/Apnea	Respiratory rate drops below preset level/apnea period exceeds preset period	Fatigue, medication
FiO_2	FiO_2 drift from preset range	Central O_2 supply level low, disconnected from O_2 source, circuit break
Fighting with ventilator	Not synchronizing with MV	Pain, disorientation, under sedation, ischemia

CONCLUSION

Mechanical ventilation is a life support system. It has become an integral part of the ICUs. It is a sophisticated machine. Handling a ventilator needs a substantial knowledge about the respiratory physiology as well as understanding of the machine. This knowledge has to be applied in the context of the patient's disease.

FURTHER READING

1. Al Ashry HS, Modrykamien AM. Humidification during mechanical ventilation in the adult patient. Biomed Res Int. 2014;2014:715434.
2. Downs JB, Klein EF Jr, Desautels D, Modell JH, Kirby RR. Intermittent mandatory ventilation: a new approach to weaning patients from mechanical ventilators. Chest. 1973;64(3):331-5.
3. Gurevitch MJ, Van Dyke J, Young ES, Jackson K. Improved oxygenation and lower peak airway pressure in severe adult respiratory distress syndrome. Treatment with inverse ratio ventilation. Chest. 1986;89(2):211-3.
4. Heenan TJ, Downs JB, Douglas ME, Ruiz BC, Jumper L. Intermittent mandatory ventilation; is synchronization important? Chest. 1980;77(5):598-602.
5. Shapiro BA, Harrison RA, Walton JR, Davison R. Intermittent demand ventilation (IDV): a new technique for supporting ventilation in critically ill patients. Respir Care. 1976;21(6):521-5.
6. West JB. Respiratory Physiology—The Essentials, 7th edition. Baltimore MD: Lippincott Williams & Wilkins; 2008.
7. World Federation of Societies of Anaesthesiologists. [online] Available from www.wfsahq.org [Last accessed February, 2025].

CHAPTER 11

Renal Replacement Therapy

Ranajit Chatterjee, Lalit Gupta

INTRODUCTION

Renal failure is a serious condition where the kidneys can no longer filter waste and excess fluid from the blood. The renal failure can be either acute or chronic. As renal function declines, treatment becomes necessary to replace the vital blood-filtering function of these organs. Renal replacement therapy (RRT) refers to the various treatment modalities used for this purpose. The main types of RRT in critical care are hemodialysis or continuous renal replacement therapy (CRRT). Hemodialysis on the other hand can be intermittent hemodialysis or slow low-efficiency daily dialysis (SLEDD). Hemodialysis uses an artificial kidney machine to filter blood. Peritoneal dialysis is another method where the patient's own peritoneum acts as the filter interface.

Renal replacement therapy helps restore fluid and electrolyte balance, remove waste, and provide life support in kidney failure patients. However, it cannot fully replace normal kidney functions. This chapter provides an overview of RRT in critical care, including the indications, modalities, and procedures.

INDICATIONS

The main indications for starting RRT are included in **Box 1**.

BOX 1: Indications of renal replacement therapy.

- Severe kidney failure [glomerular filtration rate (GFR) <15 mL/min/1.73 m^2)]
- Fluid overload unresponsive to diuretics
- Electrolyte and acid-base abnormalities refractory to medical therapy
- Uremic symptoms such as nausea, vomiting, encephalopathy, and pericarditis
- Toxic ingestions where dialysis can remove the toxin

Selecting the optimal RRT modality for a patient with kidney failure depends on several key factors. Both hemodialysis and CRRT require specific machines and other infrastructure and trained staff:

- Patient preference and ability to engage in self-care are important, as options such as home hemodialysis and peritoneal dialysis require more involvement than in-center hemodialysis.
- Access to resources such as reliable transportation for hemodialysis or supplies for home dialysis also affect modality decisions.
- The presence of certain comorbid illnesses may favor one modality over others based on treatment goals.
- Additionally, the expertise of the care team and the availability.

A collaborative decision between patients, their families, and the nephrology care team allows for personalized RRT management. In general, peritoneal dialysis may be preferred in children and younger patients, while hemodialysis is more common in end-stage renal disease (ESRD) patients.

Kidney transplantation is the optimal form of RRT when a donor kidney is available.

OVERVIEW OF RENAL REPLACEMENT THERAPY MODALITIES

There are four main types of RRT:

1. *Intermittent hemodialysis:* The patient's blood is pumped through an external filter called a dialyzer to remove wastes and extra fluid. This is typically performed once a day lasting about 4 hours and can be timed as per the requirement of the patient.
2. *CRRT:* CRRT is a machine used specifically in the critical care units for maintaining fluid and solute balances. There may be several different modalities of CRRT:
    a. *SCUF:* Slow continuous ultrafiltration
    b. *CVVH:* Continuous veno-venous hemofiltration
    c. *CVVHD:* Continuous veno-venous hemodialysis
    d. *CVVHDF:* Continuous veno-venous hemodiafiltration.
3. *SLEDD:* This is a slow dialysis using conventional hemodialysis machines. It has some advantages in hemodynamically unstable patients.
4. *Peritoneal dialysis:* A cleansing fluid called dialysate is infused into the patient's abdominal cavity to draw wastes and extra fluid from the blood into the peritoneal membrane. This can be done continuously via an indwelling catheter or intermittently by exchanging fluid 4–5 times/day.

Differences between the Different Modalities

Understanding these disparities is crucial in tailoring RRT to individual patient needs, taking into account factors such as lifestyle, medical conditions, treatment preferences, and available facilities **(Table 1)**.

PROVIDING HEMODIALYSIS

The key steps in providing hemodialysis include:

1. *Vascular access:* A central venous catheter, arteriovenous fistula, or graft is required to connect the patient to the dialysis circuit. The access should be checked for patency before each treatment.
2. *Anticoagulation:* Heparin or other anticoagulants are administered to prevent clotting in the dialysis circuit.

TABLE 1: Different modes of hemodialysis.

Mode	*Advantage*	*Disadvantage*
Hemodialysis	• Less labor intensive • Best mode for urgent correction of hyperkalemia	Difficult to run on a hemodynamically unstable patient
CRRT	• Labor intensive • Expensive • Better in hemodynamically unstable patients (though there is no outcome benefit)	• More hemorrhagic complications • Less efficient in the correction of hyperkalemia
SLEDD	• Better for hemodynamically unstable patients • Less hemorrhagic complications than CRRT	• Less efficient than hemodialysis • No outcome benefit

(CRRT: continuous renal replacement therapy; SLEDD: slow low-efficiency daily dialysis)

The dose is titrated to keep the activated clotting time within the desired range.

3. *Initiation:* The patient is connected to the dialysis machine by attaching blood tubing to the vascular access. Extracorporeal blood flow is initiated and increased gradually.
4. *Treatment prescription:* Settings such as blood flow rate, dialysate flow rate, and duration are programmed based on the patient's prescription. Fluid removal rates are set based on clinical assessment of volume status.
5. *Monitoring:* Patients are monitored continuously for any signs of intolerance such as hypotension or arrhythmias. Electrolytes, fluid status, and anticoagulation are also monitored.
6. *Termination:* Blood flow is slowed and stopped when treatment is complete. Saline flushes are done to clear the circuit, and access is closed with pressure to achieve hemostasis.
7. Key hemodialysis prescription parameters **(Table 2)**.
8. Hemodialysis is associated with several possible complications and problems including:
   a. *Hypotension:* Due to rapid fluid shifts. Managed by adjusting ultrafiltration rate and medications. (Less with CRRT but without mortality benefit)
   b. *Muscle cramping:* Caused by electrolyte shifts. Treated with stretching exercises or electrolyte adjustments.
   c. *Nausea and vomiting:* Related to dialysis disequilibrium syndrome. Improved by slower blood flow rates.
   d. *Bleeding:* From the vascular access site or due to anticoagulation. Apply pressure and adjust the heparin dose.
   e. *Infection:* Vascular access infections are a common source of bacteremia. Requires close monitoring and early antibiotic therapy.
   f. *Clotting:* Clots can occur in the dialysis circuit or vascular access. Check patency and proper anticoagulation.
   g. *Medicine dose adjustment:* Many medicines require dose adjustment with dialysis and CRRT.

TABLE 2: Hemodialysis prescription parameters.

Parameter	*Typical target range*
Blood flow rate	300–500 mL/min
Dialysate flow rate	500–800 mL/min
Frequency and duration	3 sessions/week, 3–5 hours each
Fluid removal rate	8–10 mL/kg/h maximum
Dialysate temperature	36–37°C
Dialysate electrolyte levels	K^+, Ca^{++}, Na^+, etc. customized to patient

Regular monitoring and timely interventions help mitigate these risks during hemodialysis sessions. Patient education on possible complications improves reporting and compliance.

CHAPTER 12

The Role of Nurses in the Care of Extracorporeal Membrane Oxygenation Patients

Rahul Anil Pandit, Arindam Kar

INTRODUCTION

Extracorporeal membrane oxygenation (ECMO) is a critical life-support technology used for patients with severe cardiac and respiratory failure who have not responded to conventional treatments. It is a complex and resource-intensive therapy that can bridge the gap until the patient's heart or lungs recover, or until a more definitive treatment, such as a heart or lung transplant, is available. While ECMO is a highly specialized procedure, nurses play an essential role in the multidisciplinary team that provides care to ECMO patients. Their responsibilities span across all phases of ECMO therapy: Initiation, maintenance, and eventual removal. This chapter discusses the critical role of nurses in the management of ECMO patients, emphasizing general nursing principles such as back care, skin care, and patient monitoring, as well as providing specific insights into each phase of the ECMO process.

THE ROLE OF NURSES DURING EXTRACORPOREAL MEMBRANE OXYGENATION INITIATION

The initiation of ECMO therapy is a complex process, requiring careful preparation, coordination, and assessment. Nurses are integral to the initiation process, which typically involves multidisciplinary collaboration, including doctors, perfusionists, respiratory therapists, and intensivists. It is during this phase that nurses must demonstrate strong clinical knowledge and technical skills to ensure the success of the procedure.

Preparation and Setup

Prior to ECMO initiation, nurses must prepare both the patient and the environment. The preparation process involves verifying ECMO equipment, ensuring the presence of all necessary supplies, and setting up the ECMO circuit. This includes:

- Checking the ECMO machine, alarms, and circuits for proper function
- Preparing medications and ensuring that sedatives, paralytics, and anticoagulants are available
- Ensuring that the patient is positioned appropriately for cannulation

Nurses must also provide emotional support to patients and families, as ECMO initiation is often associated with significant anxiety. Nurses communicate effectively to explain the procedure, answer questions, and offer reassurance to both patients and their loved ones.

Cannulation and Initiation

Cannulation is the process of inserting the cannula into the patient's veins or arteries, a crucial step that requires a high level of expertise. While the physician or surgeon usually performs the cannulation, nurses play an essential role in assisting with patient positioning, monitoring vital signs, and administering sedatives or paralytics as required.

Once the cannula is in place, nurses closely monitor the patient for any signs of complications, such as bleeding, infection, or hemodynamic instability. The nursing team is also responsible for tracking the ECMO pump flow rate, oxygenator function, and circuit pressures to ensure optimal operation.

THE ROLE OF NURSES IN EXTRACORPOREAL MEMBRANE OXYGENATION MAINTENANCE

Once ECMO is initiated, the maintenance phase begins, and nurses take on a critical role in ensuring the continued functioning of the ECMO system and managing the patient's clinical condition.

Monitoring and Assessment

During ECMO therapy, nurses must vigilantly monitor a range of clinical parameters, including:

- *Hemodynamic monitoring:* Nurses assess blood pressure, heart rate, central venous pressure (CVP), and other relevant parameters to ensure the ECMO system is adequately supporting the patient's circulation and oxygenation. Changes in these values may indicate issues with the ECMO machine or the patient's condition.
- *Arterial and venous blood gas (ABG) monitoring:* Frequent ABG measurements are necessary to assess oxygenation, acid-base balance, and the effectiveness of ECMO. Nurses must be skilled at interpreting these results and adjusting the ECMO settings as needed.
- *Laboratory values:* Nurses monitor coagulation profiles, including activated clotting time (ACT) and international normalized ratio (INR), to manage anticoagulation therapy, which is crucial in preventing clot formation in the ECMO circuit while avoiding bleeding complications.

Managing Complications

Extracorporeal membrane oxygenation patients are at high risk for various complications, and nurses must be vigilant in identifying and addressing these issues promptly. Common ECMO-related complications include:

- *Bleeding:* Due to anticoagulation therapy, bleeding is a significant risk. Nurses must monitor the patient for signs of excessive bleeding, assess laboratory results, and intervene when necessary (e.g., adjusting anticoagulant therapy or administering blood products).
- *Infection:* ECMO patients are at risk for infections, particularly due to central venous catheters, arterial cannulas, and other invasive devices. Nurses implement strict infection control protocols, including daily dressing changes, meticulous hand hygiene, and monitoring for signs of infection such as fever or elevated white blood cell count.
- *Organ dysfunction:* Patients on ECMO are vulnerable to kidney, liver, and lung dysfunction. Nurses must monitor urine output, liver enzymes, and other indicators of organ function. Early recognition of deteriorating organ function allows for timely intervention.
- *Cannula site and peripheral pulsation monitoring:* It is imperative that nurses have a vigil on the cannula insertion site for bleeding and any signs of infection. Specific care is important for the monitoring of distal pulses of limbs,

especially if femoral arterial cannulation is performed.

General Nursing Principles in Extracorporeal Membrane Oxygenation Maintenance

In addition to specific monitoring, nurses caring for ECMO patients adhere to key general nursing principles, which contribute significantly to the patient's overall well-being and recovery.

- *Back care:* Prolonged immobility is common in ECMO patients, and careful attention to back care is essential in preventing pressure ulcers. Nurses ensure that the patient is repositioned regularly, using support surfaces such as pressure-relieving mattresses to reduce the risk of skin breakdown. Repositioning should be done carefully to avoid dislodging cannulas or compromising the ECMO circuit.
- *Skin care:* Skin integrity is a priority, especially in patients who are immobilized or sedated for long periods. Nurses perform daily skin assessments, paying particular attention to areas prone to pressure sores. Proper hydration, moisture management, and the use of barrier creams are essential to prevent skin breakdown. Additionally, nurses monitor and care for the insertion sites of cannulas, ensuring that they are clean and dry to reduce the risk of infection.
- *Nutrition:* Nutrition is a critical aspect of ECMO care. Nurses collaborate with dietitians to ensure that patients receive adequate caloric intake, as nutritional support can impact wound healing and recovery. This is especially important in ECMO patients who may be critically ill and require enteral or parenteral nutrition.

THE ROLE OF NURSES IN EXTRACORPOREAL MEMBRANE OXYGENATION WEANING AND REMOVAL

The final phase of ECMO therapy involves weaning and eventual removal of the ECMO circuit. Weaning is a delicate process that requires careful assessment of the patient's cardiovascular and respiratory status. Nurses play a crucial role in this phase, working closely with the ECMO team to determine when the patient is ready to be weaned.

Weaning Process

The weaning process typically begins when the patient's heart or lungs show signs of recovery. The process includes reducing the ECMO flow rates and gradually decreasing support. Nurses monitor the patient's response to these changes by carefully observing vital signs, arterial blood gases, and oxygen saturation. If the patient is unable to tolerate the reduction in support, the ECMO settings are adjusted accordingly.

Removal of Extracorporeal Membrane Oxygenation

Once the patient is stable and able to maintain adequate oxygenation and circulation without ECMO support, the decision to remove the ECMO system is made. Nurses assist with the removal process, ensuring that all equipment is safely discontinued and that the patient is monitored for any signs of complications, such as bleeding or hemodynamic instability.

After ECMO removal, nurses continue to provide close monitoring and care. Patient's vital signs, including blood pressure and heart rate, are closely watched to detect any signs of decompensation. Nurses also provide ongoing support for respiratory function, particularly if the patient has been on ECMO due to respiratory failure.

CHALLENGES IN EXTRA-CORPOREAL MEMBRANE OXYGENATION NURSING CARE

While the role of nurses in ECMO care is both critical and rewarding, it is also fraught with challenges. The complexity of ECMO technology, the intensive nature of care, and the potential for rapid deterioration all contribute to the demanding nature of ECMO nursing.

Emotional and Psychological Impact

Nurses often act as a support system for families who are experiencing emotional turmoil due to their loved one's critical condition. Being on ECMO is a serious intervention, and many families may feel a sense of fear and uncertainty. Nurses must be able to provide clear, compassionate communication and support during this difficult time.

Maintaining Technical Competence

Extracorporeal membrane oxygenation technology is continually evolving, and nurses must stay up to date on new devices, protocols, and evidence-based practices to ensure the best outcomes for their patients. This requires ongoing education and training, as well as strong communication with the multidisciplinary team.

Workload and Fatigue

Extracorporeal membrane oxygenation care is intensive, and nurses may face long shifts and high patient acuity. Managing fatigue while maintaining high standards of care is a significant challenge. Ensuring that adequate staffing and support systems are in place is crucial for nurse well-being and optimal patient care.

CONCLUSION

Nurses are essential to the care of ECMO patients throughout all phases of the therapy, from initiation to weaning and removal. Their role goes beyond just monitoring and operating ECMO equipment; they provide critical assessments, support, and interventions that can make a significant difference in patient outcomes. General nursing principles, such as back care and skin care, are integral to the patient's overall well-being and recovery. By balancing technical expertise with compassionate care, nurses help ensure that ECMO patients receive the highest level of care possible while also supporting families through one of the most challenging times of their lives.

FURTHER READING

1. Bergeron A, Holifield L. Extracorporeal membrane oxygenation: The nurse's role in patient care. Nursing Critical Care. 2020;15:6-14.
2. Melnikov S, Furmanov A, Gololobov A, Atrash M, Broyer C, Gelkop M, et al. Recommendations form professional advisory committee on Nursing Practice in the care of ECMO-Supported Patients. Crit Care Nurse. 2021;41(3):e1-8.
3. Puslecki M, Dabrowski M, Baumgart K, Ligowski M, Dabrowska A, Ziemak P, et al. Managing patients on extracorporeal membrane oxygenation support during the COVID-19 pandemic - a proposal for a nursing standard operating procedure. BMC Nurs. 2021;20:214.

SECTION

4 Systems

Section Editor: *Reshu Gupta Khanikar*

13. **Cardiac Critical Care**
Ritesh Shah, Ankur Bhavsar, Vitrag Shah, Ronak Patel

14. **Critical Care Neurology and Neurosurgery**
Urvi Shukla, Sachin Tambhare

15. **Pulmonary Critical Care Nursing**
Sharmili Sinha, Alisha Chaudhury

16. **Emergencies in Gastroenterology**
Reshu Gupta Khanikar, Rakhee Baruah

17. **Care of a Patient Undergoing Major Surgery**
Vivek Dave, Anish Joshi

18. **Endocrine Emergencies**
Gunjan Chanchalani, Seema S Tekwani

19. **Trauma and Burns**
Ashutosh Bhardwaj, Quadri SM

CHAPTER 13

Cardiac Critical Care

Ritesh Shah, Ankur Bhavsar, Vitrag Shah, Ronak Patel

ACUTE CORONARY SYNDROME AND HEART FAILURE

WHAT IS ACUTE CORONARY SYNDROME?

Acute coronary syndrome (ACS) is one of the leading emergencies requiring admission in the intensive care unit (ICU). This term is used for cessation or stopping [acute myocardial infarction (MI)] or severely reduced blood supply to the heart muscles (unstable angina). The myocardial infraction is defined in **Table 1** and the clinical symptoms and signs are given in **Table 2**. The diagnoses of the various coronary syndromes are given in **Table 3**. A typical electrocardiogram (ECG) complex of ST elevation MI is shown in **Figure 1**.

TABLE 1: Definition.

Acute myocardial infarction	*Unstable angina*
It is an event of myocardial necrosis caused by unstable ischemic syndrome. In this type of ACS, blood supply to certain part of heart stops. *Two patterns:* 1. *STEMI:* ST-segment elevation myocardial infarction (MI) 2. *NSTEMI:* Non-ST-segment elevation MI	• Unstable angina is an event where there is reduction of blood flow and oxygen to certain part of the heart. It may progress to myocardial infarction. There is no necrosis of myocardium and hence, there is no release of cardiac biomarkers • Patient presentation may be similar to STEMI or NSTEMI

Nursing Considerations

Patient may present with above said symptoms. Many a time, it is common to describe such symptoms as acidity or upset stomach and ignoring anginal pain leading to catastrophic results.

History of premorbid illness is necessary like hypertension, diabetes, etc. Most importantly, the medication history is important to be documented. Many a time, medications are modified considering the present illness. If not documented, it may result into either unwanted medications given to patient or important medication being missed (medication error).

The ECG changes (ST elevation) in different leads may indicate different territory involvement of the heart. It may also give

TABLE 2: Diagnosis.

Signs and symptoms	*Clinical examination*
• Retrosternal chest pain • Epigastric pain • Perspiration • Chest pain radiation to left arm, jaw • Giddiness • Breathing difficulty • Nausea and vomiting • History of syncope	• Tachycardia • Bradycardia • Hypertension • Hypotension • Tachypnea • Cold, clammy skin • Crepitations on auscultation • Hypoxia

TABLE 3: Electrocardiogram (ECG) changes.

STEMI	*NSTEMI*	*Unstable angina*
• ST-segment elevation • New ST-segment elevation at the J point in two contiguous leads with the cutoff point greater than 0.1 mV in all leads other than V2 or V3 • Cardiac biomarkers are elevated	• No classical ST-segment elevation • ECG may be showing transient ST elevation, ST depression, new T wave inversion • Cardiac biomarkers are elevated	• Hyperacute T wave • Flattening of T wave • Inverted T waves • ST depression • Cardiac biomarkers are usually not elevated

(NSTEMI: non-ST-segment elevation myocardial infarction; STEMI: ST-segment elevation myocardial infarction)

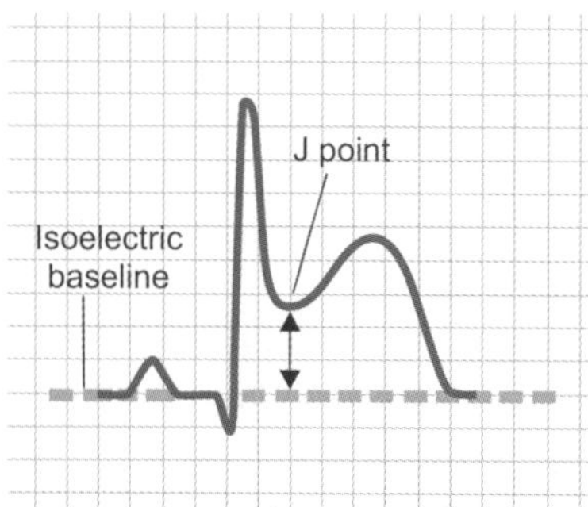

Fig. 1: ST-segment elevation.

us some prediction of coronary artery involvement **(Table 4)**.

Cardiac Biomarkers for Myocardial Necrosis

These are the substances in human body, which are released in blood circulation whenever there is damage or stress to the heart.

Commonly used cardiac biomarkers for cardiac injuries are creatine kinase MB (CK-MB) and cardiac troponins. Cardiac troponins are very sensitive and accurate and currently recommended for the diagnosis of ACSs. Even if patient is having classical signs/symptoms/ECG changes of MI, these biomarkers may be negative initially. So, we need to repeat after 4–12 hours.

Management of Acute Coronary Syndrome

- *ABC (Airway-Breathing-Circulation):*
  - *A and B:* Supplemental oxygen, if peripheral oxygen saturation (SpO_2) is <94%; secure airway if required.
    Do not use oxygen in a patient who does not have hypoxemia.
  - *C:* If hypotensive, give intravenous (IV) fluids or inotropes/vasopressors as per instruction of the cardiologist.
- Inform the cardiologist and activate cardiac catheterization laboratory.
- Get all pre-angiography workup, i.e., viral markers, creatinine, coagulation parameters, other basic blood tests (do not wait for further management till blood reports are available).
- In all the patients with STEMI, the target remains an early reperfusion. This can be done either by a percutaneous coronary balloon angioplasty with stenting, or pharmacologically by a process called thrombolysis. A strong fibrinolytic agent is injected in the system to break down the fibrin in the clot that blocked a coronary artery and caused the STEMI. Angioplasty is the treatment of choice, provided the facility is available and the time from the patient presenting at the hospital to the

TABLE 4: Electrocardiogram (ECG) changes and respective anatomical lesions.

Location of myocardial infarction (MI)	*Specific leads*	*Which vessel?*	*ST-segment*
Anterior wall	V2 to V4	Left anterior descending artery (LAD)—diagonal branch	Elevation
Septal wall	V1 and V2	Left anterior descending artery (LAD)—septal branch	Elevation
Lateral wall	I, aV_L, V5, V6	Left coronary artery (LCA)—circumflex branch	Elevation
Inferior wall	II, III, aV_F	Right coronary artery (RCA)	Elevation
Posterior wall	V1 to V4	Left coronary artery (LCA)—circumflex branch Right coronary artery (RCA)—posterior descending branch	Depression

start of the procedure (called the door to the needle time) is <120 minutes. In NSTEMI patients, there is no benefit with pharmacological thrombolysis and the angioplasty is done in some selected patients.

- *Pharmacological management:*
  - Antiplatelet agents like aspirin, clopidogrel , prasugrel, or ticagrelor as per instructions from the cardiologist; usually dual antiplatelet agents are loaded. Aspirin 300 mg with prasugrel 60 mg or ticagrelor 180 mg or clopidogrel 300 mg is given as loading dose. Subsequently, aspirin 75 mg with prasugrel 10 mg or ticagrelor 90 mg twice daily or clopidogrel 75 mg daily is continued.
  - Atorvastatin is also started immediately with a dose of 80 mg/day daily.
  - Pain relief (fentanyl or paracetamol)
  - IV metoprolol in the patient with STEMI was a routine medicine used before the days of primary percutaneous intervention (PPCI) or thrombolysis.
    - Do not give in patients with heart failure (HF) or in cardiogenic shock or if systolic blood pressure (BP) <120 mm Hg.
  - *Reperfusion therapy:*
    - *Patient with diagnosis of STEMI:*
      - PPCI
      - Fibrinolysis therapy is administered if PPCI is not possible within 120 minutes of diagnosis. Among below-mentioned agents, rTPA (recombinant tissue plasminogen activator) agents are preferable because of the less side effects and ease of administration.
      - Streptokinase
      - Urokinase
      - rTPA
      - Tenecteplase
      - Reteplase

The medicines used in ACSs is summarized in **Table 5**.

- *Patient with working diagnosis of NSTEMI-ACS:*
  - Invasive therapy is recommended.
  - An immediate invasive intervention is recommended if VERY HIGH RISK feature is present.
    - Hemodynamically unstable patient or cardiogenic shock

TABLE 5: Medications used in acute coronary syndrome (ACS).

Medication	*Dose (loading)*	*Dose (maintenance)*
Aspirin	150–300 mg	75–100 mg OD
Clopidogrel	• 300–600 mg • 300 mg when fibrinolysis is done (75 mg if age >75)	75 mg OD
Prasugrel	60 mg	• 10 mg OD • 5 mg OD (weight <60 kg) • Use with caution in age >75 • Contraindicated in prior stroke patients
Ticagrelor	180 mg	90 mg BD
Tirofiban	• 25 µg/kg over 3 minutes • Over 5 minutes if CrCl <60	• 0.15 µg/kg/min up to 18 hours • CrCl <60, 0.075 µg/kg/min for up to 18 hours *Contraindicated*: • Prior ICH • Stroke within 30 days • Fibrinolysis • Platelet <1 Lac
Heparin	70–100 U/kg	Infusion to be titrated with target aPTT 60–80 seconds (1.5–2.5 times)
Enoxaparin	1 mg/kg SC BD for 2 days	Till clinical stabilization CrCl <30—1 mg/kg OD
Fondaparinux	• 2.5 mg SC OD • During PCI—Single dose Heparin • Avoid if CrCl <20	
Thrombolytic agents	***Indication***	***Dose***
Alteplase (rt-PA)	STEMI	• >67 kg: 100 mg IV total (15 mg bolus over 2 minutes, then 50 mg over 30 minutes then 35 mg over 60 minutes) • ≤67 kg: Maximum 100 mg (15 mg bolus over 2 minutes then 0.75 mg/kg over 30 minutes then 0.5 mg/kg over 60 minutes)
Reteplase	STEMI	10 units IV push over 2 minutes; repeat in 30 minutes
Streptokinase	STEMI	1.5 MU over 60 minutes
Tenecteplase	STEMI	• <60 kg: 30 mg IV bolus • 60–69 kg: 35 mg IV bolus • 70–79 kg: 40 mg IV bolus • 80–89 kg: 45 mg IV bolus • ≥90 kg: 50 mg IV bolus

(CrCl: creatinine clearance; ICH: intracranial hemorrhage; IV: intravenous; PCI: percutaneous coronary intervention; SC: subcutaneous; STEMI: ST-segment elevation myocardial infarction)

- Recurrent or ongoing chest pain refractory to medical therapy
- Acute HF presumed to be due to myocardial ischemia
- Life-threatening arrhythmias or cardiac arrest after presentation
- Mechanical complications
- Recurrent dynamic changes suggestive of ischemia

- An early (within 24 hours) invasive strategy should be considered if any HIGH RISK features are present.
  - Confirmed diagnosis of NSTEMI based on ESC (European society of cardiology) algorithms
  - GRACE risk score >140 (Global Registry of Acute Cardiac Events)
  - Transient ST segment elevation
  - Dynamic ST segment or T wave changes

Nursing Considerations

- Medication must be given as per the protocol and after a consultation with the doctor.
- Strict monitoring of BP, pulse, respiration, and neurological signs
- *Monitor rhythm*: Ventricular dysrhythmias may occur with reperfusion.
- Assess neurological status frequently, neurological change may indicate intra-cranial bleeding.
- Watch for hematuria, hematemesis, bleeding from mucous membranes, epistaxis, ecchymosis and melena in the first 24 hours after treatment.
- Unnecessary needle pricks, nasogastric (NG) tube insertion, intramuscular injections per urethral catheterization should be avoided in the first 24 hours after treatment.

HEART FAILURE

Universal Definition

Heart failure is a clinical syndrome with current or prior symptoms and signs caused by a structural and/or functional cardiac abnormality and corroborated by at least one of the following:

- Elevated natriuretic peptide
- Objective evidence of pulmonary or systemic congestion

The symptoms and signs of HF are shown in **Table 6**. The stages of HF are shown in **Figure 2**. The classification of HF syndromes are summarized in the **Table 7**.

Stages of Heart Failure

Figure 2 illustrates the stages of HF.

Diagnosis of Heart Failure

- Clinical signs and symptoms indicating HF
- Past history of ischemic heart disease (may or may not be there)
- Raised biomarkers like BNP (B-type natriuretic peptide) and NT-proBNP (N terminal proBNP)

TABLE 6: Signs and symptoms of heart failure.

Signs and symptoms	*Clinical examination*
• Shortness of breath at rest or exertional • Orthopnea • Swelling of legs • Palpitation • Chest pain • Fatigue and weakness • Decreased urine output • Decreased appetite	• Distension of neck veins • Weak, rapid, thready pulse • Wheezing • Ascites • Anasarca • Tachycardia • Hypertension (more common) • Crepitations on auscultation • Hypoxia

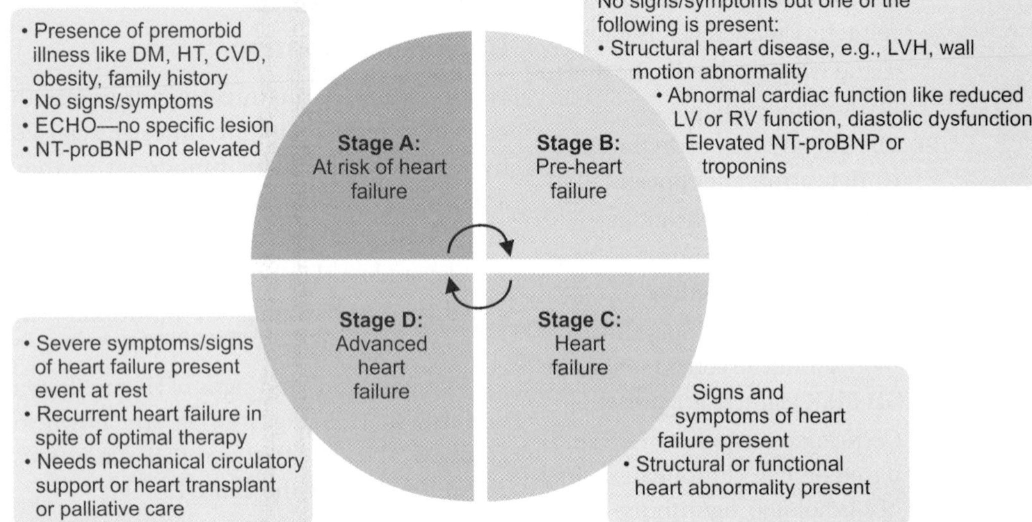

Fig. 2: Stages of heart failure. (CVD: cardiovascular disease; DM: diabetes mellitus; ECHO: echocardiogram, LV: left ventricle; LVH: left ventricular hypertrophy; HT: hypertension; NT-proBNP: N-terminal pro-B-type natriuretic peptide; RV: right ventricle)

TABLE 7: Classification of heart failure.

Terminology	*Ejection fraction (EF%)*
HF with reduced EF (HFrEF)	Left ventricular ejection fraction (LVEF) ≤40%
HF with mildly reduced EF (HFmrEF)	LVEF 41–49%
HF with preserved EF (HFpEF)	LVEF ≥50%
HF with improved EF (HFimpEF)	Baseline EF ≤40%, a ≥10% point increase from baseline EF and second measurement >40%

- 2D echocardiogram (ECHO) [measuring ejection fraction (EF)]

Clinical Profiles in Acute Decompensated Heart Failure

Figure 3 illustrates the clinical profiles in acute decompensated heart failure (ADHF).

Management of ADHF:

- Assess and stabilize ABC.
- Treat life-threatening arrhythmias as per Advanced Cardiac Life Support (ACLS) protocol
- Check the vitals, SpO_2 monitoring
- Head up position
- Secure two wide-bore IV cannulas.
- Send investigations including complete blood count (CBC), electrolytes, creatinine, arterial blood gas (ABG) cardiac biomarkers (NT-proBNP if needed)
- Start oxygen if hypoxia (SpO_2 <90–95%)
- Start noninvasive ventilation (NIV) if respiratory distress and intubation if too unstable or NIV fails
- Do ECG and ECHO
- Cardiologist's referral
- Start diuretics as early as possible (Inj. furosemide 40 mg or torsemide 20 mg IV stat followed by SOS infusion or intermittent bolus as per institutional protocol).
- *Treat triggering etiology for ADHF:*
    - ACS
    - Uncontrolled hypertension

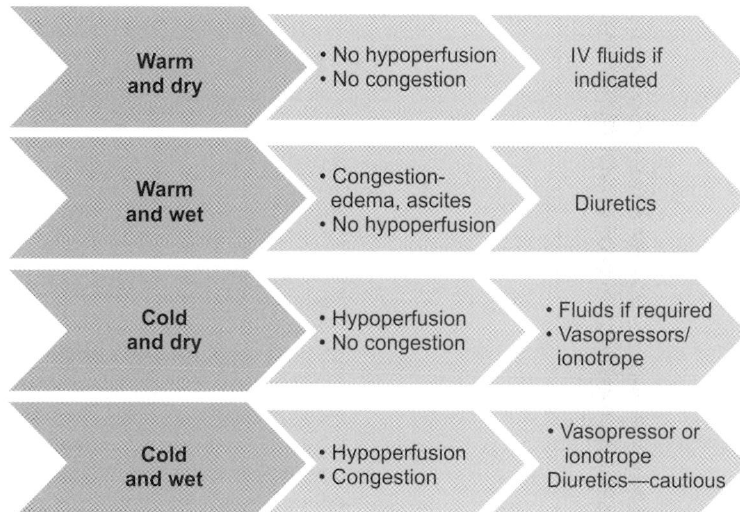

Fig. 3: Clinical profiles in acute decompensated heart failure (ADHF). (IV: intravenous)

- Control rate if tachycardia or tachyarrhythmia.
- Direct cardioversion if new-onset atrial fibrillation with rapid ventricular rate and hemodynamic unstability
- Find and treat infection if any
- Check diet and medication compliance.
- Correct anemia.
- Check and correct hypo- or hyperthyroidism.
- Cardiac surgeon consultation if acute severe mitral or aortic regurgitation or aortic dissection

Some specific situations and their management strategies are summarized in the **Table 8**.

Therapeutic end points:

- Target mean arterial pressure (MAP) >65 [>70 in chronic kidney disease (CKD) and other selected patients] to support adequate organ perfusion.
- Optimization of pre- and afterload to maximize stroke volume
- Mixed venous oxygen saturation >60%
- Adequate urine output to ensure a negative fluid balance
- Correction of metabolic acidosis and electrolytes
- Treatment for persisting ischemia if present as seen in ECG
- Adequate oxygenation to relieve respiratory distress

The various medicines used in HF are shown in the **Table 9**.

General Nursing Considerations

- Do not delay the diagnosis if a patient is having classical symptoms. Inform the doctor immediately as time is muscle.
- ABC is the key to save any patient.
- 12-lead ECG should always be taken.
- Once diagnosed, activate the catheterization laboratory and inform the cardiologist immediately whenever applicable.
- Never leave the patient's side as patient's condition may worsen anytime.
- Drug therapy is crucial to administer and monitor as they may cause significant side effects.

TABLE 8: Specific considerations as per patient's condition.

Severe ADHF (pulmonary edema) and hypotension or signs of shock	***ADHF with fluid overload but adequate end-organ perfusion [normal or elevated blood pressure (BP)]***
• Start vasopressor (norepinephrine) • With inotrope (dobutamine or milrinone) if BP permits • Assess need for mechanical support [intra-aortic balloon counter pulsation (IABP)]	• *Nitroglycerin (NTG):* If response to diuretics is inadequate, start NTG infusion at 5–10 µg/min • Titrate every 3–5 minutes as per mean arterial blood pressure or SBP to a dose range of 10–200 µg/min • Diuretics
Systolic HF—HFrEF with ADHF and shock	***Diastolic HF—HFpEF with ADHF and shock***
• Discontinue chronic beta blocker therapy • Give an IV inotrope (dobutamine or milrinone) and/or mechanical support (intra-aortic balloon counter pulsation)	• Consider possibility of acute MR/AR and cardiac surgeon referral • If possible, left ventricular outflow obstruction, treat with beta blocker, IV fluid (unless pulmonary edema), and IV vasopressor • Do not give inodilator or vasodilator

(ADHF: acute decompensated heart failure; AR: aortic regurgitation; HF: heart failure; HFpEF: HF with preserved ejection fraction; HFrEF: HF with reduced ejection fraction; IV: intravenous; MR: mitral regurgitation; SBP: systolic blood pressure)

TABLE 9: Drug-related nursing considerations.

MOA	***Adverse reaction***	***Nursing considerations***
Epinephrine	• Unwanted cardiac stimulation • Hyperglycemia • Increased metabolic rate • Splanchnic hypoperfusion • Increase serum lactate level	• *Extravasation:* Injection site—tissue sloughing; change injection sites if blanching or vasoconstriction occurs • Strict HR, BP monitoring; intra-arterial BP is preferable. Should be diluted in 5% dextrose
Norepinephrine	• Local tissue necrosis from drug extravasation • With high dose intense vasoconstriction with organ dysfunction • Hyperglycemia • Bradycardia	• *Extravasation:* Injection site—tissue sloughing; change injection sites if blanching or vasoconstriction occurs. • Strict HR, BP monitoring; intra-arterial BP is preferable; should be diluted in 5% dextrose; avoid bolus dose
Dobutamine	• Tachycardia • Ectopic beats	• Incompatible with alkaline solution like $NaHCO_3$, furosemide • Watch for arrhythmia
Dopamine	• Sinus tachycardia • Atrial fibrillation • Increased IOP • Splanchnic hypoperfusion • Delay gastric emptying	• *Extravasation:* Injection site—tissue sloughing; so use central line preferably • Correct hypovolemia before starting dopamine
Vasopressin	• Excessive vasoconstriction • Excessive water retention • Hyponatremia	Watch for BP, arrhythmias, signs of water intoxication

Contd...

Contd...

MOA	Adverse reaction	Nursing considerations
Nitroglycerin	• Hypotension • Increased ICP	Watch for BP, tolerance for drugs can occur after 24–48 hours of continuous infusion—give 6 hours drug-free interval in case of tolerance
Nitroprusside	• Cyanide intoxication • Thiocyanate intoxication—renal dysfunction	Watch for BP, progressive increase in requirement of nitroprusside to maintain desired BP may indicate cyanide intoxication

(BP: blood pressure; HR: heart rate; ICP: intracranial pressure; IOP: intraocular pressure)

- Document whatever medications are given.
- Document all regular medications that patient is on before admission and clearly document as well as instruct other co-nurses which medications are to be continued or not.
- Check/confirm the consent if any invasive intervention is planned.
- Keep assuring the patient.
- Communication is the key to save a life.

FURTHER READING

1. Bozkurt B, Coats AJ, Tsutsui H, Abdelhamid M, Adamopoulos S, Albert N, et al. Universal Definition and Classification of Heart Failure: A Report of the Heart Failure Society of America, Heart Failure Association of the European Society of Cardiology, Japanese Heart Failure Society and Writing Committee of the Universal Definition of Heart Failure. J Card Fail. 2021;S1071-9164(21)00050-6.
2. Byrne RA, Rossello X, Coughlan JJ, Barbato E, Berry C, Chieffo A, et al.; ESC Scientific Document Group. 2023 ESC Guidelines for the management of acute coronary syndromes. Eur Heart J. 2023;44(38):3720-826.
3. Collins SR. Elsevier's 2024 Intravenous Medications: A Handbook for Nurses and Health Professionals, 40th edition. Amsterdam: Elsevier; 2023.
4. O'Gara PT, Kushner FG, Ascheim DD, Casey DE Jr, Chung MK, de Lemos JA, et al. 2013 ACCF/AHA guideline for the management of ST-elevation myocardial infarction: a report of the American College of Cardiology Foundation/American Heart Association Task Force on Practice Guidelines. American Heart Association & American College of Cardiology Guidelines. Circulation. 2013; 127(4):e362-425.
5. Skidmore-Roth L. Mosby's 2024 Nursing Drug Reference, 37th edition. St. Louis: Elsevier; 2023.
6. Thygesen K, Alpert JS, Jaffe AS, Simoons ML, Chaitman BR, White HD, et al.; Joint ESC/ACCF/AHA/WHF Task Force for the Universal Definition of Myocardial Infarction. Third universal definition of myocardial infarction. Circulation. 2012;126(16):2020-35.
7. Thygesen K, Alpert JS, Jaffe AS, Simoons ML, Chaitman BR, White HD, et al. Third universal definition of myocardial infarction. J Am Coll Cardiol. 2012;60:1581-98.
8. Webb A, Angus D, Finfer S, Gattinoni L, Singer M. Oxford Textbook of Critical Care, 2nd edition. Oxford: Oxford University Press; 2016.

CHAPTER 14

Critical Care Neurology and Neurosurgery

Urvi Shukla, Sachin Tambhare

INTRODUCTION

Neurological emergencies commonly present in the emergency department and intensive care. These emergencies need a multidisciplinary team of emergency physicians, neurologists, intensivists, and critical care nurses. In this chapter, we review a few common neurological emergencies such as acute stroke, traumatic brain injury, status epilepticus, meningitis/encephalitis, and comatose patients of unknown cause. The chapter is written in a format that is easy to understand and read. It may be used as a ready reckoner to help the reader in an emergency.

STROKE

A stroke can occur when blood flow to the brain is stopped. Stroke is a medical emergency; it can cause lasting brain damage, disability, and even death. Treatment for stroke needs to be done in a time-bound fashion, and there is strong evidence that ischemic stroke should be thrombolyzed if the onset of symptoms is within 3–4.5 hours.

Across the world, stroke is recognized as an emergency and hospitals have designed their processes to recognize stroke early, to do brain imaging early and thrombolyze a patient early. The pneumonic explained here is one of the ways to help early identification of a stroke patient. The rest of the stroke treatment pathway is explained in a tabular format **(Table 1)**.

INTRACEREBRAL/ INTRAPARENCHYMAL BLEED

This is a hemorrhagic stroke. The patient presents with symptoms similar to ischemic stroke but in this case, there is a bleed in the parenchyma of the brain. Without a computed tomography (CT) scan, it is difficult to clinically differentiate between ischemic and hemorrhagic stroke. Thrombolysis is contraindicated in this type of stroke **(Table 2)**.

SUBARACHNOID HEMORRHAGE

These can be life-threatening bleeds in the brain. This bleeding happens between the arachnoid membrane and the pia mater (the innermost lining of the brain). This happens suddenly and is associated with the rupture of an aneurysm of large intracerebral arteries. This blood can easily track into the cerebrospinal fluid (CSF) spaces and ventricles. There are multiple complications associated with vasospasm, obstructive hydrocephalus, cerebral ischemia, coma, and sometimes even death **(Table 3)**.

STATUS EPILEPTICUS

It is a seizure with 5 minutes or more of continuous clinical and/or electrographic seizure activity or recurrent seizure activity without recovery between seizures. It is recognized as a medical emergency as prolonged seizures may be associated with brain damage and status epilepticus (SE) gets more difficult to treat as seizure activity is prolonged **(Table 4)**.

TABLE 1: Stroke.

Condition	*Acute ischemic stroke*
Symptoms: This pneumonic BEFAST is a quick and easy way to remember the symptoms of stroke	• B = Loss of *B*alance • E = Loss or blurry or double vision (*EYES*) • F = *F*acial deviation • A = *A*rm drop or weakness • S = Slur in *S*peech • T = last known well *T*ime
Signs	• HR >90 or <60 beats/min • SBP = N or >140 mm Hg • Loss of balance, hemiplegia, or hemiparesis may be present • In posterior circulation stroke, there may be diplopia, vomiting, ataxia, loss of balance, or sudden onset coma (*Note:* All or a few signs may be present.)
What you need to do	• A clear *last-known well* time has to be documented • When stroke is suspected, a stroke code is to be announced • NIHSS scoring has to be done bedside • Stroke mimics have to be ruled out • They are hypoglycemia, drug intoxication, acute alcohol intoxication, OPP poisoning, and postictal TODD's palsy • NIHSS scoring should not take more than 10 minutes. If the patient has come to the hospital within 3 hours of the onset of stroke symptoms, the patient should be urgently scanned to decide eligibility for thrombolysis • If NIHSS <5, no need for thrombolysis • If NIHSS 6–15, thrombolyze the patient if in a window period • If NIHSS >15, the risk of post-thrombolysis bleeding is very high and a neurologist should be consulted before a decision is made • Do ECG and ABG • Send CBC, urea/creatinine, and electrolytes • Ideally a platelet count and serum creatinine should be available before thrombolysis but thrombolysis cannot wait till the laboratory is ready
Primary treatment	• O_2 support via Hudson mask to keep SpO_2 >95% • Titrate SBP to 160–180 mm Hg and diastolic BP to <100 if the patient is for thrombolysis • Urgently do a CT brain/MRI brain (limited study) as per neurologist • Take consent for thrombolysis • Injection tenecteplase 0.25 mg/kg should be given as a quick bolus. It should be followed by a flush of 50 mL water for injection or a running NS pint • Another drug that can be used for thrombolysis is injection alteplase 0.9 mg/kg. Of which 0.1 mg/kg is given as a bolus, and the rest as an infusion over 1 hour • The patient should not receive any IM injections, no Foley's catheter insertion for at least 6–8 hours post-thrombolysis • The patient should be transferred to the ICU for further monitoring and care

(ABG: arterial blood gas; CBC: complete blood count; CT: computed tomography; ECG: electrocardiogram; HR: heart rate; ICU: intensive care unit; IM: intramuscular; MRI: magnetic resonance imaging; OPP: organophosphate; SBP: systolic blood pressure; SpO_2: oxygen saturation)

TABLE 2: Intracerebral/intraparenchymal.

Condition	*Intracranial bleed*
Symptoms	• B = loss of *B*alance • E = loss or blurry or double vision (*EYES*) • F = *F*acial deviation • A = *A*rm drop or weakness • S = slur in *S*peech • T = last known well *T*ime Headache, dizziness, and unconsciousness
Signs	• HR >90 or <60 beats/min • SBP = N or >140 mm Hg • Loss of balance, hemiplegia or hemiparesis, and loss of speech may be present • In posterior circulation bleed, there may be diplopia, vomiting, ataxia, loss of balance, or sudden onset coma (*Note:* All or few signs may be present.)
What you need to do	• Urgent CT brain is indicated • Ask for a history of drug use such as warfarin, NOACs, acitrom, steroids, and recreational drugs. Ask for a history of previous hypertension (HTN), compliance to anti-HTN medicines
Primary treatment	• O_2 support via Hudson mask to keep SpO_2 >95% • Titrate SBP to 140–150 mm Hg and diastolic BP to <100. Lowering BP is an emergency. Injection labetalol 5–10 mg bolus followed by infusion of 2–4 mg/hour is recommended • Lowering BP prevents expansion of hematoma and therefore reduces brain damage • Urgently do a CT brain • Involve a neurosurgeon if the bleed volume >30 mL or there is a posterior fossa bleed or GCS <8, or the patient is on anticoagulant drugs • Send PT/INR and APTT for all patients. Hold all anticoagulant and antiplatelet drugs. Ask the time when the last dose was taken • If there is a suspicion of an overdose of these medicines, consider doing MLC • If the patient's GCS >8, no need for early intubation • If the patient's GCS <8, early intubation is needed to prevent the risk of aspiration and hypoxemia • However, intubation should be done once BP is well controlled and by a senior member of the team

(APTT: activated partial thromboplastin time; CT: computed tomography; GCS: Glasgow Coma Scale; HR: heart rate; INR: international normalized ratio; NOACs: new oral anticoagulants; PT: prothrombin time; SBP: systolic blood pressure; SpO_2: oxygen saturation)

TABLE 3: Subarachnoid hemorrhage.

Condition	***Subarachnoid hemorrhage***
Symptoms	• *Sudden severe headache:* Thunderclap headache, which may be associated with vomiting, loss of consciousness, seizures, or focal neurological deficit • Other symptoms include decreased focus or alertness, confusion, dizziness, photophobia, blind patches in vision, double vision, and transient blindness
Signs	• HR >90 *or* <60 beats/min • SBP = N *or* >140 mm Hg • Hemiplegia, hemiparesis, loss of consciousness, nuchal rigidity, diplopia, blurring of vision, dizziness, and vomiting
What you need to do	• Urgent CT brain plain is indicated • Ask for a history of smoking, alcohol intake, cocaine or methamphetamine use, history of hypertension, connective tissue disorders, head trauma, and family history of aneurysm rupture • Send CBC, PT/INR, and APTT along with routine laboratory investigations
Primary treatment	• O_2 support via Hudson mask to keep SpO_2 >95% • Target SBP <160 mm Hg, MAP >75 mm Hg • Injection labetalol 10–20 mg IV every 10–15 minutes as needed • Give tablet nimodipine 60 mg Q4H and begin therapy within 96 hours of SAH • Reducing BP prevents further hematoma and decreases the chances of re-bleeding • If patient's GCS >8, no need for early intubation • If patient's GCS <8, early intubation is needed to prevent the risk of aspiration and hypoxemia • However, intubation should be done once BP is well controlled and by a senior member of the team • Urgently do CT brain angiography if aneurysmal rupture is suspected • Correct coagulation abnormality if any • Involve neurosurgeon, neurophysician, and interventional radiologist urgently for aneurysmal clipping or coiling in patients with aneurysm rupture and Hunt and Hess grades 1–3. For grades 4–5 surgery can be delayed if there is no spontaneous clinical improvement or the patient does not respond to therapy for decreasing intracranial pressure (ICP) • External ventricular drain (EVD) can be placed if a patient develops a hydrocephalus • These patients have a prolonged ICU stay; hence, general intensive care nursing such as thromboprophylaxis, the elevation of the head end of the bed, keeping the head in the midline position, nutrition, preventing bed sores, and oral hygiene play an important role in ICU outcomes

(APTT: activated partial thromboplastin time; CT: computed tomography; CBC: complete blood count; GCS: Glasgow Coma Scale; HR: heart rate; INR: international normalized ratio; PT: prothrombin time; MAP: mean arterial pressure; SAH: subarachnoid hemorrhage; SBP: systolic blood pressure; SpO_2: oxygen saturation)

TABLE 4: Status epilepticus (SE).

Condition	*Status epilepticus*
Types of status epilepticus	• *Convulsive status epilepticus (CSE):* Characterized by prolonged seizures that have physical abnormal movements • *Nonconvulsive status epilepticus (NCSE):* Characterized by prolonged and continuous electrical seizure activity in the brain which results in behavioral changes, altered mental status, coma, and evident on the EEG • Both types of seizure activity have either generalized or partial involvement
What you need to do	• A person who is convulsing needs the following done immediately • Roll the person onto their side when possible • Attach a cardiac monitor • O_2 support if SpO_2 <94% • Try to get two large bore IV access, if IV is established, send blood samples • If the patient's GCS <8, early intubation is needed to prevent the risk of aspiration and hypoxemia • Check finger glucose level, hypoglycemia can be the most easily treatable cause of seizures • Send CBC, RFT, LFT, SR, calcium, magnesium, ABG, toxicology screening (blood and urine) if drug abuse is suspected • IV access should be used for antiseizure medicines and antiepileptic medicines • Patients may need supportive investigations such as CT scan or MRI, or a lumbar puncture if infectious pathology is suspected • If seizures do not stop after a full dose of antiepileptic medicine or last more than 10 minutes, then this is classified as refractory status epilepticus. In such situations, electroencephalographic (EEG) monitoring may be helpful
Primary treatment	• *Stage 1:* Early SE (0 to 10 minutes): Injection lorazepam 0.1 mg/kg IV diluted slow push at 2 mg/min. If the seizure persists, repeat another 2 mg bolus dose of injection lorazepam • *Stage 2:* Established SE (10–30 minutes): Injection phenytoin infusion 15 mg/kg *or* injection sodium valproate 25 mg/kg IV infusion *or* injection levetiracetam 1 g IV infusion f/b 10 mg/kg IV BD
	• *Stage 3: Refractory SE*: Continuous seizures despite treatment after 30–60 minutes. General anesthesia is recommended such as midazolam/thiopental/propofol infusion

(ABG: arterial blood gas; CBC: complete blood count; CT: computed tomography; GCS: Glasgow Coma Scale; IV: intravenous; LFT: liver function test; RFT: renal function test; MRI: magnetic resonance imaging; SpO_2: oxygen saturation)

COMA OF UNKNOWN CAUSE

Multiple reasons can cause a coma in patients arriving in the emergency/ICU. These conditions are associated with an increased risk of death, but currently, there are no treatment guidelines **(Table 5)**.

TABLE 5: Coma of unknown cause.

Condition	*Coma of unknown cause*
What is coma	• Unresponsive state in which patients do not respond to any external stimuli or internal needs • Objectively it is defined as a Glasgow Coma Scale (GCS) <8
What you need to do	• Immediate evaluation and concurrent stabilization and assessment are required • Try to do a head-to-toe neurological examination before you intubate this patient • Patients with a GCS <8 will need intubation and mechanical ventilation • *A:* Airway (intubation) and cervical spine stabilization • *B:* Ensure appropriate and adequate ventilation • *C:* Optimize hemodynamics • *D:* Neurological deficit evaluation • Check pupillary and brain stem reflexes • Collateral history and head-to-toe examination • Do a random finger prick BSL, send CBC, blood and urine toxicology screening, LFT, RFT, PT/INR. Electrolytes, calcium, magnesium, ABG, and ECG • *Neuroimaging:* CT/MRI brain • Fundoscopy to rule out raised ICP and papilledema • EEG to rule out status epilepticus • CSF study if strong suspicion of Meningitis or encephalitis
Primary treatment	• Injection mannitol 1–1.5 g/kg if suspicion of raised ICP • Injection dextrose 50% if hypoglycemia • Injection thiamine 500 mg IV bolus if history of alcohol abuse • Injection naloxone 0.01 mg/kg IV if suspicion of opioid overdose (Do not exceed 10 mg) • Injection flumazenil 0.2 mg every 15–30 seconds, maximum dose of 3 mg/h if suspected benzodiazepine poisoning • Anticonvulsant if suspicion of NCSE • Antibiotics for meningitis or septic shock • Gastric lavage if suspicion of intoxication
Some medical conditions that can cause coma	• Cardiac arrest • Stroke • Brain tumors • Vasculitis • Airway obstruction • Hypoglycemia • Overdose/drug abuse • Hypotension • Anaphylaxis • Hyperkalemia • Myocardial infarction • Sepsis • Alcohol withdrawal • Metabolic problems • Status epilepticus

(ABG: arterial blood gas; BSL: blood sugar level; CBC: complete blood count; CSF: cerebrospinal fluid; CT: computed tomography; ECG: electrocardiogram; EEG: electroencephalogram; ICP: intracranial pressure; INR: international normalized ratio; LFT: liver function test; PT: prothrombin time; MRI: magnetic resonance imaging; NCSE: nonconvulsive status epilepticus; RFT: renal function test)

FURTHER READING

1. Aroor S, Singh R, Goldstein LB. BE-FAST (Balance, Eyes, Face, Arm, Speech, Time): Reducing the proportion of stroke missed using the FAST mnemonic. Stroke. 2017; 48(2):479-481.
2. Braun M, Schmidt WU, Möckel M, Römer M, Ploner CJ, Lindner T. Coma of unknown origin in the emergency department: implementation of an in-house management routine. Scand J Trauma Resusc Emerg Med. 2016;24:61.
3. Mehta Y, Sharma J, Mehta C. In: Bansal AR, More A, Fonseca AJ, Kapadia F, Badgurjar RK (Eds). Textbook of Critical Care including Trauma & Emergency Care, 2nd edition. Jaypee Brothers Medical Publishers (P) Ltd; 2022. p. 1072.
4. Ogbebor O, Tariq S, Jaber T, Super J, Bhanot N, Rana S, et al. Neurological Emergencies in the Intensive Care Unit. Crit Care Nurs Q. 2023;46(1):17-34.
5. Tenny S, Thorell W. Intracranial Hemorrhage. In: StatPearls. Treasure Island (FL): StatPearls Publishing; 2024.
6. Wylie T, Sandhu DS, Murr N. Status Epilepticus. In: StatPearls. Treasure Island (FL): StatPearls Publishing; 2024.
7. Ziu E, Khan Suheb MZ, Mesfin FB. Subarachnoid Hemorrhage. In: StatPearls. Treasure Island (FL): StatPearls Publishing; 2024.

CHAPTER 15

Pulmonary Critical Care Nursing

Sharmili Sinha, Alisha Chaudhury

INTRODUCTION

The respiratory system is primarily involved in gaseous exchange in humans. Both the upper and lower respiratory tracts play an important role. Appropriate knowledge about anatomical landmarks and physiology is important for a good clinical assessment to diagnose pathologies.

ANATOMY OF THE RESPIRATORY TRACT

The anatomy of the respiratory tract is given as follows:

- The upper respiratory tract comprises of nose, sinuses, mouth, pharynx, and the larynx. It extends from the anterior nares to the true vocal cords. It is involved in **(Fig. 1)**:
    - Heating and cooling of the inspired gases to the body temperature
    - Filtering the inspired gases
    - Humidifying the gases to 100% relative humidity
    - Act of phonation
- The lower respiratory tract extends from true vocal cords to the alveoli. It is involved in:
    - Ventilation and exchange of gases
    - Mucociliary mechanisms for clearance of invading organisms
- The tracheobronchial tree is divided into **(Fig. 2)**:
    - *Conducting zone:* It extends from trachea to the terminal bronchioles (0–16 generations). It is also called

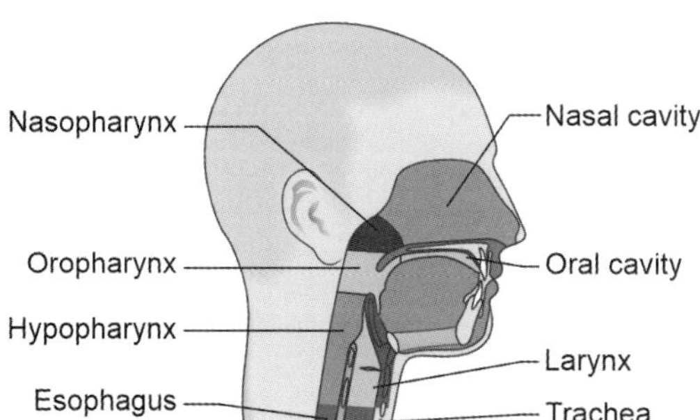

Fig. 1: Anatomy of upper respiratory tract.

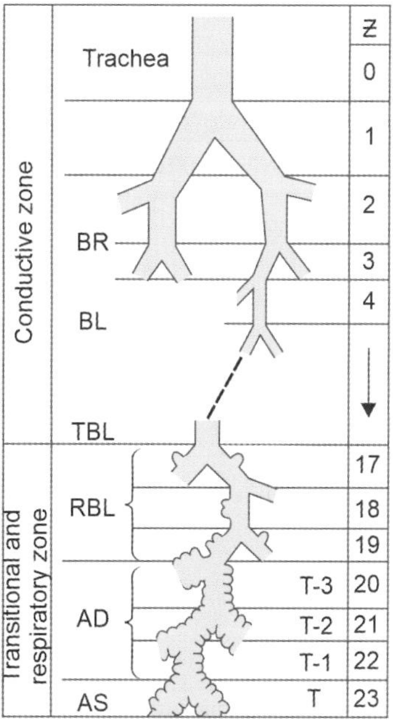

Fig. 2: Anatomy of tracheobronchial tree.

dead space as no gaseous exchange takes place here.
    - *Respiratory zone:* It extends from respiratory bronchioles to the alveolar sacs (17–23 generations).
- The alveolar capillary membrane comprises capillary endothelium, interstitial space, alveolar epithelium, and surfactant layer, which is responsible for reduction of surface tension and facilitates gaseous exchange.
- Muscles of respiration are:
    - *Inspiration:* Diaphragm is the major muscle supported by external intercostals. Accessory muscles are sternocleidomastoid and scalenes.
    - *Expiration:* During quiet exhalation, there is little or no muscle contraction. During forceful exhalation, the major muscles involved are abdominal wall muscles (rectus abdominis, transverse abdominis, external oblique, and internal oblique muscles).

PHYSIOLOGY OF RESPIRATORY SYSTEM

The physiology of the respiratory tract is as follows:

- Ventilation is the process by which gas is inspired into and expelled from the lung. Understanding lung volumes, lung compliance, and ventilation-perfusion is essential for clinical application of respiratory physiology in critical care.
- The body can readily meet its usual requirements with a typical tidal ventilation of 4–8 mL/kg. When necessary (such as during exercise), the body possesses a mechanism to produce additional ventilation in the form of an expiratory reserve volume and an inspiratory reserve volume **(Fig. 3)**.
- A person's vital capacity breath (normal 4–5 liters) occurs when they take a full inspiratory breath after tidal expiration and then expire to reserve volume.
- Residual volume is the volume in the lungs that is present after a vital capacity

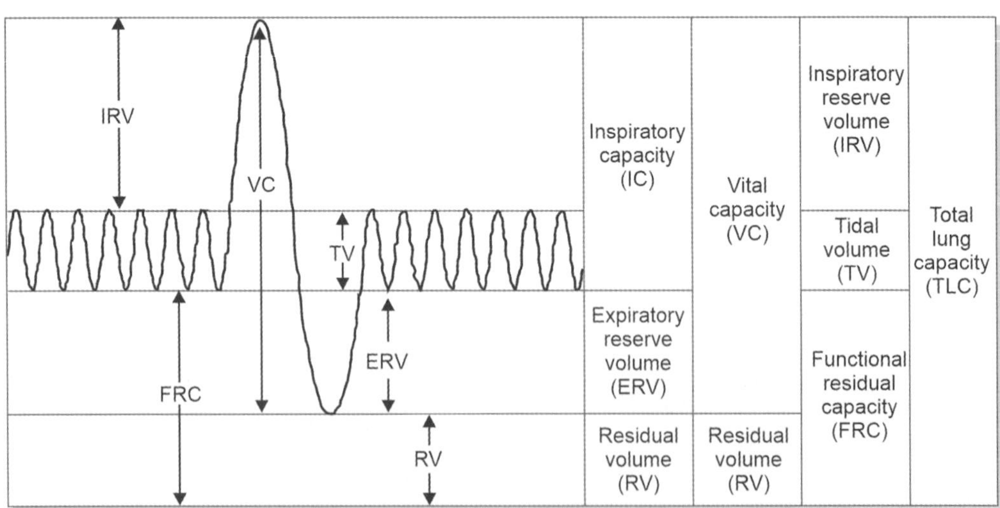

Fig. 3: Demonstration of static lung volumes.

breath. This prevents the alveoli from collapsing.

- Functional residual capacity (FRC) is the residual volume with expiratory reserve volume. FRC is essentially the volume of air remaining in the lungs following a normal expiration. Not only do the gases in the lungs after expiration stop alveolar collapse, but they also keep the pulmonary blood moving through the capillaries during this phase oxygenated. Changes in body weight, anesthesia, and position can all affect FRC. This reserve known as FRC is what increases the nonhypoxic apnea period during intubation. FRC values range from 2.8 to 3.1 L when in a standing position, but some variations may occur.
- Alveolar ventilation is the part of minute ventilation that enters alveoli and participates in gas exchange. About 5 L/min is the normal value of alveolar ventilation, which is comparable to the amount of blood passing through the lung (5 L/min for cardiac output). Alveolar ventilation to perfusion ratio is therefore roughly one.

APPROACH TO PATIENT WHO IS HYPOXEMIC

A general algorithm for approaching a patient who is hypoxemic is given in **Flowchart 1**.

NEBULIZED DRUGS AND MACHINES

Nebulized drugs and machines include the following:

- Aerosol therapy is a routine procedure in pulmonary critical care. The devices used can be divided into nebulizers and pressurized metered dose inhalers (pMDIs).
- Nebulizers used in the intensive care unit (ICU) are of three types: (1) Jet, (2) ultrasonic, and (3) mesh.
  1. *Jet nebulizers* convert liquids into aerosols that can be inhaled by patients into the lungs. It functions on

Flowchart 1: Algorithmic approach to a hypoxemic patient.

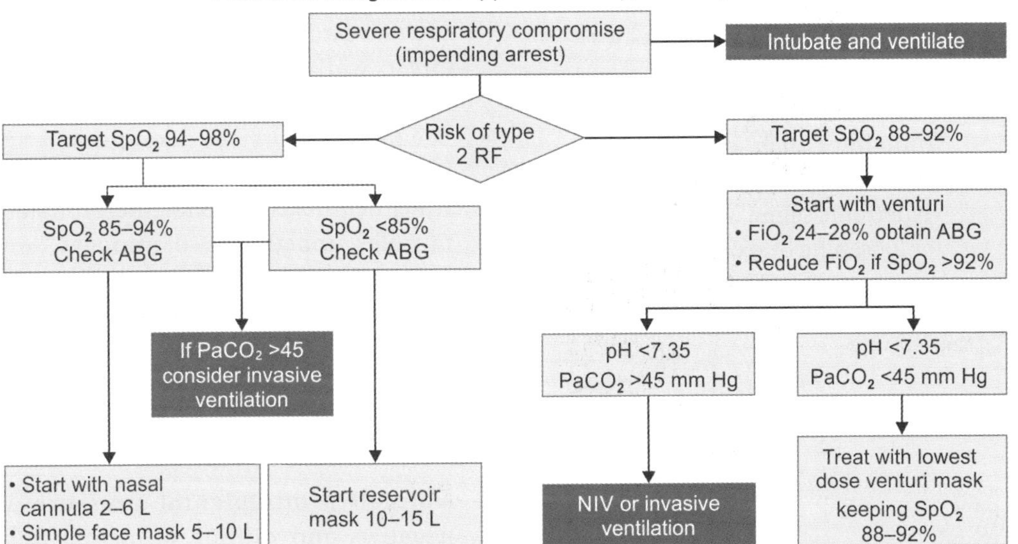

(ABG: arterial blood gas; FiO_2: fraction of inspired oxygen; NIV: noninvasive ventilation; $PaCO_2$: partial pressure of carbon dioxide; RF: respiratory failure; SpO_2: oxygen saturation)

the Bernoulli's principle, which uses compressed air or oxygen passing through a narrow orifice at 6–8 L/minute to suck drug solution from a reservoir into a feed tube.

2. *Ultrasonic nebulizers* use a piezoelectric transducer that produces ultrasonic waves that pass through the liquid medication in the nebulizer cup and generate aerosols at the surface of the solution, which get delivered to a patient either with the inspiratory flow or with the help of a fan in the nebulizer.
3. *Mesh nebulizers* can be divided into two categories: (1) Active and (2) passive (static). Although active mesh nebulizers have a vibrating mesh with multiple apertures, passive (static) mesh nebulizers use a vibrating horn with piezoelectric crystal to generate aerosols **(Fig. 4)**.

- Optimal nebulizer position is proximal before the Y-piece adapter, which showed a two-fold higher lung dose than positions next to the ventilator.
- Various nebulized drugs used in ICU are:
  - Bronchodilators like salbutamol and ipratropium bromide
  - Antibiotics such as tobramycin and colistin
  - Hypertonic saline or N-acetyl cysteine for loosening of secretions

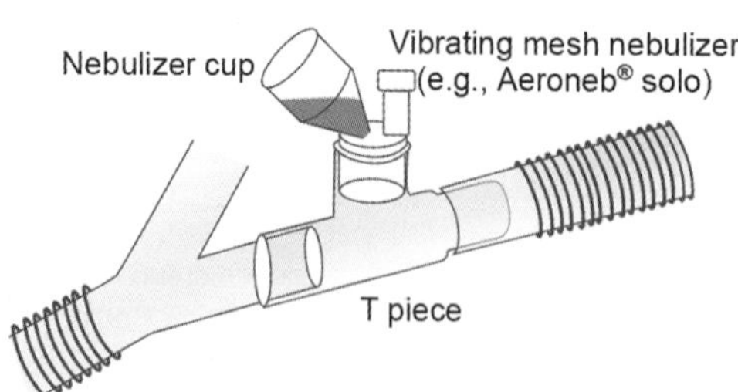

Fig. 4: Vibrating mesh nebulizer.

CHEST PHYSIOTHERAPY

- Manual techniques such as percussion and vibration are to drain the secretions by loosening the mucus in the lung. Postural drainage method helps to drain secretions based on the lobe involved **(Figs. 5A and B)**.
- Monitoring of vitals or any sign of discomfort is mandatory during the procedure as it can result in a drop in saturation and lead to respiratory distress. Preprocedure hand wash by the healthcare provider and postprocedure oral care for the patient should be done.
- Percussion involves striking the chest wall in a rhythmic fashion with cupped hands over the chest segment that needs to be drained. The wrist movement is accordingly managed so as to make the procedure painless.
- Vibration is the application of manual compression or tremors with the use of vibrating devices to the chest wall during the exhalation phase of respiration.
- Physiotherapy is contraindicated in cases of acute cardiac illnesses, pneumothorax, chest wall diseases, or pulmonary hemorrhage.
- Breathing exercises like pursed lip breathing are also a part of physiotherapy, which help in strengthening the respiratory muscles, mostly the diaphragm, and reduce the work of breathing, especially in patients with chronic obstructive pulmonary disease (COPD).

CARE OF PATIENT WITH CHEST DRAINAGE SYSTEMS

- Normally, intrapleural pressure is negative, and <10 mL of pleural fluid is present in the intrapleural space between the parietal and visceral pleura

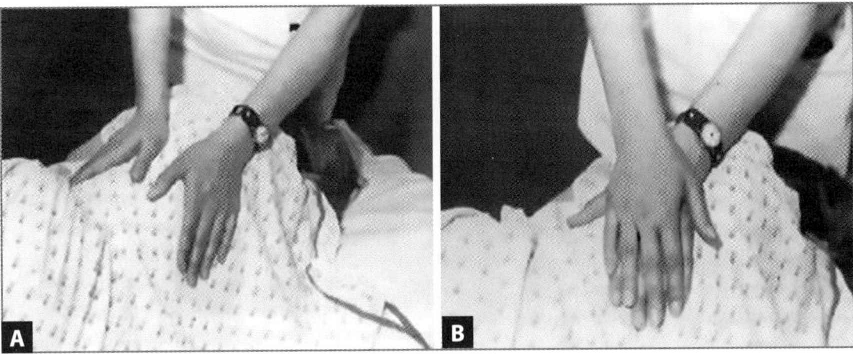

Figs. 5A and B: Percussion and vibration methods of chest physiotherapy.

for lubrication. Accumulation of air or fluid into this space creates a positive pressure that requires drainage based on the clinical condition to promote lung expansion, maintain normal intrathoracic pressure, and facilitate normal respiratory mechanics.

- *Indications:*
  - Pneumothorax
  - Complicated pleural effusions or empyema
  - Postsurgery
  - Hemothorax
  - Malignant effusions planned for pleurodesis
- Chest tubes are used for this purpose and the location determines the type of drain expected, for example, it is placed higher in case of a pneumothorax, and to drain fluid it is placed in dependent areas. In cases of loculated collections, the pocket should be localized with the help of imaging for placement of the tube. Ideal site is the 5th intercostal space midaxillary line called the "safe triangle".
- The chest tube is then attached to an underwater seal system, which can be a single chamber or three chambers. For single-chamber systems, water needs to be filled to the required level as indicated **(Figs. 6A and B)**.
- After the tube is inserted, vitals are monitored, assessed for pain, and auscultated for lung sounds. The drain output needs to be measured carefully at the end of every shift and documented.
- Insertion site needs to be checked daily and dressing change should be done in case it gets soiled. The chest tube connection and patency need to be checked in every shift, and care should be taken to prevent dislodgement during any movement.
- Removal should be done as per the doctors' advice usually after the lung has fully expanded on chest-X ray and drain output has come to <100 mL. After explaining the procedure in detail, analgesia should be given, sutures should be removed, and the tube should be removed after the patient takes a deep breath in the state of full inspiration followed by appropriate dressing.

RELEVANCE OF IMAGING

Relevance of imaging is given as follows:

- *Chest X-ray:*
  - It is the most commonly performed radiological investigation in ICUs and hospitals. It can be used to diagnose various lung conditions and to

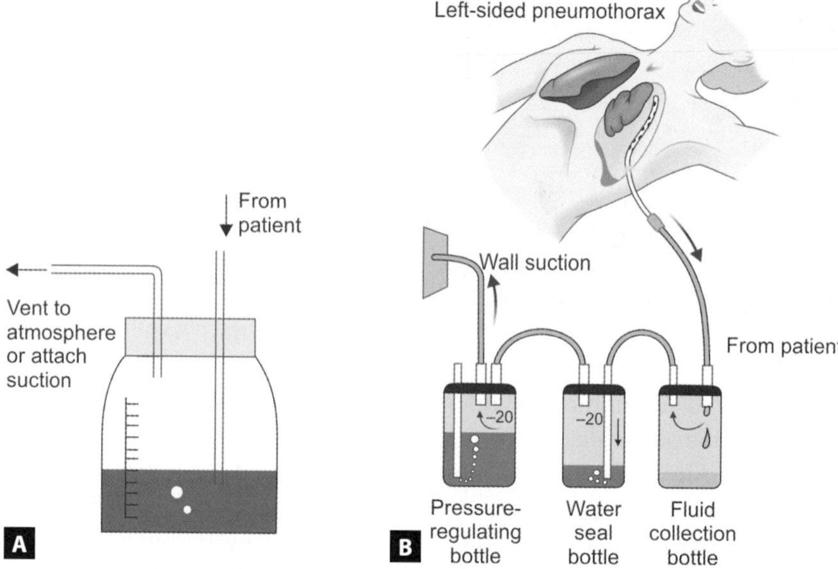

Figs. 6A and B: Single and triple chamber chest drainage systems.

monitor post placement of central lines, intercostal drainage systems (ICDs), and endotracheal tube position.
- In the ICU, mostly anteroposterior (AP) views are obtained as it is more feasible since sick patients cannot be mobilized. Ideal view recommended is posteroanterior view.
- In the AP view, the heart appears enlarged, and mediastinal widening can be noted.

- *Ultrasonography (USG):*
  - It is a quick bedside, noninvasive, and radiation-free imaging modality to evaluate the lung and pleura **(Fig. 7)**.
  - It is mainly used for procedures like pleural fluid aspiration, lung or pleural biopsies, and emergencies like pneumothorax postintervention.

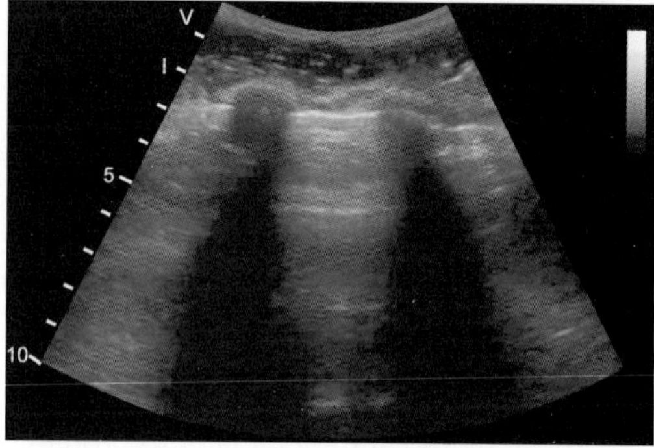

Fig. 7: Ultrasound of normal lung and pleura.

- *Computed tomography (CT) scans:*
  - It uses X-ray beams to take internal images of the heart, lungs, ribs, lymph nodes, and airways, and with the help of contrast, blood vessels can be visualized too **(Fig. 8)**.

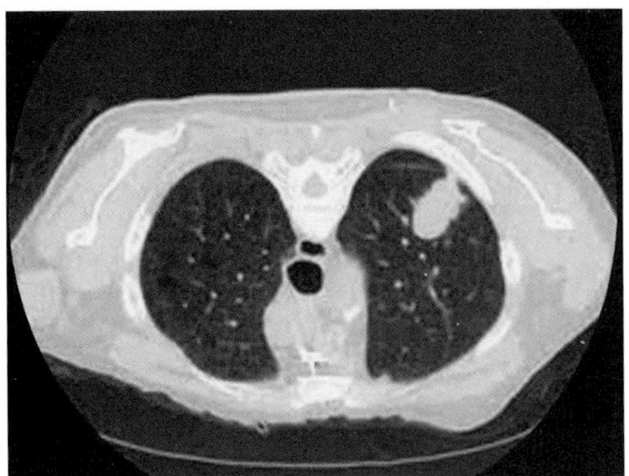

Fig. 8: Computed tomography (CT) scan of lungs showing a mass.

- It can be used to detect pulmonary nodules, mass lesions, pulmonary embolisms, or complicated pneumonias.

CONCLUSION

Nursing care of a patient suffering from a pulmonary disease depends on care of the airway, oxygenation (both have been dealt with in Chapter 20) and providing proper nebulization, chest physiotherapy, etc. The nurses should also be aware of the imaging technics and the approach to a patient in respiratory distress.

FURTHER READING

1. Chatburn R. Understanding mechanical ventilators. Expert Rev Respir Med. 2010;4(6):809-19.
2. Hellyer TP, Ewan V, Wilson P, Simpson AJ. The Intensive Care Society recommended bundle of interventions for the prevention of ventilator-associated pneumonia. J Intensive Care Soc. 2016;17(3):238-43.
3. Kiefer T. Chest Drains in Clinical Practice. Cham: Springer; 2017.
4. Lutfi MF. The physiological basis and clinical significance of lung volume measurements. Multidiscip Respir Med. 2017;12:3.
5. McCool FD, Rosen MJ. Nonpharmacologic airway clearance therapies: ACCP evidence-based clinical practice guidelines. Chest. 2006;129(1 Suppl):250S-9S.
6. O'Driscoll BR, Howard LS, Earis J, Mak V; British Thoracic Society Emergency Oxygen Guideline Group; BTS Emergency Oxygen Guideline Development Group. BTS guideline for oxygen use in adults in healthcare and emergency settings. Thorax. 2017;72(Suppl 1):ii1-ii90.
7. Rochwerg B, Brochard L, Elliott MW, Hess D, Hill NS, Nava S, et al. Official ERS/ATS clinical practice guidelines: Noninvasive ventilation for acute respiratory failure. Eur Respir J Aug. 2017;50(2):1602426.

CHAPTER

16 Emergencies in Gastroenterology

Reshu Gupta Khanikar, Rakhee Baruah

INTRODUCTION

Emergencies in gastroenterology may include conditions such as gastrointestinal (GI) bleeding, bowel obstruction, severe abdominal pain, pancreatitis, liver failure, and acute diarrhea or vomiting leading to dehydration. Nurses play a crucial role in assessing patients, monitoring vital signs, administering medications, providing comfort measures, and assisting with the procedures such as endoscopy or colonoscopy in emergency situations. They also collaborate closely with the medical team to ensure timely and appropriate interventions to stabilize patients and optimize outcomes.

The emergencies in gastroenterology can be listed as following:

- Acute pancreatitis
- Gastrointestinal bleeding
- Bowel obstruction
- Acute liver failure (ALF)
- Perforated peptic ulcer (or any other hollow viscus perforation)
- Diverticulitis
- Ischemic colitis
- Acute cholecystitis
- Acute appendicitis
- Intestinal ischemia

These conditions often require urgent medical attention and may necessitate interventions such as endoscopy, surgery, or supportive care in hospital setting.

ACUTE PANCREATITIS

- *Definition:* Acute pancreatitis (AP) is an inflammatory condition of the pancreas characterized by sudden onset upper abdominal pain.
- *Causes:* The most common causes include gallstones and excessive alcohol consumption. Other causes include certain medications, trauma, infections, high blood calcium levels, high lipid levels, and genetic factors.
- *Symptoms:* Symptoms include severe abdominal pain that may radiate to the back, nausea, vomiting, fever, and abdominal tenderness.
- *Diagnosis:* Diagnosis is typically made through a combination of medical history, physical examination, blood tests (amylase and lipase levels), and imaging studies such as ultrasound, CT scan, or MRI.
- *Complications:* AP can lead to serious complications such as pancreatic necrosis, pseudocysts, abscesses, organ failure, and systemic inflammation response syndrome (SIRS).
- *Treatment:* Treatment often involves hospitalization, pain management, intravenous fluids, and supportive care. In severe cases, interventions such as endoscopic retrograde cholangiopancreatography (ERCP), surgery, or drainage procedures may be necessary **(Flowchart 1)**.

Flowchart 1: Algorithm for the medical management of acute pancreatitis (AP).

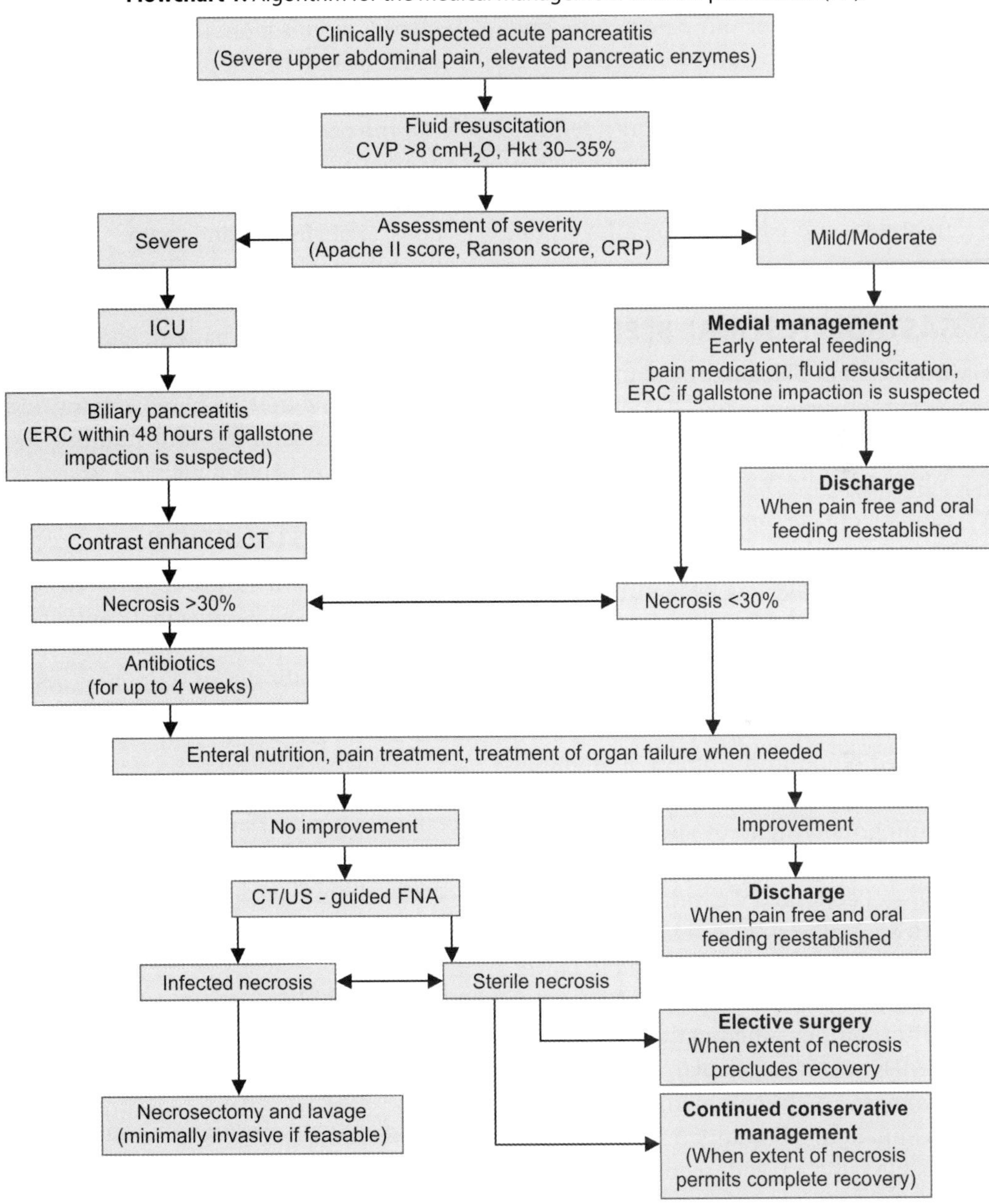

(CRP: C-reactive protein; CVP: central venous pressure; ERC: endoscopic retrograde cholangiography; FNA: fine needle aspiration; ICU: intensive care unit; US: ultrasound)

- *Prevention:* Prevention strategies include maintaining a healthy diet, limiting alcohol consumption, managing conditions such as gallstones, and avoiding certain medications known to trigger pancreatitis.

- *Prognosis:* Prognosis varies depending on the severity of the pancreatitis and any associated complications. Mild cases typically resolve with supportive care, while severe cases may require intensive treatment and have a higher risk of mortality. Prompt diagnosis and treatment are essential for a favorable outcome.

GASTROINTESTINAL BLEEDING

Gastrointestinal bleeding refers to bleeding that occurs anywhere in the GI tract, from the esophagus to the rectum.

It is categorized into two—upper and lower:

1. Upper GI bleed—any bleeding above the ligament of Treitz
2. Lower GI bleed—any bleed below the ligament of Treitz

- *Symptoms:* Hematemesis (vomiting blood), melena (black, tarry stools), hematochezia (bright red or maroon-colored blood in the stool), abdominal pain or discomfort, weakness, dizziness, fainting, and signs of shock in severe cases.
- *Causes:* Peptic ulcers, gastritis, esophageal varices, Mallory-Weiss tears, angiodysplasia, diverticulosis, inflammatory bowel disease, malignancies, arteriovenous malformations, medications (such as NSAIDs or anticoagulants).
- *Diagnosis:* Clinical history, physical examination, laboratory tests (hemoglobin, hematocrit), endoscopic procedures (esophagogastroduodenoscopy, colonoscopy), imaging studies (CT angiography, nuclear medicine scans) **(Flowchart 2)**.
- *Treatment:* Management depends on the cause and severity of bleeding. Interventions may include supportive care, blood transfusions, intravenous fluids, proton pump inhibitors (for peptic ulcers), endoscopic therapies (such as cauterization or clipping), angiographic embolization, or surgery **(Flowchart 3)**.
- *Complications:* Hemorrhagic shock, anemia, rebleeding, need for repeat interventions, transfusion-related complications, organ failure, and death.

Prompt evaluation and management are crucial to identify the source of bleeding, stabilize the patient, and prevent complications. Treatment strategies aim to control bleeding, restore blood volume and hemodynamic stability, and address the underlying cause of bleeding.

BOWEL OBSTRUCTION

Bowel obstruction is a condition where the normal passage of intestinal contents is blocked.

- *Symptoms:* Abdominal pain, cramping, bloating, constipation, vomiting, inability to pass gas or stool.
- *Causes:* Adhesions from surgery, hernias, tumors, impacted feces, volvulus (twisting of the intestine), and intussusception (telescoping of the intestine).
- *Diagnosis:* Physical examination, imaging tests (X-ray, CT scan), and blood tests **(Flowchart 4)**.
- *Treatment:* NPO (nothing by mouth), IV fluids, nasogastric suction, and surgery in severe cases
- *Complications:* Perforation, sepsis, electrolyte imbalances, and bowel ischemia. Prompt medical attention is crucial for proper diagnosis and management.

ACUTE LIVER FAILURE

- *Definition:* ALF is defined as severe acute liver injury for fewer than 26 weeks duration with encephalopathy and

Flowchart 2: Algorithm for investigation of GI bleed.

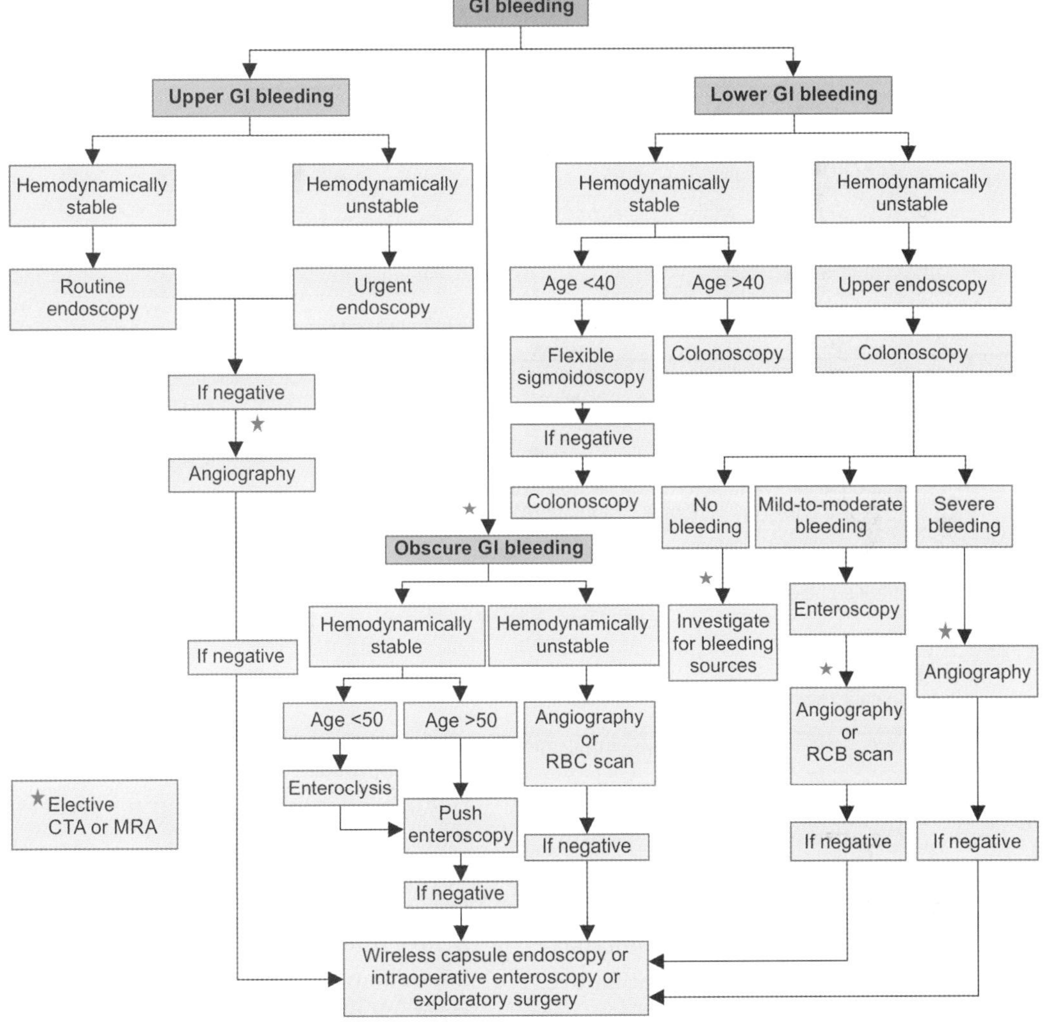

(GI: gastrointestinal; RBC: red blood cell)

impaired synthetic function (INR >1.5) in a patient without cirrhosis or preexisting liver disease.

- *Causes:* Hepatotoxicity, acute viral hepatitis, autoimmune hepatitis, acute steatosis syndromes, toxins, vascular, metabolic, malignancy, and miscellaneous
- *Symptoms:* Jaundice, ascites, peripheral edema, encephalopathy (confusion, flapping tremor, and constructional apraxia); cerebral edema, coagulopathy, upper gastrointestinal bleeding, acute kidney injury, sepsis, and previously normal liver function
- *Diagnosis:* CBC, serology (HBsAg, IGM anti-HBc, IGM anti-HEV, IGM anti-HAV, anti-HCV, anti-HDV, anti-HIV), copper studies, autoimmune markers, and USG
- *Treatment:* Measures to decrease ICP (elevate head end 30–45°,

Flowchart 3: Management of upper GI bleed.

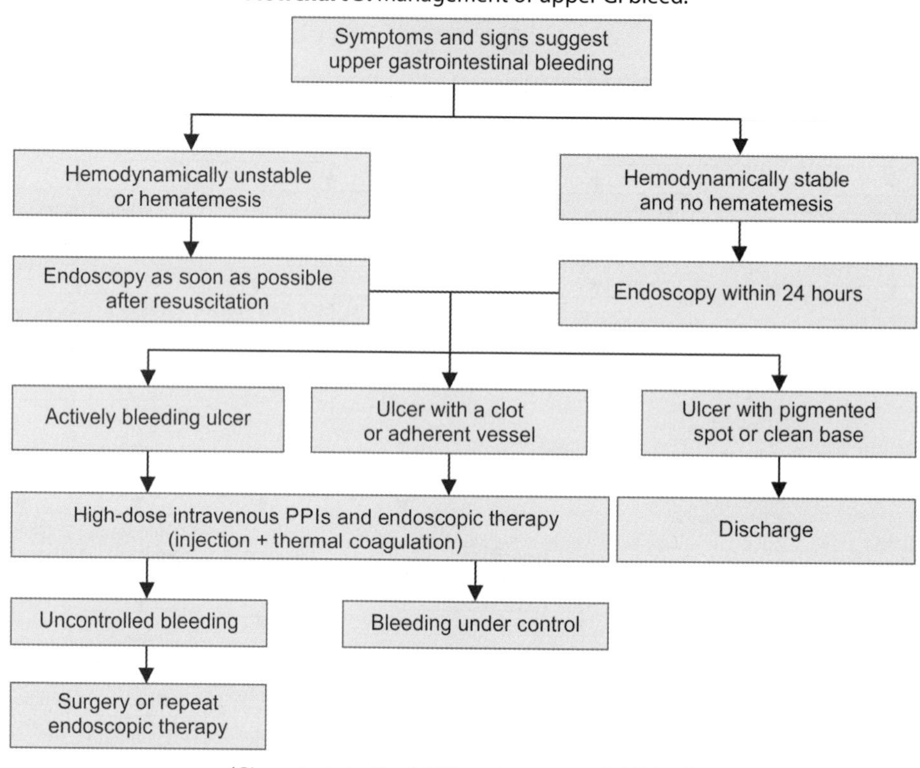

(GI: gastrointestinal: PPI: proton pump inhibitor)

avoid hyperthermia, avoid vigorous endotracheal suction, and sedation). Correct fluid and electrolytes status, maintain adequate nutrition, sepsis control with prophylactic antibiotics and antifungals, IHD/CRRT in renal failure, fresh frozen plasma (FFP), platelet transfusion in select patient in bleeding, seizure prophylaxis.

PERFORATED PEPTIC ULCER

Perforated peptic ulcer is a serious complication of peptic ulcer disease where there is a hole in the stomach or duodenal lining.

- *Symptoms:* Sudden, severe abdominal pain, often radiating to the back or shoulders, abdominal tenderness, rigidity, guarding, rebound tenderness, nausea, vomiting, and fever
- *Causes:* Chronic peptic ulcer disease (most commonly caused by *Helicobacter pylori* infection or nonsteroidal anti-inflammatory drugs), which weakens the stomach or duodenal lining, leading to perforation.
- *Diagnosis:* Clinical presentation, abdominal X-ray (may show air under the diaphragm), CT scan, and blood tests (elevated white blood cell count) **(Flowchart 5)**.
- *Treatment:* Immediate surgical intervention is usually necessary to repair the perforation, remove any infected tissue, and control peritonitis. Antibiotics and intravenous fluids are administered to treat infection and restore fluid balance.

Flowchart 4: Flow diagram for diagnostic assessment of bowel obstruction.

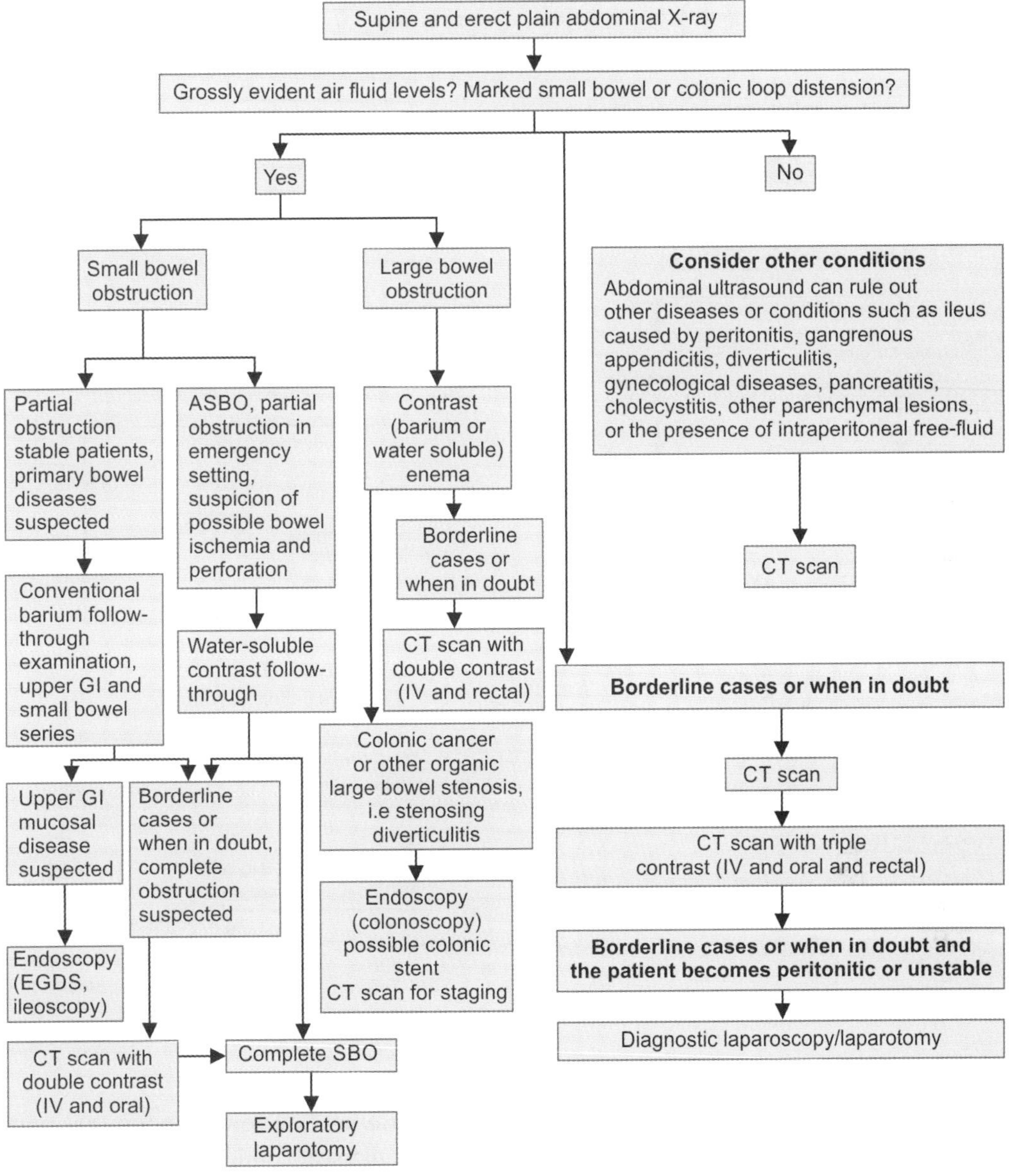

(ASBO: adhesive small bowel obstruction; EGDS: esophagogastroduodenoscopy; GI: gastrointestinal; IV: intravenous; SBO: small bowel obstruction)

Figure 1 shows the determinants of the outcomes of patients with perforated peptic ulcer.

- *Complications:* Peritonitis (inflammation of the abdominal cavity), sepsis, abscess formation, and organ failure

Flowchart 5: Algorithm of suggested selective treatment of a duodenal ulcer that has perforated.

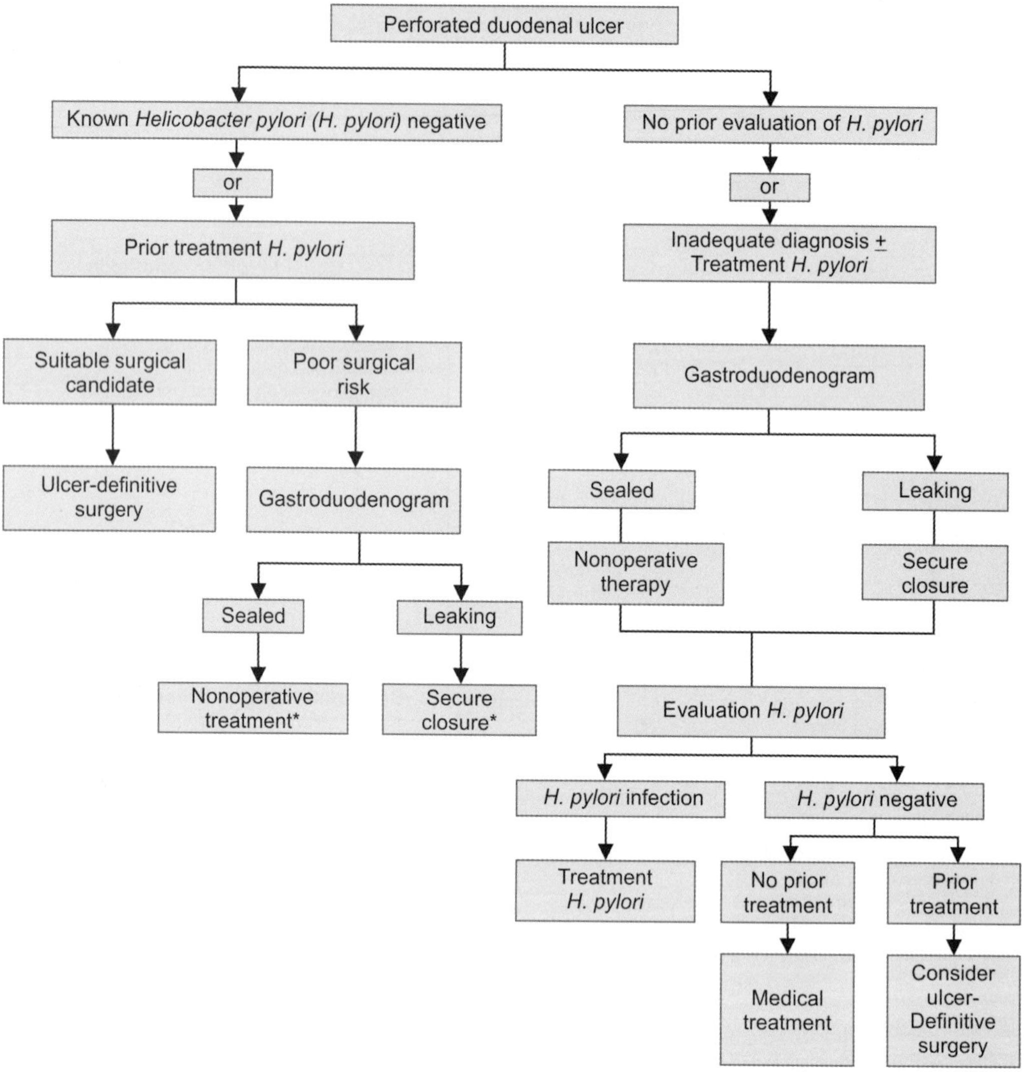

Perforated duodenal ulcer

Known *Helicobacter pylori (H. pylori)* negative

or

Prior treatment *H. pylori*

Suitable surgical candidate

Ulcer-definitive surgery

Poor surgical risk

Gastroduodenogram

Sealed

Nonoperative treatment*

Leaking

Secure closure*

No prior evaluation of *H. pylori*

or

Inadequate diagnosis ± Treatment *H. pylori*

Gastroduodenogram

Sealed

Nonoperative therapy

Leaking

Secure closure

Evaluation *H. pylori*

H. pylori infection

Treatment *H. pylori*

H. pylori negative

No prior treatment

Medical treatment

Prior treatment

Consider ulcer-Definitive surgery

Perforated peptic ulcer requires prompt recognition and surgical management to prevent life-threatening complications.

DIVERTICULITIS

Diverticulitis is inflammation or infection of small pouches that form in the wall of the colon, known as diverticula.

- *Symptoms:* Left lower abdominal pain, fever, nausea, vomiting, change in bowel habits, bloating, constipation, or diarrhea
- *Risk factors:* Aging, a low-fiber diet, obesity, lack of exercise, smoking, and certain medications
- *Diagnosis:* Clinical history, physical examination, blood tests (elevated white

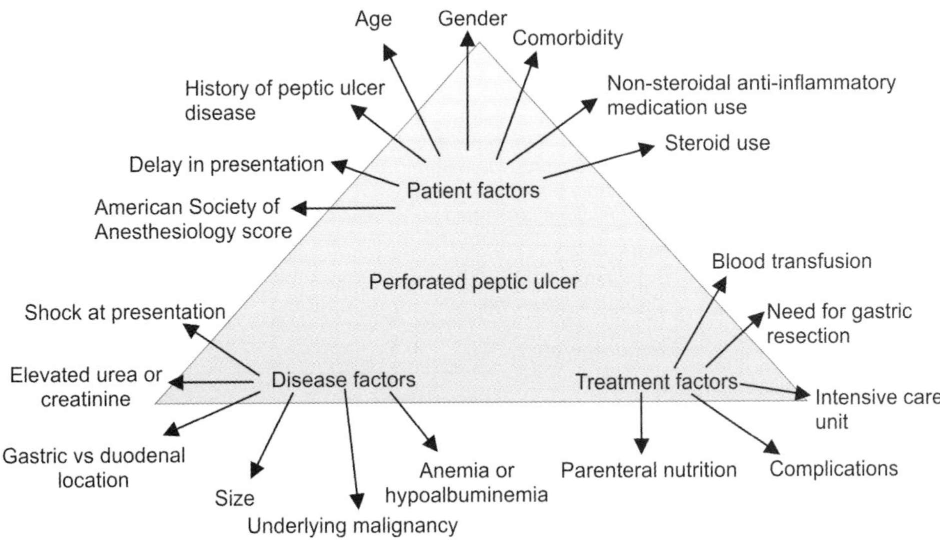

Fig. 1: Determinants of outcomes in patients with perforated peptic ulcer.

blood cell count), imaging studies (CT scan is most accurate), and colonoscopy may be done after the acute episode resolves **(Flowchart 6)**.

- *Treatment:* Mild cases may be managed with rest, clear liquid diet, antibiotics, and pain relievers. Severe cases or complications may require hospitalization, intravenous antibiotics, bowel rest (NPO), and, in some cases, surgery to remove the affected portion of the colon.
- *Complications:* Abscess formation, perforation of the colon, fistula formation (abnormal connections between organs), bowel obstruction, and peritonitis

Preventive measures include maintaining a high-fiber diet, staying hydrated, exercising regularly, and avoiding smoking and excessive use of nonsteroidal anti-inflammatory drugs (NSAIDs).

ISCHEMIC COLITIS

Ischemic colitis (IC) occurs when blood flow to the colon is reduced, leading to damage or injury to the tissue.

- *Symptoms:* Sudden onset of abdominal pain (often on the left side), cramping, tenderness, urgency to defecate, bloody diarrhea (may be bright red or maroon), nausea, vomiting, and fever
- *Risk factors:* Older age, atherosclerosis, cardiovascular disease, diabetes, hypertension, hypercoagulable disorders, vasculitis, and certain medications (e.g., vasoconstrictors, estrogen therapy)
- *Diagnosis:* Clinical presentation, physical examination, blood tests (elevated white blood cell count, elevated lactate), imaging studies (CT angiography is preferred), and colonoscopy (may show areas of ischemia or ulceration)
- *Treatment*: Mild cases may resolve with bowel rest, intravenous fluids, and antibiotics. Severe cases may require hospitalization, supportive care, and sometimes surgery if there is bowel necrosis or perforation **(Flowchart 7)**.
- *Complications*: Bowel infarction, perforation, peritonitis, sepsis, stricture formation, and chronic IC

Flowchart 6: The management flowchart for diverticular disease.

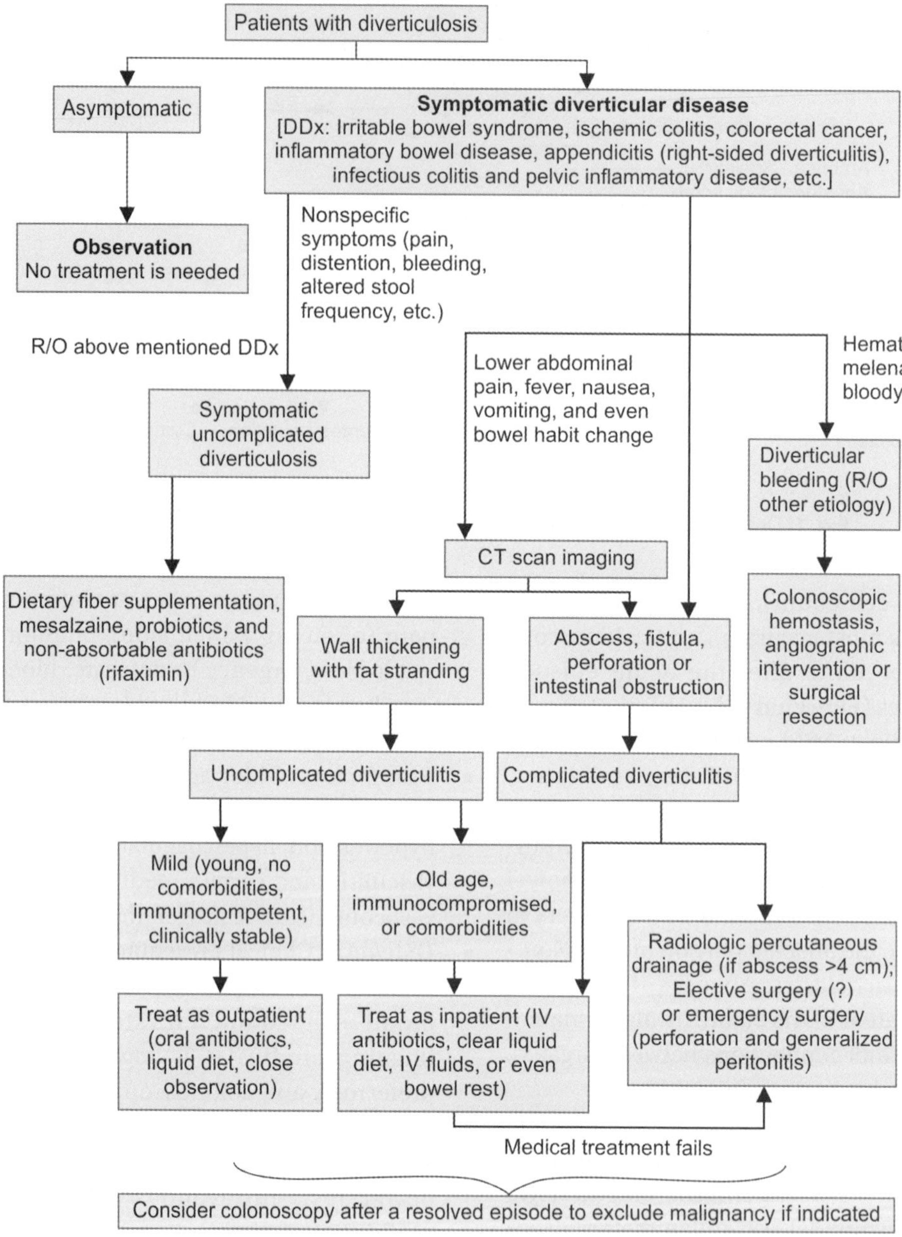

Patients with diverticulosis

Asymptomatic

Observation
No treatment is needed

Symptomatic diverticular disease
[DDx: Irritable bowel syndrome, ischemic colitis, colorectal cancer, inflammatory bowel disease, appendicitis (right-sided diverticulitis), infectious colitis and pelvic inflammatory disease, etc.]

Nonspecific symptoms (pain, distention, bleeding, altered stool frequency, etc.)

R/O above mentioned DDx

Symptomatic uncomplicated diverticulosis

Dietary fiber supplementation, mesalzaine, probiotics, and non-absorbable antibiotics (rifaximin)

Lower abdominal pain, fever, nausea, vomiting, and even bowel habit change

CT scan imaging

Wall thickening with fat stranding

Uncomplicated diverticulitis

Mild (young, no comorbidities, immunocompetent, clinically stable)

Treat as outpatient (oral antibiotics, liquid diet, close observation)

Old age, immunocompromised, or comorbidities

Treat as inpatient (IV antibiotics, clear liquid diet, IV fluids, or even bowel rest)

Abscess, fistula, perforation or intestinal obstruction

Complicated diverticulitis

Radiologic percutaneous drainage (if abscess >4 cm); Elective surgery (?) or emergency surgery (perforation and generalized peritonitis)

Medical treatment fails

Hematochezia, melena, bloody stool

Diverticular bleeding (R/O other etiology)

Colonoscopic hemostasis, angiographic intervention or surgical resection

Consider colonoscopy after a resolved episode to exclude malignancy if indicated

Preventive measures include managing risk factors such as controlling hypertension, diabetes, and hyperlipidemia, quitting smoking, and maintaining a healthy lifestyle. Prompt medical attention is crucial to prevent complications and ensure appropriate management.

Flowchart 7: Algorithm for the treatment of ischemic colitis (IC).

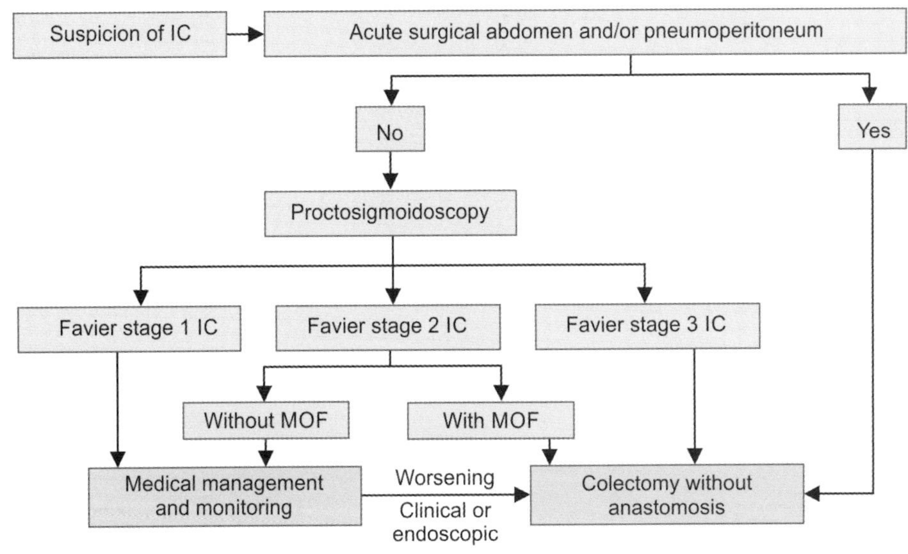

(MOF: multiorgan failure)

ACUTE CHOLECYSTITIS

Acute cholecystitis is inflammation of the gallbladder, usually caused by gallstones blocking the cystic duct.

- *Symptoms:* Severe right upper quadrant abdominal pain, fever, nausea, vomiting, and tenderness over the gallbladder
- *Risk factors:* Gallstones, obesity, rapid weight loss, female gender, and older age
- *Diagnosis:* Clinical history, physical examination, ultrasound, and blood tests (e.g., elevated white blood cell count, liver enzymes)
- *Treatment:* NPO (nothing by mouth), IV fluids, antibiotics, pain management, and cholecystectomy (surgical removal of the gallbladder) in severe cases
- *Complications:* Gangrene or perforation of the gallbladder, abscess formation, and bile duct obstruction

Timely diagnosis and intervention are essential to prevent complications and resolve symptoms.

ACUTE APPENDICITIS

Acute appendicitis is inflammation of the appendix, usually caused by obstruction of the appendiceal lumen.

- *Symptoms:* Right lower quadrant abdominal pain (McBurney's point), which starts as vague discomfort and progresses to severe, sharp pain, nausea, vomiting, anorexia, low-grade fever, rebound tenderness, and guarding.
- *Diagnosis:* Clinical history, physical examination (including the McBurney's point tenderness test), blood tests (elevated white blood cell count), and imaging studies (ultrasound or CT scan).
- *Treatment:* Surgical removal of the appendix (appendectomy) is the standard treatment. In uncomplicated cases, laparoscopic surgery is often preferred for its shorter recovery time and lower complication rates.
- *Complications:* Perforation of the appendix leading to peritonitis, abscess

TABLE 1: Emergencies in gastroenterology with their diagnosis and management.

Sl. No.	*Condition*	*Features*	*Causes*	*Diagnosis*	*Treatment*
1	Acute pancreatitis	Severe abdominal pain that may radiate to the back, nausea, vomiting, fever, and abdominal tenderness	Gallstones, excessive alcohol consumption. Other causes include certain medications, trauma, infections, high blood calcium levels, high lipid levels, and genetic factors	Medical history, physical examination, blood tests (amylase and lipase levels), and imaging studies such as ultrasound, CT scan, or MRI	Hospitalization, pain management, intravenous fluids, and supportive care. In severe cases, interventions such as endoscopic retrograde cholangiopancreatography (ERCP), surgery, or drainage procedures may be necessary
2	Upper GI bleeding	Shock, orthostatic hypotension, profuse active bleeding, hematocrit decrease by more than 10%	Peptic ulcer disease, drug-associated, esophagitis, Mallory–Weiss tear, gastric/esophageal varices, stress ulceration, gastritis/gastric erosions; hemorrhagic gastritis, *tumors*: Gastric; esophageal, Cameron ulcers within hiatus hernia, swallowed blood from nasal bleeding	CBC, UGI endoscopy, USG	• *Nonvariceal bleed*: Injection therapy (adrenaline 1:10,000 to 1:20,000), mechanical therapy with hemostatic clip, thermal therapy (heater and bipolar probe), argon plasma coagulation, Coagrasper • *Variceal bleed*: Injection therapy (glue for gastric varix) and mechanical therapy, e.g., EVL
3	Lower GI bleeding	Abdominal pain, painless bleeding, bloody diarrhea, rectal pain, constipation	• Small bowel diverticular disease, intussusception • Mesenteric infarction • Large n bowel (colonic diverticular disease, arteriovenous malformations, colitis)	CBC, digital rectal examination to rule out anorectal pathology, colonoscopy, USG, angiography, radionuclide scintigraphy	Endoscopic treatment modalities (injection adrenaline 1:10,000 to 1:20,000), contact or noncontact thermal coagulation, mechanical devices such as metallic clips and band ligation, surgery for life-threatening bleeding not responding to hemostatic techniques

Contd...

Contd…

Sl. No.	Condition	Features	Causes	Diagnosis	Treatment
4	Bowel obstruction	Abdominal pain, cramping, bloating, constipation, vomiting, inability to pass gas or stool	Adhesions from surgery, hernias, tumors, impacted feces, volvulus (twisting of the intestine), intussusception (telescoping of the intestine)	Physical examination, imaging tests (X-ray, CT scan), blood tests	NPO (nothing by mouth), IV fluids, nasogastric suction, surgery in severe cases
5	Perforated peptic ulcer	Sudden, severe abdominal pain, often radiating to the back or shoulders, abdominal tenderness, rigidity, guarding, rebound tenderness, nausea, vomiting, fever	Chronic peptic ulcer disease (most commonly caused by *Helicobacter pylori* infection or nonsteroidal anti-inflammatory drugs), which weakens the stomach or duodenal lining, leading to perforation	Clinical presentation, abdominal X-ray (may show air under the diaphragm), CT scan, blood tests (elevated white blood cell count)	• Immediate surgical intervention is usually necessary to repair the perforation, remove any infected tissue, and control peritonitis • Antibiotics and intravenous fluids are administered to treat infection and restore fluid balance
6	Acute liver failure	Jaundice, ascites, peripheral edema, encephalopathy (confusion, flapping tremor, constructional apraxia); cerebral edema, coagulo-pathy, upper GI bleeding, AKI, sepsis, previously normal LFT	Hepatotoxicity, acute viral hepatitis, autoimmune hepatitis, acute steatosis syndromes, toxins, vascular, metabolic, malignancy, miscellaneous	CBC, serology (HBsAg, IGM anti-HBc, IGM anti-HEV, IGM anti-HAV, anti-HCV, anti-HDV, anti-HIV), copper studies, autoimmune markers, USG	Measures to decrease ICP (elevate head end 30–45°, avoid hyperthermia, avoid vigorous endotracheal suction, sedation), correct fluid and electrolytes status, maintain adequate nutrition, sepsis control with prophylactic antibiotics and antifungals, IHD/CRRT in renal failure, FFP, platelet transfusion in select patient in bleeding, seizure prophylaxis

Contd…

Contd...

Sl. No.	*Condition*	*Features*	*Causes*	*Diagnosis*	*Treatment*
7	Diverticulitis	Left lower abdominal pain, constipation, or diarrhea, bloating, nausea, vomiting	Smoking, obesity, lack of exercises, low-fiber diet, aging, certain medications	• History and physical examination, routine blood tests, imaging studies (CT scan most accurate) • Colonoscopy after resolution of acute episode	• Mild—rest, IVF, antibiotics, pain relievers • Severe—IV antibiotics, NPO, surgery in select cases to remove affected colon
8	Ischemic colitis	Cramping, tenderness, urgency to defecate, sudden onset left-sided abdominal pain, bloody diarrhea, fever	Atherosclerosis, hypercoagulable disorder, vasculitis, old age, certain medications (vasoconstrictors, estrogen therapy)	History and physical examination, routine blood tests (elevated WBC, elevated lactates), CT angiography, colonoscopy	• Mild cases—bowel rest, intravenous fluids, and antibiotics • Severe cases—hospitalization, supportive care, and sometimes surgery if there is bowel necrosis or perforation
9	Intestinal ischemia	Severe abdominal pain, often out of proportion to physical findings, cramping, tenderness, nausea, vomiting, diarrhea (which may be bloody), rectal bleeding, fever, signs of shock in severe cases	Atherosclerosis, embolism (e.g., from atrial fibrillation or thrombus), arterial thrombosis, hypotension, vasculitis, hypercoagulable states, cardiac diseases	Clinical suspicion based on symptoms, physical examination, blood tests (elevated lactate, metabolic acidosis), imaging studies (CT angiography is preferred, but angiography may be needed for definitive diagnosis)	Immediate restoration of blood flow is essential. This may involve fluid resuscitation, vasopressors to support blood pressure, anticoagulation, thrombolysis or embolectomy for arterial occlusions, and surgery (revascularization or bowel resection) in severe cases

(AKI: acute kidney injury; CBC: complete blood count; CRRT: continuous renal replacement therapy; EVL: endoscopic variceal ligation; FFP: fresh frozen plasma; GI: gastrointestinal; IHD: intermittent hemodialysis; LFT: liver function test; UGI: upper gastrointestinal; USG: ultrasound)

formation, sepsis, bowel obstruction, and adhesions

- *Management:* Antibiotics may be given before surgery if perforation or abscess is suspected, but surgery remains the definitive treatment. In cases of appendiceal abscess or localized perforation, percutaneous drainage may be attempted before surgery.

Early recognition and prompt surgical intervention are crucial to prevent complications such as perforation and peritonitis.

INTESTINAL ISCHEMIA

Intestinal ischemia occurs when blood flow to the intestines is compromised, leading to tissue damage and potentially life-threatening complications.

- *Symptoms:* Severe abdominal pain, often out of proportion to physical findings, cramping, tenderness, nausea, vomiting, diarrhea (which may be bloody), rectal bleeding, fever, and signs of shock in severe cases
- *Types:* Acute mesenteric ischemia (sudden decrease in blood flow), chronic mesenteric ischemia (gradual decrease in blood flow due to atherosclerosis), and nonocclusive mesenteric ischemia (blood flow reduction without vessel occlusion)
- *Risk factors:* Atherosclerosis, embolism (e.g., from atrial fibrillation or thrombus), arterial thrombosis, hypotension, vasculitis, hypercoagulable states, and cardiac diseases
- *Diagnosis:* Clinical suspicion based on symptoms, physical examination, blood tests (elevated lactate, metabolic acidosis), and imaging studies (CT angiography is preferred, but angiography may be needed for definitive diagnosis)
- *Treatment:* Immediate restoration of blood flow is essential. This may involve fluid resuscitation, vasopressors to support blood pressure, anticoagulation, thrombolysis or embolectomy for arterial occlusions, and surgery (revascularization or bowel resection) in severe cases.
- *Complications:* Bowel infarction, perforation, peritonitis, sepsis, and multiorgan failure.

Early diagnosis and intervention are crucial to improve outcomes and reduce morbidity and mortality associated with intestinal ischemia.

The common emergencies in gastroenterology are summarized in **Table 1**.

FURTHER READIN

1. Barkun A, Bardou M, Marshall JK; Nonvariceal Upper GI Bleeding Consensus Conference Group. Consensus recommendations for managing patients with nonvariceal upper gastrointestinal bleeding. Ann Intern Med. 2003;139:843-57.
2. Chen YC, Tseng CW, Wu CC, Hsieh YH, Tseng KC, Hung TS. (2016). Colonic diverticular disease and diverticulitis: Symptoms, treatment options and long-term health outcomes. [online] Available from https://novapublishers.com/wp-content/uploads/2019/01/Colonic-Diverticular-Disease-and-Diverticulitis.pdf [Last accessed February, 2025].
3. Chung KT, Shelat VG. Perforated peptic ulcer - an update. World J Gastrointest Surg. 2017;9(1):1-12.
4. Mayerle J, Simon P, Lerch MM. Medical treatment of acute pancreatitis. Gastroenterol Clin N Am. 2005;33(4):855-69, viii.
5. Moszkowicz D, Mariani A, Trésallet C, Menegaux F. Ischemic colitis: The ABCs of diagnosis and surgical management. J Visc Surg. 2013 Feb;150(1):19-28.
6. O'Grady JG, Schalm SW, Williams R. Acute liver failure: redefining the syndromes. Lancet. 1993;342(8866):273-5.

CHAPTER 17

Care of a Patient Undergoing Major Surgery

Vivek Dave, Anish Joshi

INTRODUCTION

Nurses are one of the pillars of effective patient care in the intensive care unit (ICU). They have a variety of roles and functions associated with patient's surgical management. Nurses provide care for a patient before, during, and after surgery. It is collectively known as perioperative nursing care. Nursing care plans are very much essential for patients undergoing surgery, as they help in proper optimization of the patients which leads to comprehensive and effective care throughout the perioperative time. Surgical intervention may be needed to diagnose the underlying condition, as a source control, to correct a deformity, to restore a functional process, or to reduce the level of dysfunction. The surgical procedures are sometimes elective or preplanned or, in potentially life-threatening conditions, emergency surgical interventions are to be done.

NURSING PERSPECTIVES ON PATIENTS UNDERGOING SURGERIES

- To evaluate the patient's overall clinical status, identify the risk factors and contraindications for surgery.
- To establish and follow comprehensive perioperative plan for the patient, including preoperative preparation and postoperative care.
- To give emotional and psychological support to the patient posted for surgical intervention.
- To administer preoperative medications as per the prescription including anxiolytics and prophylactic antibiotics.
- To ensure proper informed consent is obtained prior to the surgical procedure.
- To monitor patient's vital signs, including blood pressure, heart rate, and oxygen saturation throughout the perioperative period.
- To assist with positioning the patient appropriately during surgery and provide necessary support and comfort.

Nursing Care during the Preoperative Period

It starts from the consent taking and it ends when the patient is transferred to the operation room. The surgeon explains the pathology, surgical approach, need for amputation, possible functional alterations; explains whether the surgery is urgent or not, the objectives, methods, expected benefits, potential dangers, inconvenience, probabilities of complications, and makes a prognosis to make decision. Preoperative anesthesia assessment is an integral part of preoperative care and the anesthesiologist will assess the patient and explain the entire anesthesia process in detail to the patient. The nurse on duty should be present during the explanations and should be fully aware of the explanations. Nurses are responsible for correct preoperative medications and preoperative preparation.

Personal Antecedents

It is important to know of allergies to medications or other agents, such as antiseptics, foods; in the case of any of them existing, this must be made visible to the patient and in the clinical chart, also, medications being taken (for diseases or through habit), including over-the-counter drugs, many are adjusted before surgery either by surgeon or by anesthetist. It is essential to inquire about the family history of any anesthesia problems or bleeding, in the case of female patient, regarding pregnancy, and also regarding past surgical history and trauma. Uncontrolled blood pressure and sugar levels must have to be optimized before shifting the patient to the operating room.

Informed Consent

It is a legal document that defines the obligations of the parties involved in the act or the procedure. It comes under the responsibility of the nursing staff to check all the documents regarding consent. This document is signed by the relative or the caregiver or the companion who agrees about the said procedure or surgery.

Preparation of Skin and Shaving

Suppressing the bacterial flora is the most important aspect of eliminating one of the sources of surgical infection. This can be achieved by proper bathing and asepsis of the surgical area. The presurgical bath to be done with antiseptic soap, focusing on contaminated areas such as navel, inguinal folds, perineum, and arm pits on previous day and on the day of surgery, including washing of hair with shampoo. If the procedure is in the head, two baths with 4% chlorhexidine solution are recommended. The current trend of cleaning the operative area, consists of making sparse trichotomy, avoiding shaving which may cause lacerations. This is because the lacerations may be the focus for infection. It should be done with an electric razor after testing for the sensitivity, 2 hours before surgery and outside the operative room.

Preoperative Fasting

Proper duration of nil by mouth is important to prevent risk of aspiration after anesthesia. General anesthesia increases the danger of bronchial aspiration when the surgical intervention is an emergency and the fasting time is unknown. Fasting of clear liquids must be 2 hours and from all liquids to normal diet, fasting duration varies from 4 to 8 hours.

Hematic Products

In procedures or surgeries where blood loss is expected, blood bank must be well informed by sending a cross match sample and products must be preserved in advance. The patient's relatives or caregivers must be explained regarding the process of replacement of the blood products as well.

Patency of Venous Line/Catheters

A good quality venous access is to be secured. In a patient where high alert medicines are going on such as potassium chloride, inotropic agents, etc., central venous catheter is supposed to be secured in advance. In conscious and well-cooperative patients, indwelling urinary catheter should be avoided.

Preparation of the Colon

An elective surgery on the colon requires mechanical preparation. The objective is to arrive at the operation table with an empty gastrointestinal tract and free from pathogenic germs. If required, it will be ordered by the treating surgeon for its preparation.

Safety Indicators

It is always essential and necessary from the nursing perspective to verify the patient, the exact surgical procedure and the correct surgical site (e.g., identifying the right or the left leg) to prevent any untoward events.

Education for the Postoperative

The educational interventions have positive effects on knowledge, satisfaction, physical, mental, social aspects, quality of life, and knowledge of self-care practices. It plays an important role in the patient's recovery and these must be taught alongside breathing exercises, passive exercises of upper and lower limbs, changes of position, and early mobilization.

Emotional Preparation

It helps to get rid of negative thought process from the mind of the patient and it must be simultaneously started at the moment the surgical procedure has been planned. For some patients, surgical intervention can lead to anxiety and apprehension throughout the perioperative period, which can also be based on the fear of pain and anesthesia. With proper counseling, it can give proper relief, hope, and inner peace during the entire process. Emotional and psychological support is quite important.

Nursing Care in the Transoperative Period

Prophylactic Antibiotics

The risk of infection depends on the magnitude of the surgery and the host's resistance. It is paramount to make efforts to control the sterile technique, but host and procedural factors make it a problem. The prophylactic antibiotic is selected according to the spectrum, hospital antibiogram, pharmacokinetics, and possible adverse drug reactions keeping in mind. The hospital infection control committee at each hospital formulates its own protocols and methods to carry out the practice. Note that the antibiotic should be administered in such a time that it achieves bactericidal concentration by the time the knife touches the skin.

Patient's Preparation in the Surgical Room

Thorough preparation of the surgical area for the procedure is performed separately to avoid microorganisms in the incision site. Each institute creates its own policies for the antiseptics used, their concentrations, and areas where these are used.

Anesthesia

For the procedure, the patient must be subjected to some type of anesthesia; general, regional, or local. Under general anesthesia, the patient is unconscious throughout the surgical procedure. Local anesthesia is used to anesthetize a small area of the body, while with regional anesthesia the body area is broader. With local and regional anesthesia, the patient is awake during the procedure, probably sedated.

Venous and Arterial Lines

Looking to patient's general condition and comorbidities, in some surgical procedure the patient may require invasive hemodynamic monitoring intraoperatively for effective management. Central venous catheter, invasive arterial line insertion and sometimes pulmonary artery catheter in case of complex cardiac procedures will be required. Generally, once the patient is anesthetized, catheters are inserted after thorough aseptic precautions.

Inadvertent Hypothermia

It is a preventable surgical complication (temperature below 37°C). Hypothermia is associated with the alteration of the metabolism of medications, infection at the surgical site, increased risk of bleeding, paralytic ileus, and postoperative cardiovascular events. The nurse should look for hypothermia particularly in the elderly and after a long surgery.

Nursing Care during the Postoperative Period

It starts as soon as the patient is shifted to the postanesthesia recovery ward and one has to observe for the vitals of the patient closely. The patient has not completely recovered from the anesthesia sometimes and has to be cared by specialized nursing staff and doctors. The patient from this area is either shifted to ward or discharged once they are stable. It is managed by anesthesiologist when there is an emergency or there is a requirement. Simulation should be done to teach any emergencies that can arise in the postoperative period by animated videos, flowcharts, and diagrams. There should be multipara monitor, crash cart for any emergencies including advanced airway equipment, infusion pumps, defibrillator, and an invasive ventilator.

Shifting of the patient from the operation theater out: Anxiety is very common once the patient is out of the anesthesia and detailed hand over has to be given by the operation theater nurse to the recovery area nurse, mentioning comorbidities, allergies, antibiotics and blood products given, type of anesthesia, total intravenous (IV) fluids given, and blood loss if any, and any complications that may have happened inside the operation theater.

CLINICAL IMPORTANCE OF POSTANESTHETIC WARD (BOX 1)

Respiratory System

Airway reflexes may not have been fully developed and these patients are more prone for aspiration. Some patients have an endotracheal or laryngeal mask airway in situ which needs to be removed once the patient is fully awake and out of the anesthesia. The nursing team should be able to identify hypoxemia and be able skilled enough to do adequate suctioning and monitor vital parameters including capnography for such patients. One in five patients are prone to develop pulmonary complications.

Cardiovascular

Cardiovascular depression may be present due to anesthesia effect as well as blood loss in major surgeries. Noninvasive blood pressure monitoring and electrocardiogram (ECG) should be mandatory. Some patients do

BOX 1: Five essential points to remember.

1. Patients should be fully informed about the procedure, postoperative recovery, and discharge to home
2. Psychological and physiological care of preoperative patients is important
3. The special needs of children and patients with a learning disability or mental health issues must be addressed
4. Nursing staff must adhered to the national and local guidelines, assessment tools and hospital policies/protocols established toward patient centric care
5. Patient privacy, dignity, and comfort must be maintained

have invasive lines in situ along with central venous lines which have to be zeroed and care of such lines is of utmost importance.

Nausea and Vomiting in Postoperative Period

One-third of patients do have nausea and vomiting, which may result in an extended stay in the recovery area.

Pain Management

Pharmacological and nonpharmacological methods should be used to give maximum patient comfort. Epidural administration of the drugs and patient controlled anesthesia are few techniques which are considered better over fixed dosages of intravenous analgesics. Side effects of opioid analgesics should be known by the nursing staff to avoid complications such as respiratory depression or motor weakness.

Patients with Special Needs

Pediatric and geriatric patients require specialized care and specific algorithms and protocols have to be followed for these patients. Such patients recover better when they have their relatives by the bedside, which decreases the anxiety and stress of the patient and gives better nursing outcomes.

CONCLUSION

Care during entire perioperative period is a complex process of relationship between the patient and his/her companions with healthcare staff. Therefore, within this context, utmost patient safety must be present in every care provided from the preoperative period to the postoperative period. Hence, the nursing staff must be aware regarding all the details in care so that the passage of patients through this context is as fruitful and beneficial as possible.

CHAPTER 18

Endocrine Emergencies

Gunjan Chanchalani, Seema S Tekwani

INTRODUCTION

The endocrine system is a complex network of glands, which secrete hormones important for regulating metabolism, tissue function, growth and development.

Awareness of the potential endocrine emergencies is important for a critical care nurse. The role of a nurse in managing endocrine emergencies includes identifying the patients at risk, assessing the patient who presents or develops signs and symptoms, implementing treatment modalities to correction and restore normal function, and to take measures to prevent further complications. The majority of endocrine emergencies are related to diabetes, however emergencies related to pituitary, thyroid, and adrenal are also common.

PHYSIOLOGY

The endocrine system consists of the hypothalamus-pituitary axis, thyroid and parathyroids, adrenals, pancreas, and the reproductive organs **(Table 1)**.

TABLE 1: Physiology of endocrine system.

Releasing organ	*Hormone*	*Target tissue*	*Role/function*
Hypothalamus	Thyrotropin-releasing hormone (TRH), gonadotropin-releasing hormone (GnRH), growth hormone-releasing hormone (GHRH), corticotropin-releasing hormone (CRH), somatostatin, and dopamine	Anterior pituitary	TRH, CRH, GHRH, GnRH stimulate the anterior pituitary to release the respective hormones—thyroid-stimulating hormone (TSH), adrenocorticotropin hormone (ACTH), growth hormone (GH), follicle-stimulating hormone (FSH), and luteinizing hormone (LH). Somatostatin inhibits release of GH and TSH. Dopamine inhibits release of prolactin
	Oxytocin and vasopressin	Stored in posterior pituitary	Stored in posterior pituitary
Anterior pituitary	TSH	Thyroid gland	Stimulates the thyroid gland to release the thyroid hormones
	GH	All body tissues	Stimulates growth of all tissues, increases protein synthesis
	ACTH	Adrenal cortex	Stimulates secretion of the glucocorticoids

Contd...

Contd…

Releasing organ	*Hormone*	*Target tissue*	*Role/function*
	Prolactin	Mammary glands and gonads	Stimulates mammary gland growth and milk production
	FSH	Ovaries, testes	In females, stimulates growth and development of follicles in the ovary and secretion of estrogens. In males, important for spermatogenesis
	LH	Ovaries, testes	In females, triggers ovulation and stimulates the secretion of progesterone by the corpus luteum. In males, stimulates testosterone secretion
Posterior pituitary	Antidiuretic hormone (ADH) or vasopressin	Vascular smooth muscle	Causes vasoconstriction and increases the blood pressure
		Renal tubules	Promotes reabsorption of water
	Oxytocin	Mammary glands, uterus	Stimulates milk ejection from breast. Stimulates uterine contraction during labor
Pineal gland	Melatonin	Hypothalamus	Maintains circadian rhythm
Thyroid	Triiodothyronine T3	All body tissues	Regulates the metabolism of the body cells
	Thyroxine T4	All body tissues	Inactive form—precursor of T3
Parathyroid	Parathyroid hormone	Bone and kidney	Regulates the calcium and phosphate levels in the body
Pancreas	Insulin—from β cells	All body tissues	Glucose metabolism—improves glucose utilization by the tissue and decreases blood sugar levels
	Glucagon—from α cells	All body tissues	Increases blood glucose levels
Adrenal cortex	Glucocorticoids/cortisol	All body tissues	Maintains blood pressure (BP), suppresses the immune system
	Mineralocorticoids/ aldosterone	Kidney	Regulates fluid, sodium, and potassium balance
	Adrenal androgens—dehydroepiandrosterone (DHEA) and DHEA sulfate	Genital	Androgenic properties
Adrenal medulla	Epinephrine	α and β adrenergic receptors	Responses related to flight and fright – tachycardia, increased stroke volume, dilates pupils, constricts blood vessels, relaxes bronchial smooth muscle, hyperglycemia
	Norepinephrine	α and β adrenergic receptors	Same as epinephrine

INITIAL EVALUATION AND MANAGEMENT OF A PATIENT PRESENTING WITH ENDOCRINE EMERGENCY

Most patients with endocrine emergencies present with fatigue, weakness, mental status changes, and polyuria and polydipsia.

Care begins with stabilization of airway, breathing, and circulation (ABC), and neurological assessment. It is important to look for the precipitating factor and should be treated accordingly. Specific treatment should be directed as per the diagnosis.

Specific Conditions

In this chapter we will discuss, diabetic emergencies, thyroid emergencies, and acute adrenal crisis.

Diabetic Emergencies

There are three major emergency conditions which can occur in the diabetic patient: (1) Hypoglycemia, (2) Diabetic ketoacidosis (DKA), and (3) hyperosmolar hyperglycemic state (HHS).

Hypoglycemia: Hypoglycemia is a more common, life-threatening emergency in the diabetics. Hypoglycemia is defined as blood sugar levels <60 mg/dL, however many authors define it as below 80 mg/dL. Signs and symptoms are more common at blood sugar levels <40 mg/dL.

Precipitating/risk factors of hypoglycemia are—missed meal after taking diabetic medications such as insulin or oral hypoglycemic agents (OHAs), excess alcohol intake, and chronic liver conditions. There may be rarer conditions precipitating hypoglycemia in patients who are not on any hypoglycemic drugs, such as insulinomas, Addison's disease, pituitary insufficiency, sepsis, and due to some medicines such as quinine, fluoroquinolones, etc. Sometimes, worsening renal condition interferes with drug clearance and may increase the level of antidiabetic drugs and hence precipitate hypoglycemia. Ingestion or injection of an antidiabetic medicine in excess amount, both unintentionally and intentionally may precipitate hypoglycemia.

Pathophysiology of hypoglycemia is as follows. Glucose is one of the two vital nutrients for the brain. And a drop in blood sugar levels leads to reduce level of alertness, cognitive problems, and if prolonged can lead to seizures, coma, and death.

Symptoms of hypoglycemia include hunger, uneasiness, tremor, headache, sweating, impaired vision, weakness, palpitations, acute confusion, and coma.

On examination—any patient with altered level of mentation or consciousness, blood sugar levels should be immediately checked. There may also be: Pallor, confused state, tachycardia, sweating, and sometimes isolated hemiparesis or hemiplegia (stroke mimic).

Laboratory findings are low blood sugar levels in the capillary blood glucose testing done at the bedside. To confirm, a laboratory sample should be sent to the lab. A metabolic screen should be sent to look for renal and hepatic function.

Treatment of a patient with hypoglycemia: Often the patients need rapid administration of intravenous (IV) glucose, dextrose 25% or 50%, 100 mL intravenously immediately.

Glucagon may be given intramuscular in patients with recurrent episodes, or who have taken a long-acting drug, notably sulfonylureas. Once patient is conscious and able to swallow well, oral feed can be given. Frequent monitoring of the blood sugar—every 1-2 hourly should be done. While correcting a blood sugar level one needs to watch out for hypokalemia.

Complications: Most patients respond to glucose administration in 10–20 minutes, if the neurological signs persist, further evaluation should be done to look for any neurological pathology. Prolonged hypoglycemia can lead to permanent brain injury.

Diabetic ketoacidosis: It is a potentially life-threatening condition, although seen more often in patients with type 1 diabetes mellitus (DM), it can also happen in the patients of type 2 DM. It can be the presenting complaint in some previously undiagnosed patients.

Precipitating factors—infection, myocardial infarction, stroke, pregnancy, missed dose of insulin, and other stressors. Now a days new antidiabetic drugs like sodium glucose cotransporter inhibitors may uncommonly precipitate DKA.

Pathophysiology—the stressors increase gluconeogenesis and severe hyperglycemia. The excess glucose gets excreted in urine causing osmotic diuresis, leading dehydration, with loss of water as well as electrolytes. Due to absolute deficiency of insulin, this excess glucose is not utilized and thus the fat and muscle is mobilized for energy leading to lipolysis and production of fatty acids and ketones, thus leading to ketoacidosis.

Clinical features: DKA usually develops over 2–3 days. It is seen relatively more often in young adults. It presents with polyuria, polydipsia, fatigue, weakness, and abdominal pain.

In severe cases there may be altered consciousness levels, confusion, and coma.

On examination, the patient usually has normal blood pressure, there is rapid, deep breathing (Kussmaul's respiration). The skin is dry, there is diminished skin turgor and the mucous membranes are dry. There may be a typical fruity smell in the breath due to acetone in the breath. In severe cases there may be hypotension shock, oliguria or anuria etc. There may be cardiac arrhythmias, sometimes fatal, often precipitated by electrolyte imbalances.

The laboratory work up shows sugar levels are high, >250 mg/dL and arterial blood gas (ABG) shows metabolic acidosis (pH <7.3), with a high anion gap. Serum ketones are high, urinary acetone or blood β-hydroxybutyrate can be measured.

Blood urea nitrogen (BUN) and creatinine may be raised. Serum potassium may be low or high. Usually, there is extracellular shift of potassium due to acidosis and body potassium is usually depleted. The anion gap is high.

Management: The four major interventions in DKA are correction of dehydration, control of blood sugar, correction of hypokalemia, and removal of the precipitating cause if any. IV fluid replacement should be started immediately with 1–2 liters of normal saline given over the first hour and ultimately an adult patient may require 8–10 L of fluid in the first 12 hours. Fluid replacement should be carefully titrated, with monitoring of urine output. The choice of fluid is initially normal saline, which should be changed to 5% dextrose water, once the blood sugar is <250 mg%.

Regular insulin should be given as a bolus of 0.1 U/kg started as an infusion at 0.1 U/kg/hour to allow a steady decrease in the serum glucose levels at the rate of 50–75 mg/dL/hour. Blood sugar should be monitored every 1 hourly. Insulin infusion should be continued till the anion gap is closed serum electrolytes should be monitored 3–6 hourly and corrected accordingly. If serum potassium is <3.5 mmol/L, insulin should be withheld till it is corrected.

Magnesium and phosphorus should be replaced as needed. Acidosis gets corrected with fluid replacement and insulin therapy. Routine use of bicarbonate for correction of acidosis should be discouraged.

It is important to send markers of infection, cultures, check ECG, and take a proper drug history, and look for the precipitating factor. Potential complications include hypoglycemia, hypokalemia with cardiac dysrhythmias, and cerebral edema in case the sugar drops rapidly. Hence, frequent monitoring of vitals with neurological status is important.

Hyperosmolar hyperglycemic state: Also known as hyperosmolar hyperglycemic nonketotic coma, it is another life-threatening emergency in diabetics, more common in type 2 DM, with marked elevation in the blood sugar levels, with hyperosmolarity with little or no ketosis. The mortality in the HHS ranges from 10 to 50%.

The precipitating factors for HHS are acute myocardial infarction and stroke. Other causes include noncompliance to medications, infection, etc. Most patients are elderly with >50 years of age.

Pathophysiology of HHS is severe hyperglycemia causing osmotic diuresis, leading to severe dehydration, with loss of water as well as electrolytes. There is often hypernatremia and hyperosmolarity as water is lost more than the sodium. Urine output often decreases causing prerenal azotemia. However, there is sufficient circulating insulin to avert production of ketones.

The onset is of HHS is insidious, developing over days to weeks. It is seen more often in elderly, alcoholics, etc. The presentation is with polyuria, polydipsia, and vague abdominal pain. Neurological symptoms are more common with headache, blurred vision, and confusion which progresses to altered consciousness, seizures, and even coma.

On examination there is dry skin, diminished skin turgor, and dry mucous membranes. Sensorium is usually down and there is oliguria/anuria.

Laboratory findings are as follows. Sugar levels are high—usually >500 mg/dL or higher. Serum osmolarity >320 mOsm/kg. ABG shows pH >7.3. BUN and creatinine are usually raised, serum sodium is usually high—depending on the level of dehydration, serum potassium may be low or high.

Management—stabilizing the airway, breathing, and circulation should be done immediately and some patients even require intubation for airway protection.

Treatment should focus on the correction of dehydration, gradual correction of sugar levels, maintenance of electrolytes, treatment of underlying illness, and close monitoring of neurological status. IV fluid replacement should be started immediately—with 1–2 liters of crystalloid over the first hour. Fluid replacement should be carefully titrated, to prevent complications. In spite of hypernatremia, the first few liters of fluid replacement should be done by normal saline. After the blood glucose levels reach 250–300 mg/dL, 5% dextrose should be infused. Regular insulin should be given as a bolus of 0.05 U/kg started as an infusion at 0.05 U/kg/hour to allow a steady decrease in the serum glucose levels at the rate of 50–75 mg/dL/hour. Blood sugar should be monitored every hourly. Insulin infusion should be continued till the HHS is resolved. Serum electrolytes should be monitored 3–6 hourly and corrected accordingly. If serum potassium is <3.5 mmol/L, insulin should be withheld till it is corrected. Magnesium and phosphorus should be replaced as needed.

TABLE 2: Differences between DKA and HHS.

Diabetic ketoacidosis (DKA)	*Hyperglycemic hyperosmolar state (HHS)*
More common in type I DM, younger patients	More common in type 2 DM, older patients
Acute or subacute onset <24 hours	Insidious onset over several days
Blood sugar level >250 mg/dL	Blood sugar level >500 mg/dL
Marked acidosis and ketosis	Mild ketosis, no acidosis per se
Pain abdomen vomiting	Drowsiness

It is important to send cultures, check ECG, and look for the precipitating factor.

Potential complications include hypoglycemia, hypokalemia with cardiac dysrhythmias, and cerebral edema in case the sugar drops rapidly. Hence, frequent monitoring of vitals with neurological status is important. The salient differences between DKA and HHS are shown in the **Table 2**.

Thyroid emergencies: These are rare conditions these days, although life-threatening if they set in.

Thyroid storm: A thyroid storm occurs when the body is overwhelmed by the excess thyroid levels in the blood. Thyroid storms are precipitated by stress—infection, trauma, surgery, thyroxine overdose or cessation of therapy in hyperthyroid patients.

Pathophysiology: The excess thyroid hormones increase metabolism, affect sympathetic nervous system, thus increasing oxygen consumption, and increasing heat production and causing fluid and electrolyte derangements.

Clinical features of a thyroid storm are nausea, vomiting, diarrhea, altered mental status, restlessness, palpitations, hyperthermia, tremors, profuse sweating, fatigue, weight loss, and muscle weakness.

On examination, the patients have tachycardia may have arrhythmia, hypertension, tachypnea. The patients are dehydrated, febrile with temperature >102.2°F.

Agitated and delirious. The pulse is bounding, on auscultation there may be systolic murmur. There may be an enlarged thyroid gland. Some patients may present with cardiac failure.

Laboratory findings: ECG shows sinus tachycardia and arrhythmias like atrial fibrillation. Arterial blood gas analysis shows hypoxemia and metabolic acidosis. There may be episodes of hypoglycemia and there may be electrolyte derangement.

Management: Secure ABC, start IV fluids, start dextrose. Monitor blood pressure (BP), electrocardiogram (ECG), fluid status, and temperature. Electrolytes imbalances arrhythmias and heart failure need to be treated. This may need β-blockers, digoxin, etc. Rapid cooling may be needed in case of very high fever. The precipitating cause should be corrected.

Specific antithyroid medications are used like thyroid hormone antagonists (propylthiouracil, methimazole), β-blockers, iodine dyes, and corticosteroids.

Myxedema coma: This is a life-threatening condition, often presenting in patients with underlying hypothyroidism. Despite the name as coma, not all patients with myxedema coma are in coma.

Precipitating/risk factors: This is more common in females. It may be precipitated by infection, trauma, surgery, central nervous system (CNS) depressants, stroke, and cold weather.

Pathophysiology: Patients usually have long-standing hypothyroidism, either diagnosed or undiagnosed previously. A precipitating factor like infection may overwhelm the body. A myxedema coma happens when a low circulating thyroid hormones lead to extreme low metabolic rate.

Clinical features: Lethargy, altered mentation, cold intolerance, constipation, cardiac or respiratory failure. On examination patients may have myxedematous facies with puffiness, macroglossia, periorbital edema, coarse, sparse hair, and dry skin. There is nonpitting edema of the legs, goiter may be present. The patients are often hypothermic with temperature <95°F. Bradycardia, low cardiac output state, hypoventilation, etc., are the usual features.

Laboratory findings: ECG shows sinus bradycardia. Other features are anemia, elevated creatine phosphokinase (CPK), hypoglycemia, elevated transaminases, hyperlipidemia, hyponatremia, and respiratory acidosis. Finally, there are low T3 and T4 levels.

Management: ABC is to be secured. Intravenous fluids, vasopressors are needed. Intravenous levothyroxine (T4) is the specific treatment. Hydrocortisone should be administered until coexisting adrenal insufficiency is ruled out. Warming blankets are needed to combat hypothermia. The precipitating cause should be corrected.

Acute adrenal crisis—this is life-threatening condition, which requires a high level of clinical suspicion.

Precipitating/risk factors: This often occurs on a sudden withdrawal of steroid therapy or a failure to supplement adequate steroids in a state of physiological stress (infection, trauma, acute coronary event, etc.). Sometimes adrenal hemorrhage postpartum pituitary necrosis may also precipitate.

Pathophysiology—Patients on long-term steroids have a hypothalamus-pituitary-adrenal axis completely suppressed. Hence, when the supplementation is withdrawn, the patient is prone to develop acute adrenal crisis.

Clinical features are as follows: Acute confusion, severe discomfort, giddiness, hypotension, and shock.

On examination: The hypotension is often unresponsive to fluid resuscitation and vasopressors. That causes circulatory collapse. There is hyperkalemia, hyponatremia, elevated temperature. Skin hyperpigmentation may be present.

Laboratory findings—hyponatremia, hyperkalemia, hypercalcemia, hypoglycemia, BUN, and creatinine are elevated. The plasma cortisol levels are low.

Abdominal CT may help identify adrenal hemorrhage, calcification or metastasis, and coexisting hypothyroidism should be excluded.

Management—ABC, supplement oxygen rapid IV crystalloids, vasopressors.

Steroid supplementation is started, usually hydrocortisone 100 mg IV 6 hourly.

Dexamethasone should be given if the reason for the crisis is unknown, as it does not interfere with the subsequent testing. Fludrocortisone is given if hypotension, and electrolyte derangement persists. Dextrose 50% in case of hypoglycemia, correction of electrolytes, and correction of concurrent hypothyroidism are other sides of the treatment.

FURTHER READING

1. Bajwa SJS, Jindal R. Endocrine emergencies in critically ill patients: challenges in diagnosis and management. Indian J Endocrinol Metab. 2012;16(5):722-7.
2. Meyer G, Badenhoop K. Addison-Krise–Risiko erkennen und rasch behandeln. Addisonian Crisis-risk assessment and appropriate treatment. Dtsch Med Wochenschr. 2018;143(6):392-6.
3. Mishra A, Quinn M. Endocrine emergencies. InnovAiT. 2020;13(3):165-72.
4. Muneer M, Akbar I. Acute metabolic emergencies in diabetes: DKA, HHS, and EDKA. Adv Exp Med Biol. 2021;1307:85-114.
5. Nasrullah A, Azharuddin S, Young M, Kejas A, Dumont T. Endocrine Emergencies in the Medical Intensive Care Unit. Crit Care Nurs Q. 2022;45(3):266-84.
6. Pfadt E, Carlson DS. Acute adrenal crisis. Nursing. 2006;36(8):80.
7. Ylli D, Klubo-Gwiezdzinska J, Wartofsky L. Thyroid emergencies. Pol Arch Intern Med. 2019;129(7-8):526-34.

CHAPTER 19

Trauma and Burns

Ashutosh Bhardwaj, Quadri SM

TRAUMA

INTRODUCTION

Trauma patients present with unique challenges requiring prompt and effective nursing care. This chapter outlines essential principles for the comprehensive management of trauma patients, encompassing assessment, intervention, and ongoing care.

INITIAL ASSESSMENT

Primary survey is the quick evaluation of vital functions. Essentially, the ABCs plus the D and E.

- *Airway patency:* Chin lift, jaw thrust if not patent, with C spine immobilization.
- *Breathing:* Is patient oxygenating and ventilating adequately? If not then ventilate followed by rapid sequence intubation (RSI).
- *Circulation:* Look for signs of shock—hypotension, tachycardia, pallor, altered mental status, and poor capillary refill test (CRT). Two large bore IV cannula are attained and labs are also during this time and resuscitation is started.
- *Disability/neurologic assessment*—Assessing Glasgow Coma Scale (GCS).
- *Exposure*—Completely undress patient to rule out other injuries, keep patient warm to prevent hypothermia.

The primary survey is also meant to identify and treat life-threatening injuries, beginning with the most severe.

AIRWAY EVALUATION

- Initial steps in airway management are chin lift and jaw thrust, while at the same time stabilizing and immobilizing the cervical spine. Supplemental oxygen should also be provided.
- The adequacy of oxygenation and ventilation dictates the urgency of securing the airway.
- If oxygenation and ventilation are inadequate, gently ventilate if necessary with cricoid pressure followed by RSI (with manual in line stabilization).
- If a difficult airway is anticipated and oxygenation and ventilation is marginal, assess the possibility to topicalize the airway and perform an awake fiber optic intubation (FOI).
- Always have a cricothyrotomy kit available as well as skilled and experienced personnel around that can perform one, in case the airway cannot be secured.
- Treat all trauma patients as full stomach.
- Maxillofacial, neck injuries, and cervicofacial burns are most common trauma-related causes of difficult intubation.
- Nasotracheal tube is contraindicated in presence of basilar skull fracture.
- About 2–4% of blunt trauma patients have cervical spine injuries and of these 7–15% are unstable.
  If suspicious for C spine injury, computed tomography (CT) scans can rule out majority of injuries.

However, it is not sensitive enough to rule out ligament injuries. Scan of choice to rule out ligamentous injury is magnetic resonance imaging (MRI).

SECONDARY SURVEY

Secondary survey, is a more intense, systematic exam to uncover and identify additional injuries. It includes detailed head to toe examination of patient.

Radiographic studies such as X-rays (chest, abdomen, and pelvis) and FAST (Focused assessment with sonography for trauma: **Box 1**) are also performed at this time. CT scans are performed depending on patient stability.

Numerous injuries are possible but some common ones are: Traumatic brain injury (TBI), neck injuries involving, vascular and airway structure damage, pneumothorax, aortic injuries, liver and spleen lacerations, and pelvic injuries.

It is important to note that many injuries can be missed during the initial evaluation and to remember this, as occult injuries can be fatal. So always have a high index of suspicion for certain injuries depending on the mechanism of injury.

BOX 1: Focused assessment with sonography for trauma (FAST) exam.

FAST exam

Focused assessment with sonography for trauma:
Screens for free fluid around four areas:

1. Heart
2. Liver
3. Spleen
4. Pelvis
    - A positive FAST is defined as a dark strip (free fluid/blood) in the dependent areas of the peritoneum
    - If the FAST is positive and patient is stable, computed tomography (CT) scans usually follow
    - If the FAST is positive and patient is unstable then patient usually goes straight to operating room

COMPLICATIONS

Traumatic Brain Injury

- 40% of deaths from trauma are caused by head injury.
  The most feared consequence of a head injury is ischemia of the brain.
  The bedside scoring for traumatic brain injury is done by Glasgow Coma Scale (GCS) **(Table 1)**.
- Important goal in TBI patients is to prevent secondary injuries such as intracerebral hemorrhage (ICH), which is due to cerebral edema related to the head injury.
- Hypoxia and hypotension are very detrimental to TBI patients.

Goals in TBI patients are:

- Normalize intracranial pressure (ICP)
- Optimize cerebral perfusion pressure (CPP) (CPP = MAP–ICP); MAP—mean arterial pressure, ICP—intracranial pressure.
- Optimize oxygen delivery
- Aim for MAP >80 mm Hg, PaO_2 >110 mm Hg, ICP <20 mm Hg, and CPP 50–70 mm Hg.

Hemorrhage

Hemorrhage is the most common cause of traumatic hypotension and it is the second most common cause of mortality after head injury.

High-energy deceleration impact, falls from heights >6 meters are highly likely to produce major bleeding and damage.

Most common places for occult bleeding resulting in hypotension is in the thorax, abdomen, and retroperitoneum.

TABLE 1: Mild traumatic brain injury (TBI) [Glasgow Coma Scale (GCS) of 13–15], moderate TBI (GCS 9–12), and severe is GCS 8 or less.

Glasgow Coma Scale		
Response	***Scale***	***Score***
Eye opening response	Eyes open spontaneously	4 points
	Eyes open to verbal command, speech, or shout	3 points
	Eyes open to pain (not applied to face)	2 points
	No eye opening	1 point
Verbal response	Oriented	5 points
	Confused conversation, but able to answer questions	4 points
	Inappropriate responses, words discernible	3 points
	Incomprehensible sounds or speech	2 points
	No verbal response	1 point
Motor response	Obeys commands for movement	6 points
	Purposeful movement to painful stimulus	5 points
	Withdraws from pain	4 points
	Abnormal (spastic) flexion, decorticate posture	3 points
	Extensor (rigid) response, decerebrate posture	2 points
	No motor response	1 point

Minor brain injury = 13–15 points | *Moderate brain injury* = 9–12 points | *Severe brain injury* = 3–8 points

Rapid operative treatment for damage control is key in patients with hemorrhagic shock. The triad of complications which lead to death in trauma are shown in the **Box 2**.

As patients become hypothermic, they become more coagulopathic. Coagulopathy makes the bleeding worse. Increased/uncontrolled bleeding in turn worsens the metabolic acidosis as the body cannot keep up with the oxygen demand. The acidosis also makes the coagulopathy worse.

BOX 2: Triad of death.

In trauma patients, there is a group of interrelated conditions that leads to death. This triad consists of:
1. Hypothermia
2. Coagulopathy
3. Acidosis

Resuscitation

There is a concept of permissive hypotension in trauma patients [excluding trauma patients with TBI or spinal cord injury (SCI)], which require higher perfusion pressures.

Studies have shown that patient outcomes are better when a lower MAP (~60 mm Hg) is the target as opposed to a higher MAP.

Another reason to avoid aggressive fluid resuscitation is that it leads to dilution of coagulation factors, platelets, and also increased bleeding due to the increased blood pressure (BP).

Goals for resuscitation are:
- Systolic blood pressure (SBP) 80–100 mm Hg unless TBI or spinal cord injury (SCI)
- Core temperature >36°C
- Hematocrit 25–30%
- Normal coagulatin [prothrombin time (PT), partial thromboplastin time (PTT)]
- Platelet count >50,000

Normal ionized calcium: Should keep close eye on calcium level as the citrate (anticoagulant) in blood products can bind calcium and cause hypocalcemia. FFP is the blood product that has the most citrate out of all the blood products.

Correct acidosis via improved perfusion.

BURNS

INTRODUCTION

Burns are a global health problem, which account for an estimated 180,000 deaths annually as per WHO data. As per the available data in India, over 1,000,000 people are moderately or severely burnt every year.

A burn is an injury to the skin or other tissue caused by heat, radiation, electricity, friction, or contact with chemicals substances.

Thermal burns occur when some or all of the in the skin or other tissues are destroyed by hot liquids, hot solids, or flames.

CLASSIFICATION

First-degree burns or superficial burns affect only epidermis. Burn site is painful, red, and dry but has no blisters, e.g., mild sunburn.

Second-degree burns or partial thickness burns involve the epidermis and part of the dermis. Burn site is painful, red, blistered, and maybe swollen.

Third-degree burns or full thickness burns destroy both the epidermis and dermis. They may involve the innermost layer of subcutaneous tissue. Burn site is white or blackened and charred.

Fourth-degree burns involves both layers of the skin and underlying tissue as well as deeper tissue, involving muscle and bone. There is no feeling of pain since the nerve endings are destroyed.

The extent of the burns is estimated by the rule of 9 **(Box 3)**.

Major burns are full-thickness burns >10% of total body surface area (TBSA), partial-thickness burns >25% of TBSA in adults or over 20% at extremes of age, and burns that involve face, hands, and perineum.

Associated injuries: Knowing the mechanism of injury can help figure out associated injuries.

BOX 3: Rule of 9s.

- Size of the burned area is estimated via the rule of 9s as a fraction of the total body surface area (TBSA)
- For adults:
  - Head is 9% of TBSA
  - Upper extremities are 9% each
  - Trunk is 36%; (18% front, 18% back)
  - Lower extremities are 18% each

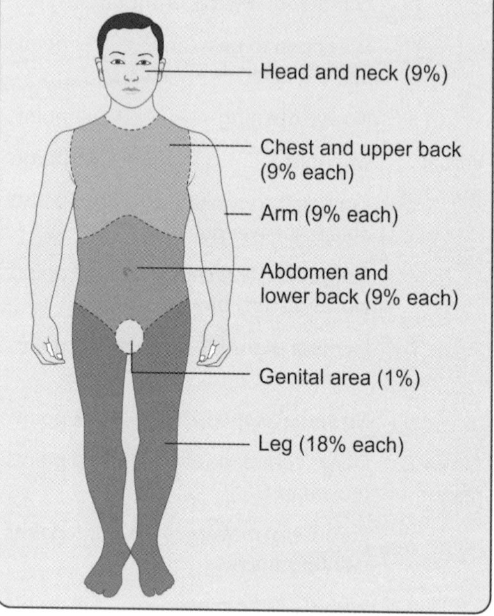

- Burns from motor vehicle accidents or industrial accidents can be associated with other traumatic injuries.
- Electrocution burns may be associated with hematomas, severe fractures, skeletal and cardiac muscle injury, leading to arrhythmias. These burns may show very little evidence of external damage.
- Thermal trauma in closed space flames is usually associated with airway damage.

Initial Fluid Resuscitation in Burns

Numerous formulas have been developed to aid in fluid resuscitating the burn patient. Fluid of choice are crystalloids, specifically Ringer lactate (RL).

The most well-known formula is the *Parkland formula*; based on the percentage of BSA burned.

- Total fluid in 1st 24 hours = 4 mL/kg BW per % burn TBSA.
- Out of which half of the fluid to be given in 1st 8 hours, rest in 16 hours. *Modified Parkland formula*
- *Initial 24 hours:* RL 4 mL/kg/% burn (adults)
- *Next 24 hours:* Begin colloid infusion of 5% albumin 0.3–1 mL/kg/% burn/16 hour

Burn wound management consists of:

- Debridement (removal of all devitalized tissue)
- Degree (depth assessment)
- Dressing selection (nonadherent films or fine mesh gauze in combination with topical antimicrobials)
- Definitive care (early burn wound excision and grafting within 72 hours)

Silver sulfadiazine: Topical sulfonamide Mechanism of action (MOA)—silver ion act on cell membrane and cell wall to produce bactericidal effects used on 2nd and 3rd degree burns.

To be spread all over burn twice a day, to be removed completely between applications to prevent pseudo-eschar formation. Pain control to be done with nonsteroidal anti-inflammatory drugs (NSAIDs), opioids, and if necessary sedation.

Special Considerations

Head and Facial Burns

- Shave area of head involved to avoid pseudo-eschar formation and monitor possible development of folliculitis.
- Avoid use of silver sulfadiazine and collagen near eyes.
- Best topical option for face is Garamycin.
- Ears have high risk of infection due to poor blood supply hence more cautious debridement.

Burns Center Referral Criteria

- Deep partial thickness burns >10% TBSA.
- Burns involving face, hands, feet, genitalia, or any major joint.
- Full thickness burns in any age group.
- Electrical burn including lightning.
- Inhalation burn requiring intubation of patient.
- Chemical burn that are deep and extensive.
- Any patient with burns and concomitant trauma in which burn injury poses the greatest risk of morbidity and mortality.

FURTHER READING

1. Cancio LC. Initial assessment and fluid resuscitation of burn patients. Surg Clin North Am. 2014;94(4):741-54.
2. Gallagher JJ, Williams-Bouyer N, Villarreal C, Heggers J, Herndon D. Treatment of infection in burns James J. Total Burn Care, 4th edition; 2012.
3. Jordan J. Approach to the Trauma Patient. [online] Available from https://www.merckmanuals.com/professional/injuries-poisoning/approach-to-the-trauma-patient/approach-to-the-trauma-patient [Last accessed February, 2025].
4. Kaafarani HMA, Velmahos GC. Damage Control Resuscitation In Trauma. Sage Journals. 2014;103(2).
5. Muthukumar V, Karki D, Jatin B. Concept of lethal triad in critical care of severe burn injury. Indian J Crit Care Med. 2019;23(5):206-9.
6. Smolle C, Cambiaso-Daniel J, Forbes AA, Wurzer P, Hundeshagen G, Branski LK, et al. Recent trends in burn epidemiology worldwide: A systematic review. Burns. 2017;43(2):249-57.

SECTION 5

General Nursing

Section Editor: *Asif Ahmed*

20. Airway Management
Ranvir Singh Tyagi

21. Oral and Eye Care in Critically Ill Patients
Lalit Singh, Dharmendra Kumar Ojha

22. Delirium and Sedation in Intensive Care Unit
Swapnabharati Moharana, Swagata Tripathy

23. Bedsore and Pressure Injuries
Durgesh Satalkar

24. Physiotherapy and Mobilization
Parshotam Lal Gautam, Rubina Khullar Mahajan, Anoopjit Kaur

25. Transferring a Critically Ill Patient
Manish Munjal, Bikram K Gupta, Preeti Singh

26. Nutrition
Sanjith Saseedharan Saroja

27. Defibrillation, Cardioversion, and Transcutaneous Pacing
Shyam Sunder Tipparaju, Shwetha Ram Chandankhede

28. Injections and Infusions
Rohit Kumar Patnaik, Nupur Karan, Tapas Kumar Sahoo

29. Transfusion Medicine
Chandrashish Chakravarty

30. Intravenous Fluid Therapy in Intensive Care Nursing
Anand Vinaykumar Joshi

31. Setting Up Trays
Sananda Chakraborty, Sudipta Mukherjee

32. Alarm Fatigue and Burn Out
Susruta Bandyopadhyay, Diptanjan Ray

33. Sample Collection
Kanwalpreet Sodhi, Manender Kumar

34. Nursing Care of the Terminally Ill
Nandhakishore Jampala, Ganshyam Jagathkar

CHAPTER 20

Airway Management

Ranvir Singh Tyagi

INTRODUCTION

Airway is defined as a passage through which the air/gas passes during respiration. The function of the airway is to help transport air to and from the external environment.

ANATOMY OF UPPER AIRWAY

Airway can be divided into two parts:

1. *Upper airway:* Nose, mouth, nasal cavity, paranasal sinuses, pharynx, and larynx.
2. *Lower airway:* Trachea, bronchi, bronchioles, alveolar ducts, and alveoli.

Airway obstruction can occur during sleep, unconsciousness, or when the person is under general anesthesia. This is due to collapsible soft tissue around the pharynx. Even before any airway protection device is used, a jaw thrust and neck extension help to create space between the epiglottis and posterior pharyngeal wall and keep the airway patent. Any swelling in the soft tissue within the bony enclosure of pharynx or a decrease in bony enclosure size (e.g., due to trauma) would result in anatomical imbalance and cause limitation of space available for airway.

AIRWAY MANAGEMENT

Maintaining an open airway is the first most important step of managing any critically ill or compromised patient, A of ABC approach (see the chapter on resuscitation).

Upper airway obstruction can be relieved with the triple maneuver—head tilt, chin lift, and jaw thrust in a supine patient **(Fig. 1)**. In suspected case of cervical spine injury, only jaw thrust is given.

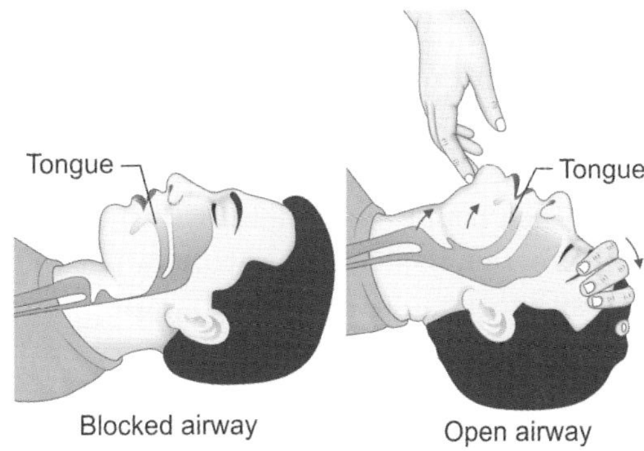

Fig. 1: Triple maneuver to relieve a blocked airway.

Respiratory Assessment

After taking a focused history, adequacy of ventilation and patent airway can be ensured by assessing:

- *Level of consciousness:* AVPU (alert, responding to voice, responding to pain, unresponsive)
- Whether patient can maintain a patent airway or not? Signs of obstruction—snoring or abnormal breathing sound, labored breathing, restlessness, etc.
- *Respiratory effort:* Rate (tachypnea), depth (shallow breathing in respiratory depression), pattern of breathing (forced breathing in asthma or chronic obstructive pulmonary disease; abnormal breathing patterns, e.g.,—Kussmaul, Cheyne Stoke's, or Biot's pattern), use of accessory muscles such as sternocleidomastoid, intercostal, and abdominal muscles.

- *Asymmetrical chest movements*—flail chest, hemothorax, pneumothorax, etc.
- Cyanosis
- Oxygen saturation <92% and elevated or very low-end tidal CO_2.
- *Auscultation:* Wheeze suggests bronchospasm, obstruction; fine rhonchi-pulmonary edema, coarse rhonchi-chest infection.

Steps of Airway Management

Assess for patient's responsiveness. If patient is unresponsive, not breathing, and carotid pulse also could not be felt in 10 seconds, activate the basic life and/or advanced life support team and cardiopulmonary resuscitation can be started.

If patient has got pulse, but there is absent breathing or gasping movements, give one rescue breaths each 5–6 seconds with a bag and mask device **(Fig. 2)** or mouth to mouth, if you are comfortable. The bag of the self-inflating bag mask device should be pressed only sufficient to get a visible chest rise. Do not over ventilate as gastric insufflation may lead to vomiting/aspiration and will also compromise the ventilation. Oxygen can also be connected to the bag through oxygen connector tubing.

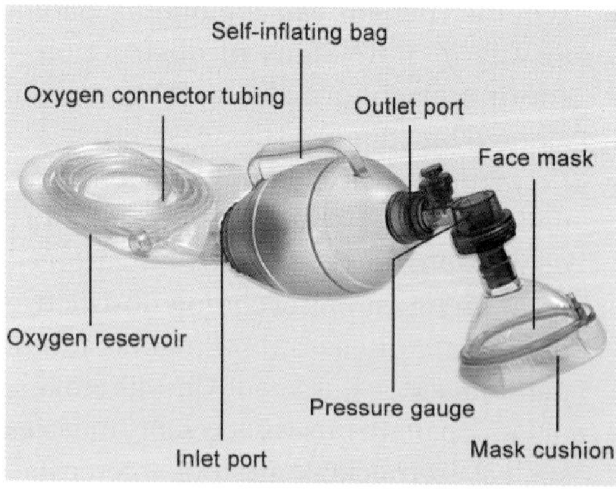

Fig. 2: Ambu bag and mask.

Face Mask

This allows administration of gases from the breathing system without introducing any apparatus into the patient. It has three parts.

1. *Body:* If it is transparent, it allows observation for secretions, condensation of exhaled gases.
2. *Seal (rim, flap):* Two types, pad and flange.
3. *Connector (orifice):* 22 mm internal diameter.

Holding the Mask

- One hand or two hands—E-C clamp; another person can bag if using both hands **(Fig. 3)**.
- Avoid pressures on eyes, soft tissues.
- Esmarch—Heiberg maneuver; This is dorsiflexion at atlanto-occipital joint and protrusion of the mandible (forward thrust on rami).
- You can use oropharyngeal airway (OPA) or nasopharyngeal airway (NPA) to aid mask ventilation.
- It is better to use the smallest mask which will do the job. As this causes less dead space.
- *Difficult mask ventilation:* Sizeable beard, obesity, an edentulous patient, history of obstructive sleep apnea, large tongue/tonsils, and abnormal facial anatomy may make mask ventilation difficult.
- If the patient has got both pulse and breathing, but oxygen saturation is low (<90%), supplementary oxygen should be started, while cause for desaturation are being explored.

Oxygen delivery systems can be divided into low flow and high flow systems. Low-flow systems provide lower oxygen flow than the actual inspiratory flow.

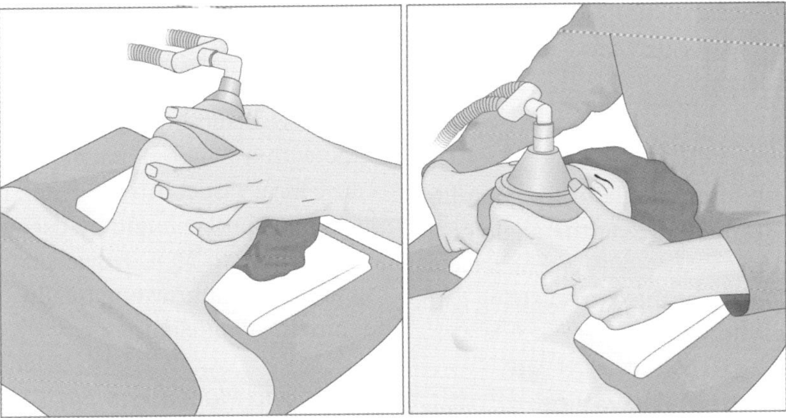

Fig. 3: Holding a mask properly one hand or two hands method.

TABLE 1: The oxygen delivery capacities of various systems.

Device	Flow (liters/min)	FiO_2 (fraction of inspired oxygen)
Nasal cannula	1–6	0.24–0.40
Simple face mask	5–10	0.35–0.60
Face tent	5–15	0.35–0.50
Venturi mask	2–15	0.24–0.60
Nonrebreathing mask	10–15	0.6–0.9
High flow nasal cannula	15–60	0.3–1.0

- Low flow system—nasal cannula, simple face mask, partial rebreathing, and nonrebreathing masks.
- High flow systems—venturi mask, high flow nasal cannula, tracheostomy collar, and face tent.

The oxygen delivery capacities of various systems are shown in **Table 1**.

AIRWAY ADJUNCTS

Oropharyngeal Airway or Oral Bite Block

- Oral airways are made of rigid plastic material, semicircular in shape, and available in sizes ranging from infants to adults (000 to 6).
- All oral airways have a *flange* to prevent over insertion, a straight *bite block* portion and a *curve section* leading to *air channel.*
- *Purpose:* Its purpose is to lift the tongue and epiglottis away from the posterior pharyngeal wall and prevent them from obstructing the space above the larynx during unconsciousness or after anesthesia or the patient having excess oral secretions, during seizures, or when the patient is biting down on oral endotracheal tubes.
- Pharyngeal and laryngeal reflexes should be depressed before insertion. It should not be put in an awake patient because it may elicit gag reflex and vomiting.
- Check for the correct size. Hold the airway by the cheek and see the airway reaches from the corner of the mouth to the angle of the mandible.
- It is inserted upside down with the tip pointing upward and then rotated 180° as it reaches the posterior pharyngeal wall into the position.
- Too small—may cause the tongue to kink and force part of it against the roof of the mouth, causing obstruction.

- Too large—obstruction by displacing the epiglottis posteriorly, and may traumatized the larynx.

Different Sizes (Fig. 4)

Correct sizing—from angle of the mandible to the nose or the flange at the angle of the mouth **(Fig. 5)**.

Best indicator for the correct sizing is the unobstructed airflow.

Nasopharyngeal Airway or Nasal Trumpet

It helps in maintaining airway patency in semiconscious patients. Nasal airways are softer and are useful in patients who are not deeply anesthetized since they tend to provoke less of a gag reflex. It is better tolerated in the patient with airway reflexes intact. It resembles a shortened tracheal tube with a flange. Phenylephrine drops to cause local vasoconstriction and lidocaine as local anesthesia should be used prior to the insertion of an NPA. However, in the acute situation, the lubricating quality of lidocaine ointment is sufficient.

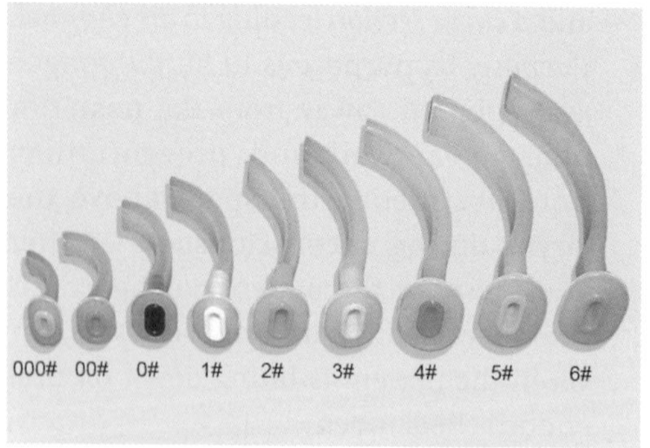

Fig. 4: Different sizes of oral airways.

Sizing and Placement (Fig. 6)

Tip of the airway is inserted perpendicular to the face and not upward toward the cribriform plate. Length of the airway is to be assessed as per the distance from the tip of the nose to meatus of the ear. The nasal airway insertion should be avoided in the presence of coagulopathy, basilar skull fractures, nasal infections, or deformities. The airway is secured to the nose with a tape to prevent displacement. Complications of these airways include bleeding. Sinusitis, and erosion of the mucous membranes. Regular checks to look for local sores or obstruction due to dried up secretions are needed. Sinusitis has been documented as a complication. The airway may be changed from one nostril to the other from time to time.

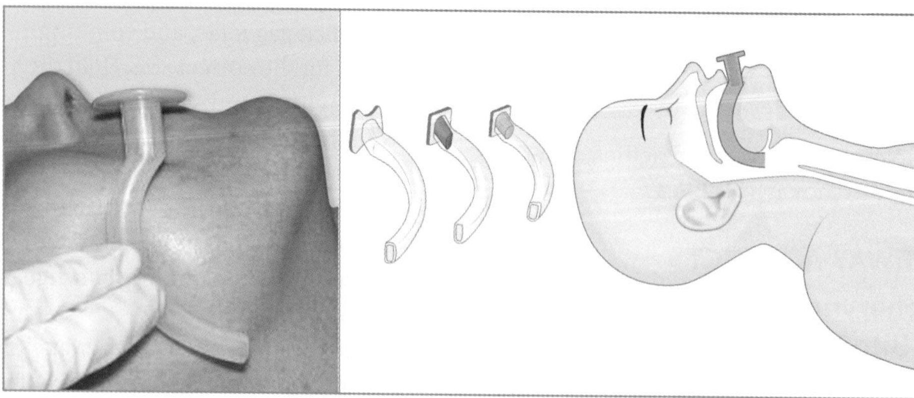

Fig. 5: Choosing the right size.

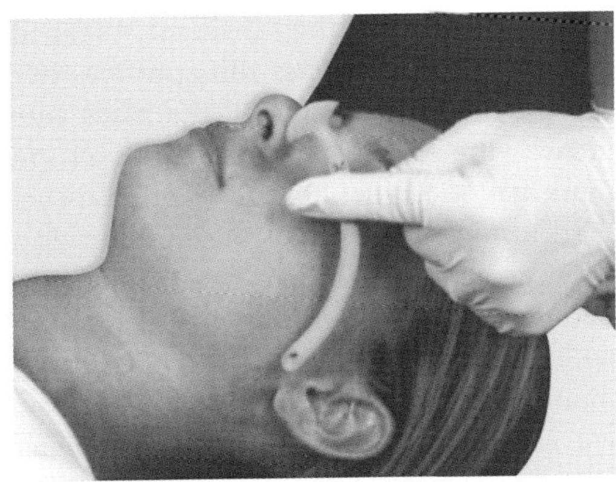

Fig. 6: Sizing and placement of nasopharyngeal airway.

Supraglottic Airway Device (Table 2)

They facilitate ventilation and oxygenation without endotracheal intubation. The supraglottic airway device (SADs) have a cuff that make a tight seal "above the glottis" when properly placed. They are divided in to first [classic, flexible. Ambu laryngeal mask airways (LMAs)] and second generations (proseal LMA and i-gel, etc.). Second generation SAD airway have an additional gastric channel and higher seal pressure, allowing higher ventilatory pressure.

TABLE 2: Choosing the correct size of the mask for the supraglottic airway device (SADs).

Mask Size	***Patient selection guidelines***	***Maximum cuff inflation volume (air)***
1	Neonates/infants up to 5 kg	Up to 4 mL
1½	Infants 5–10 kg	Up to 7 mL
2	Infants/children 10–20 kg	Up to 10 mL
2½	Children 20–30 kg	Up to 14 mL
3	Children 30–50 kg	Up to 20 mL
4	Adults 50–70 kg	Up to 30 mL
5	Adults 70–100 kg	Up to 40 mL
6	Large adults over 100 kg	Up to 50 mL

Insertion Technique for Supraglottic Airway

- A tube of appropriate size is to be selected
- Use sedative and analgesia, if required.
- The cuff is to be deflated.
- The outer cuff is to be lubricated
- *Position of the patient:* Neck flexed to 15°, head extended on neck (i.e., chin anteriorly), no lateral deviation.
- From behind the patient, the tube is to be held like a pen and inserted into the mouth, sliding the outer cuff along the palate.
- The tongue is to be pushed back until it reaches the posterior pharynx wall.
- Pressure to be applied to the device to direct it backward and downward until it reaches the back of the hypopharynx.
- The cuff is to be inflated per instruction mentioned earlier.
- The ventilation bag/machine is to be attached and ventilation started.
- A correct placement is to be corroborated by chest movement or $ETCO_2$.
- Secure with bandage or tape.

Uses of SADs—airway maintenance during routine low-risk surgery, as a conduit for intubation, and used for airway management during resuscitation/cardiac arrest (especially in cannot intubate cannot ventilate scenario) or in prehospital emergency care. They offer higher alternative to orotracheal intubation, particularly when providers are not well-trained to intubate. Contraindications to elective use of SADs include low pulmonary compliance, high airway resistance, presence of pharyngeal pathology, risk for aspiration, and/or airway obstruction below the larynx. They should not be used in a conscious or awake patient (gag reflex, laryngospasm, etc.).

Endotracheal Tube

The endotracheal tube (ETT) is a tube constructed of polyvinyl chloride (PVC) or silicon that is placed between the vocal cords through the trachea to provide oxygen and inhaled gases to the lungs. It protects the lungs from aspiration, such as gastric contents and blood. The main reasons for ETT insertion are an inability to protect the airway against aspiration, inability to maintain the patency of the airway. Failure to ventilate, failure to oxygenate, and anticipation of a deteriorating course leading to respiratory failure. Ideal size in the average female 7–7.5 mm ID, male 8–8.5 mm ID.

Equipment Required for Endotracheal Tube Insertion

- Laryngoscope (the blade size should be assessed, it should reach between the lips and larynx—size 3 for most patients)
- Cuffed endotracheal tube
- Syringe for inflating the cuff
- Monitoring to be done by end-tidal CO_2 monitor, pulse oximeter, cardiac monitor, and blood pressure machine.
- Tape
- Suction
- Ventilation bag and face mask
- Oxygen supply
- In awake patients, sedation, and short-acting muscle relaxants may be used to facilitate intubation.

Steps of intubation—after preoxygenation and administration of hypnotic, analgesics, and muscle relaxant, put the patient in sniffing the morning air position, open the mouth with dominant hand after head tilt chin lift maneuver, insert laryngoscope with nondominant hand on right angle of the mouth—displace the tongue to the left—lift the laryngoscope toward the roof after reaching the vallecula—you can visualize leafy epiglottis and then inverted V-shaped laryngeal opening. Pass the appropriately sized ETT through that till the black line crosses the laryngeal opening (19–21 cm mark at the lip in adult females and 22–24 cm mark in adult male). Following insertion of an ETT, the cuff of the tube is inflated with just enough air to create an effective seal. Confirm with five-point auscultation, $ETCO_2$ trace, maintenance of saturation, and chest X-ray, etc. After confirmation of correct placement, ETT should be properly fixed.

Aids to intubation—stylets (malleable, flexible, hollow with provision for oxygenation, and optical), Eschmann tracheal introducer or gum elastic bougie, forceps—Magills, flexible fiberoptic bronchoscope.

ETT suctioning—the endotracheal intubation prevents glottic closure and effective coughing, hence the patient needs periodic endotracheal suctioning to remove secretions. Currently, two methods are commonly used for ETT suctioning: The closed and open methods. Closed suctioning means the ventilator circuit remains closed while suctioning is performed with an in-line suction catheter device, whereas open suctioning means the ventilator circuit is opened, or removed, during suctioning.

Signs and symptoms pointing toward need for ET suctioning-secretions. In the airway, suspected aspiration, decreased breath sounds, inspiratory wheezes, or expiratory crackles, increase. In peak airway pressures, restlessness, ineffective or frequent cough, gradual or sudden decrease in PaO_2 or saturation.

Steps of Endotracheal Suctioning

- Oxygenate with 100% oxygen for minimum of 30 seconds with one of the following with ventilator or with manual breathing circuit.

- Insert catheter (closed or open system) gently until resistance is met, then pull back.
- Place the nondominant thumb over the control vent of the suction catheter to apply continuous or intermittent suction as the catheter is completely withdrawn.
- Suction should be applied only as needed and for as short a time as possible (not >10 seconds).
- Oxygenate for 30 seconds and then repeat.
- Monitor cardiopulmonary status before, during, and after suctioning.

EXTUBATION

A patient is ready to be weaned from the ventilator and extubated when he/she is breathing spontaneously and maintaining a normal arterial blood gas (ABG) with minimal to moderate amounts of oxygen administration (FiO_2 <0.50). The patient should be able to protect his/her airway, and clear pulmonary secretions.

Preparations for extubation include explaining to the patient of what to expect, the need to cough; setting up the appropriate method for delivering O_2 therapy post extubation (e.g., face mask, nasal cannula) and preparation for reintubation, if needed, and positioning the patient with the head of the bed elevated at 30–45° to improve diaphragmatic function. Suctioning of the ETT is performed prior to extubation. Hyperoxygenation with 100% oxygen for 30–60 seconds. Then ETT is removed after completely deflating the cuff. Then oxygen delivery method is immediately applied and the patient is encouraged to take deep breaths. Monitor hemodynamic and respiratory parameters following extubation.

FURTHER READING

1. Baid H, Creed F, Hargreaves J. Oxford Handbook of Critical Care Nursing. Oxford: Oxford University Press; 2016.
2. Hagberg CA. Benumof and Hagberg's Airway Management, 5th edition. Philadelphia: Elsevier Health Sciences; 2022.
3. Lloyd G. Basic Airway Management. In: Fordham S (Ed). RCEM Learning; 2020.

CHAPTER 21

Oral and Eye Care in Critically Ill Patients

Lalit Singh, Dharmendra Kumar Ojha

INTRODUCTION

The oral cavity hosts the second-largest microbial colonization site in the human body, including bacteria, fungi, viruses, and archaea. Adequate oral and eye care are integral to nursing practices in critical care, significantly impacting patient comfort, well-being, and overall health. Oral hygiene interventions, such as mechanical cleaning and topical disinfectants, can reduce hospital-acquired infections by nearly 40%. Providing consistent and effective oral and eye care minimizes complications such as ventilator-associated pneumonia (VAP), aspiration pneumonia, and other nosocomial infections.

ORAL CARE IN CRITICALLY ILL PATIENTS

Microbial Colonization and Infections

Critically ill patients are particularly vulnerable to infections due to immune compromise and inadequate oral hygiene. Common pathogens colonizing the oral tract, such as *Staphylococcus aureus*, *Streptococcus mutans*, and *Enterococcus faecalis*, are linked to VAP. Studies have shown that dental plaque serves as a reservoir for these pathogens, facilitating their transfer to the lower respiratory tract via endotracheal tubes, which can further develop biofilms.

Oral health also influences systemic conditions. Poor oral hygiene exacerbates chronic diseases such as diabetes, increasing the risk of periodontitis and poor glycemic control. Additionally, conditions such as osteoporosis and chronic kidney disease heighten the risk of complications in patients with preexisting oral issues.

Assessment and Protocols

Oral health assessments should be part of routine care to evaluate baseline conditions and implement targeted hygiene plans. Several clinical tools are used for assessing oral health in critically ill patients such as Bedside Oral Exam (BOE) **(Table 1)**, Revised Oral Assessment Guide (ROAG), General Oral Health Assessment Index (GOHAI), and Intensive Care Oral Care Frequency Assessment Scale (ICOCFAS). Tools such as the Beck Oral Assessment Scale (BOAS) and Mucosal Plaque Score are effective in assessing oral health status.

The following practices are recommended for oral care:

- Use 0.1–0.2% chlorhexidine mouthwash every 12 hours for antibacterial action.
- Employ soft-bristled toothbrushes with water for mechanical plaque removal and tissue moistening.
- Apply petroleum jelly or lanolin-based ointments to prevent dry lips in patients with prolonged mouth opening.

TABLE 1: Oral care.

Bedside oral exam (BOE)			
Numerical and descriptive ratings			
Category	***1. Normal***	***2 . Moderate dysfunction***	***3. Severe dysfunction***
Swallow	Normal swallow	Pain or difficulty with swallowing	Unable to swallow (intubated, absent gag)
Lips	Smooth, pink	Dry or cracked	Ulcerated or bleeding
Tongue	Pink, moist, papillae present	Coated or loss of papillae with thin appearance, with or without (w/o) redness	Blistered, cracked, or w/o bleeding
Saliva	Watery	Thick or ropy	Absent
Mucosal membranes	Pink, moist	Red or coated, no ulcers	Ulcers with or w/o bleeding
Gingiva	Pink, firm	Edema, with or w/o redness; with or w/o bleeding	Bleeds easily
Teeth or dentures	Clean or no teeth	Local debris (between teeth)	General debris, decay
Odor	Normal	Slightly to moderately odor	Strong foul odor

- Perform suctioning of oral and tracheal secretions every 2–4 hours using normal saline.

Despite its importance, oral care is often neglected due to staff shortages, inadequate training, and lack of standard guidelines.

EYE CARE IN CRITICALLY ILL PATIENTS

Risk Factors and Complications

Eye care is essential for preventing complications such as corneal epithelial defects, keratitis, and corneal ulcers in intensive care unit (ICU) patients. Critically ill patients are prone to ocular surface diseases (OSDs) due to impaired tear production, reduced blink rates, and inability to close the eyes completely (lagophthalmos). Muscle relaxants, sedatives, and noninvasive ventilation (NIV) further exacerbate these risks. The risk factors for developing OSD are summarized in **Table 2**.

Prevention and Protocols

Effective eye care practices can significantly reduce the incidence of ocular complications. Recommended interventions include:

- Liberal use of lubricants, such as Lacrilube ointment, to maintain hydration of the cornea
- Administration of artificial tear drops every 2 hours to prevent dryness
- Cleaning eyelids and lashes with saline-soaked cotton swabs every 6–8 hours
- Manual closure or taping of eyelids in cases of incomplete closure although this should be performed judiciously to avoid skin irritation
- Adherence to strict hand hygiene protocols among healthcare staff

TABLE 2: Risk factors for ocular surface diseases.

Category	*Risk factors in ICU patients for developing OSD*
Disease processes	*Fluid maldistribution:* Risk of facial edema, chemosis, and lid swelling
	Altered level of consciousness (low GCS): Reduces blink reflex and is associated with lagophthalmos
	• Peripheral or central neurological injury • Immunosuppression • Preexisting eye conditions
Treatment processes	*Continual positive airway pressure (CPAP) and oxygen masks:* Gas flow causes drying effects on the eye
	Use of muscle relaxants or sedation: Reduces blink rate, impairs blink reflex, and is a precursor to lagophthalmos
	Mechanical positive pressure ventilation: • Increases jugular pressure, causes conjunctival edema, increasing the risk of lagophthalmos • Associated with increased length of stay and use of sedation and muscle relaxants
	Prone position: • Direct injury during positioning • Causes conjunctival edema, increasing the risk of lagophthalmos
ICU environment	*Length of stay:* Increased length of stay associated with an increased risk of OSD
	Respiratory micro-organisms: • Increased exposure to micro-organisms (can be multiresistant organisms) • Increased risk of exposure from tracheal suctioning

(GCS: Glasgow Coma Scale; ICU: intensive care unit; OSD: ocular surface disease)

Studies emphasize the importance of structured eye care guidelines in preventing ocular complications and improving patient outcomes.

The nurse-led eye care in critical care protocol is shown in **Flowchart 1**.

BARRIERS AND RECOMMENDATIONS

The main challenges in providing oral and eye care in ICUs include inadequate staff, insufficient training, lack of proper equipment, and absence of standardized protocols.

To address these barriers:

- Develop and implement structured guidelines for oral and eye care.
- Provide specialized training for healthcare staff.
- Ensure the availability of necessary equipment and resources.
- Regularly evaluate adherence to care protocols and outcomes.

CONCLUSION

Oral and eye care are fundamental components of critical care nursing. Proper implementation of evidence-based practices

Flowchart 1: Nurse-led eye care in critical care.

Nurse-led eye care protocol

RISK ASSESS

On admission
THINK! Does your patient wear contact lenses?
Will these need to be removed?
Do regular medications need prescribing, particularly for glaucoma?

DAILY

Assess ALL ICU patients for risk of ocular surface disorder
Are any of the following risk factors present?
- Reduced blinking and/or poor eyelid closure
- Sedation +/- paralysing agents
- PEEP ≥5 cmH_2O
- Prone positioning
- Conjunctival edema
- Cardiac or renal failure

Yes → **Eye hygiene**
No → *Eye hygiene as per patient preference*

Eye hygiene
Hand hygiene using 7 step procedure, maintain ANTT
Clean eyes with sterile water soaked gauze
Each gauze singe use-Wipe inside to outside, then dispose

Observe!
Redness, swelling, discharge or lid margin crusting?
Consider ophthalmology referral
John Cooper ANP bleep 5235

4 hourly

Ocular surface protection
Hand hygiene using 7 step procedure, maintain ANTT
Apply Lacrilube to inside "V" pocket of lower eyelids
Use individual, labeled tubes (L+R) for each eye

Hints and tips
- Where able, use the minimal amount of sedation possible to protect blink reflexes
- DO NOT use saline to clean eyes
- Ensure eyes are covered when using an open suction system

(ANTT: aseptic non-touch technique; ICU: intensive care unit; PEEP: post end-expiratory pressure)

reduces the risk of nosocomial infections, enhances patient comfort, and improves overall prognosis. Addressing existing barriers through standardization of care protocols and staff training is imperative to ensure high-quality care in ICU settings.

FURTHER READING

1. Abranches J, Zeng L, Bélanger M, Rodrigues PH, Simpson-Haidaris PJ, et al. Invasion of coronary artery endothelial cells by *Streptococcus mutans*. Oral Microbiol Immunol. 2009;24(2):141-5.
2. Alpert PT. Oral health: the oral-systemic health connection. Home Health Care Manag Pract. 2017;29(1):56-69.
3. Beck S. Impact of a systematic oral care protocol on stomatitis after chemotherapy. Cancer Nurs. 1979;23(1):85-99.
4. Berry AM, Davidson PM. Beyond comfort: oral hygiene as a critical nursing activity. Intensive Crit Care Nurs. 2006;22(6):318-28.

5. Dewhirst FE, Chen T, Izard J, Paster BJ, Tanner ACR, Yu WH, et al. The human oral microbiome. J Bacteriol. 2010;192(19): 5002-17.
6. Emily Brennan, Manchester Royal Infirmary. Nurse-led eye care in the Intensive Care Unit A protocol for practice. NHS Foundation trust.
7. Grap MJ, Munro CL. Preventing ventilator-associated pneumonia: evidence-based care. Crit Care Nurs Clin North Am. 2004;16(3): 349-58.
8. Hearne BJ, Hear EG, Montgomery H, Lightman SL. Eye care in the intensive care unit. Intensive Care Soc. 2018;19(4):345-50.
9. Hearne BJ, Hearne EG, Montgomery H, Lightman SL. Eye care in the intensive care unit. J Intensive Care Soc. 2018;19(4):345-50.
10. Henriksen BM, Ambjørnsen E, Axéll T. Evaluation of a mucosal-plaque index. Spec Care Dentist. 1999;19(1):15-47.
11. Heo SM, Haase EM, Lesse AJ, Gill SR, Scannapieco FA. Genetic relationships between respiratory pathogens and dental plaque. Clin Infect Dis. 2008;47(12):1562-70.
12. Hindlekar PS. Eye care. In: Shastri P (Ed). ICU Manual for Nurses. New Delhi: Jaypee Brothers Medical Publishers; 2017. pp. 19-22.
13. Javanmard R, Mozaffari N, Iranpour S, Shamshiri M. Application of the Modified Barrow Oral Care Protocol in Patients Receiving Mechanical Ventilation. J Crit Intensive Care. 2021;12:85-90.
14. Kaneoka A, Pisegna JM, Miloro KV, Lo M, Saito H, Riquelme LF, et al. Prevention of healthcare-associated pneumonia with oral care. Infect Control Hosp Epidemiol. 2015;36(8):899-906.
15. Marshall AP, Elliott R, Rolls K, Schacht S, Boyle M. Eye care in the critically ill: clinical practice guideline. Aust Crit Care. 2008;21:97-109.
16. Safdar N, Crnich CJ, Maki DG. The pathogenesis of ventilator-associated pneumonia. Respir Care. 2005;50(6):725-739.
17. Sands KM, Twigg JA, Lewis MAO, Wise MP, Marchesi JR, Smith A, et al. Microbial profiling of dental plaque in mechanically ventilated patients. J Med Microbiol. 2016;65(2):147-59.
18. Scannapieco FA, Bush RB, Paju S. Associations between periodontal disease and risk for nosocomial bacterial pneumonia and COPD. Ann Periodontol. 2003;8(1):54-69.
19. van der Maarel-Wierink CD, Vanobbergen JNO, Bronkhorst EM, Schols JMGA, de Baat C. Oral health care and aspiration pneumonia. Gerodontology. 2013;30(1):3-9.

CHAPTER 22

Delirium and Sedation in Intensive Care Unit

Swapnabharati Moharana, Swagata Tripathy

DELIRIUM IN INTENSIVE CARE UNIT

INTRODUCTION

Delirium is a nonspecific, generally reversible manifestation of an acute illness. In the intensive care unit (ICU), it is an independent predictor of mortality, prolonged ICU and hospital stay, increased cost of care, and long-term cognitive impairment. Delirium is a syndrome of acute onset of change in mental state with features of confusion, inattention, disorganized thinking, and altered level of consciousness. According to the Diagnostic and Statistical Manual of Mental Disorders 5 (DSM-5), delirium is defined as inattention (reduced ability to focus, sustain, or shift attention) that develops over a short period with additional feature of disturbance in cognition. Delirium is a common problem in elderly populations who are critically ill, but the incidence of delirium in mechanically ventilated patients in ICU remains as high as 80%. The pathophysiology of delirium needs to be better understood. However, there is an increased risk of delirium with the use of gamma aminobutyric acid (GABA) agonists and anticholinergics. The recent theories include the role of imbalance in neurotransmitters such as GABA, acetylcholine, and dopamine in the development of delirium.

TYPES OF DELIRIUM

There are three subtypes of delirium according to the psychomotor behavior of the patients:

1. *Hypoactive delirium (24.5–43.5%):* Lethargic, withdrawn, attitude, drowsiness, apathy, confusion, decreased responsiveness, and slowed motor function
2. *Hyperactive delirium (1.6–23%):* Agitation, restlessness, emotional lability, and paranoid
3. *Mixed delirium (52.5%):* The most frequent type. Patients manifest a fluctuation of hypoactive and hyperactive delirium features.

Hyperactive delirium is more quickly diagnosed by ICU staff than hypoactive subtypes due to the noticeable clinical features. Hypoactive delirium is often diagnosed late and not given immediate attention as the patients appear calm despite having delirium. The prognosis of hypoactive delirium is the poorest. Patients affected by hypoactive delirium show increased 6-month mortality compared to patients affected by other types of delirium.

INTENSIVE CARE UNIT DELIRIUM ASSESSMENTS

As delirium is associated with worse clinical outcomes, early diagnosis or assessment is imperative to prevent long-term

Flowchart 1: Confusion Assessment Method-ICU (CAM-ICU).

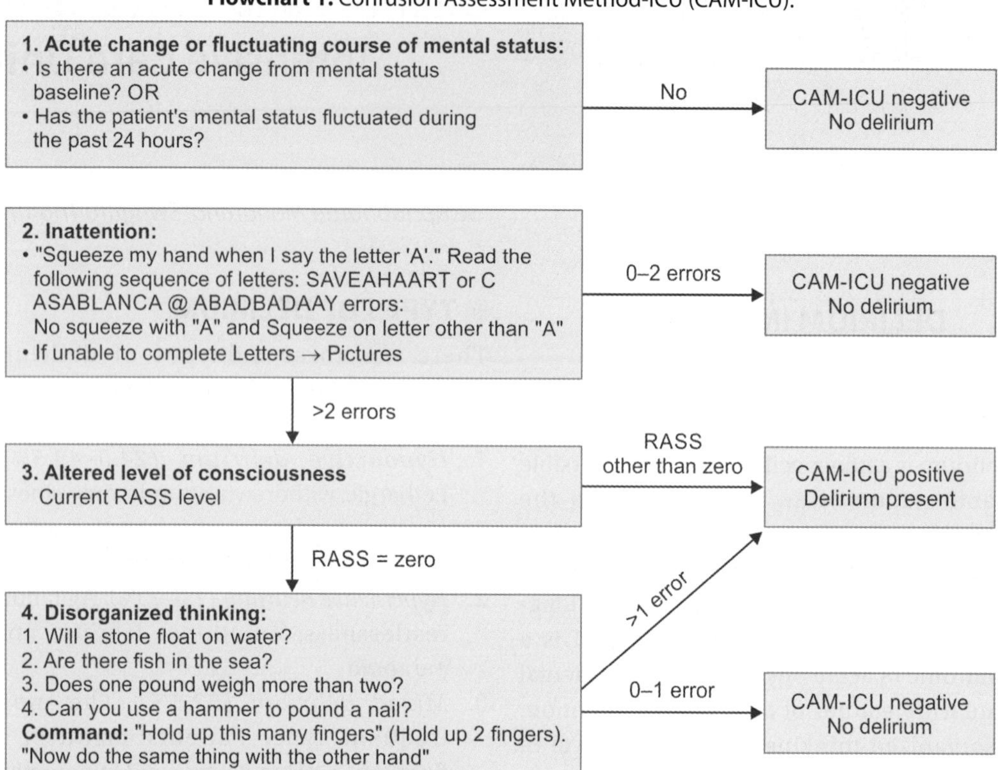

complications. Routine assessments will increase the rate of early detection of all types of delirium, and risk factors can be minimized, leading to a better prognosis. Therefore, it is recommended to do routine assessments at least once per shift as per the pain, agitation and delirium guidelines.

The Confusion Assessment Method-ICU (CAM-ICU) **(Flowchart 1)** is the most common screening tool used to diagnose delirium in the ICU.

The CAM-ICU involves a two-step assessment:

- *Step 1:* Evaluate the level of consciousness/arousal by using the Richmond Agitation Sedation Scale (RASS) **(Table 1)**.
- *Step 2:* Assess patients (moderately sedated, RASS score-3 or more alert) for four characteristics of delirium, i.e., acute onset of altered mental status, inattention, disorganized thinking, and altered level of consciousness. Three out of four features diagnose delirium.

CAUSES OF DELIRIUM

The potential causes of delirium broadly include:

- Infectious
- Alcohol/substance intoxication or withdrawal
- Hypoglycemia
- Medications
- Trauma

TABLE 1: Richmond Agitation Sedation Scale (RASS).

+4	Overtly combative, violent, and immediate danger to staff
+3	Pulls or removes tubes or catheters; aggressive
+2	Frequent nonpurposeful movement, fights ventilator
+1	Anxious, apprehensive but not aggressive
0	Alert and calm
–1	Drowsy, awakens to voice (eye opening/ eye contact) >10 seconds
–2	Light sedation, briefly awakens to voice (eye opening/eye contact) <10 seconds
–3	Moderate sedation, movement or eye opening to voice. But no eye contact
–4	Deep sedation, no response to voice, but movement or eye opening to physical stimulation
–5	Unarousable, no response to voice or physical stimulation

- Metabolic
- Hypoxia
- CNS disease
- Endocrinopathies
- Seizures
- Acute vascular
- Vitamin deficiencies
- Toxins
- Heavy metal ingestion

RISK FACTORS FOR DELIRIUM

There are numerous risk factors for delirium, and it is essential to identify the precipitating risk factors to minimize or avoid them.

Predisposing Factors

- Advanced age
- Baseline cognitive impairment
- Increased comorbid disease burden (especially respiratory disease)
- Frailty
- Alcohol and drug abuse
- High severity of illness
- Surgery (abdominal, hip, cardiac)

Precipitating Factors

Nonpharmacologic:

- Metabolic disturbances
- Hypotension
- Sepsis
- Mechanical ventilation
- Poor pain control
- Immobility (physical restraints, catheters)
- Sleep disturbances
- Reduced sensory input (blindness and deafness)
- Urinary retention or fecal impaction

Pharmacologic:

- Benzodiazepines
- Opioids
- Anticholinergics
- Steroid
- Deep sedation

COMPLICATIONS OF DELIRIUM IN INTENSIVE CARE UNIT PATIENTS

Critically ill patients in ICU who develop delirium may have various complications:

- Prolonged stay in the ICU
- Prolonged stay in hospital
- Longer duration of mechanical ventilation
- Increased incidence of ICU readmission
- Increased incidence of unintentional removal of catheters and tubes
- Risk of long-term cognitive impairment
- Increased cost of care
- Increased mortality

MANAGEMENT OF DELIRIUM

It includes prevention, nonpharmacologic interventions, and pharmacologic interventions.

Prevention of Delirium

Delirium prevention is paramount in minimizing the precipitating risk factors and decreasing the incidence and average duration of delirium.

The ABCDEF bundle checklist is a multicomponent, evidence-based guide for assessing and preventing delirium complications in the ICU **(Table 2)**. Interventions such as improving cognitive function, improving sleep hygiene, providing hearing aids and spectacles, and early mobilization should be encouraged. Pharmacologic agents are not recommended for preventing delirium in the ICU. Light sedation should be practiced for patients as it allows earlier detection of delirium and mobilization. In mechanically ventilated patients requiring sedation, dexmedetomidine infusion is recommended over benzodiazepine infusion (midazolam) to decrease the duration and incidence of delirium development.

Nonpharmacologic Interventions

- Cognitive behavior therapy includes frequent patient orientation and occupational therapy.
- Mobilization
- Family participation
- *Environmental interventions:* Noise reduction, exposure to natural bright light, and darkened lighting in the evening

TABLE 2: ABCDEF bundle checklist.

A	Assess, prevent, and manage pain
B	Both spontaneous awakening trials (SAT) and spontaneous breathing trials (SBT)
C	Choice of sedation and analgesia
D	*Delirium*: Assess, prevent, and management
E	Early mobility and exercise
F	Family engagement and empowerment

- *Restraints used in ICU:* The use of physical restraints (through any device, material, or apparatus attached to a patient's body which cannot be removed easily by the patient) in ICU is to protect the patients from self-harm, removing therapeutic devices and harm to others and restraining leads to increased risk of delirium, emotional distress for both patient and ICU staffs, damage to limbs, pressure injury and even death. So, physical restraints should be minimized, and when required, soft restraints may be used carefully for the shortest possible period and only after the failure of behavioral and pharmacologic interventions.

Pharmacologic Interventions

According to pain, agitation, and delirium guidelines:

- No single drug is effective in all types of delirium.
- There is only limited evidence that haloperidol decreases the duration of delirium in ICU patients.
- Atypical antipsychotics (e.g., olanzapine, risperidone, and quetiapine) may reduce the duration of delirium.
- Caution should be taken while using atypical antipsychotics and haloperidol in patients with QT prolongation or used with other QT interval prolonging medications.
- *Dexmedetomidine:* Continuous intravenous (IV) infusion administered for sedation in patients requiring mechanical ventilation reduces the duration of delirium.
- *Short-acting benzodiazepines*: Midazolam is helpful in patients with alcohol withdrawal.
- Rivastigmine, donepezil, and physostigmine are not recommended for delirium management in ICU.

SEDATION IN INTENSIVE CARE UNIT

The use of sedation in the ICU is a common practice. It is required to reduce physiological stress, alleviate pain, and reduce endotracheal tube tolerance, facilitate mechanical ventilation, and facilitate invasive procedures in the ICU. Appropriate sedation aims to make patients calm, comfortable, and cooperative without oversedation or undersedation.

PROBLEMS WITH OVERSEDATION

- Hypotension/bradycardia
- Immobility
- Delirium
- Failure to recognize cerebral insults
- Respiratory depression
- Poor cough
- Aspiration
- Gastroparesis
- Post-traumatic stress disorder
- Cognitive impairment
- Venous stasis

PROBLEMS WITH UNDERSEDATION

- Pain
- Hypertension
- Tachycardia
- Anxiety
- Ventilator asynchrony
- Post-traumatic stress disorder
- Agitation

MONITORING DEPTH OF SEDATION

Numerous methods are there to monitor the depth of sedation. The Richmond Agitation-Sedation Scale is the most valid, reliable, and commonly used method in ICU **(Table 1)**.

SEDATION PROTOCOLS

- Sedative medications need to be titrated to maintain light sedation rather than deep sedation in ICU patients unless clinically contraindicated according to pain agitation and delirium guidelines.
- Maintaining light sedation is associated with better clinical outcomes such as decreased delirium and decreased duration of mechanical ventilation and ICU stay.
- Nonbenzodiazepines (propofol or dexmedetomidine) should be preferred over sedation with benzodiazepines (midazolam) for better clinical outcomes in mechanically ventilated patients such as reduced duration and incidence of delirium, shortened duration of mechanical ventilation, reduced hospital, and ICU stay. **Table 3** describes the details of various sedative medications. Active metabolites of midazolam prolong sedation, especially in patients with renal failure. Avoid IV loading dose dexmedetomidine in hemodynamically unstable patients. Pain at the injection

TABLE 3: Clinical pharmacology of sedative medications.

Agent	Onset of action after IV loading dose	Elimination half-life	Active metabolites	Loading dose (IV)	Maintenance dose	Adverse effects
Midazolam (GABA agonist)	2–5 minutes	3–11 hours	Yes	0.01–0.05 mg/kg	0.02–0.1 mg/kg/h	Respiratory depression and hypotension

Contd...

Contd...

Lorazepam	15–20 minutes	8–15 hours	None	0.02–0.04 mg/kg	0.02–0.06 mg/kg q2–6 hours (≤10 mg)	Respiratory depression, hypotension, and propylene glycol-related acidosis, and nephrotoxicity
Diazepam	2–5 minutes	20–120 hours	Yes	5–10 mg	0.03–0.1 mg/kg q0.5–6 hours	Respiratory depression, hypotension, and phlebitis
Propofol	1–2 minutes	Short term use = 3–12 hours Long term use = 50 + 18/.6 hours	None	5 µg/kg/min over 5 minutes	5–50 µg/kg/min	Pain on injection, hypotension, respiratory depression, pancreatitis, and propofol infusion syndrome
Dexmede-tomidine (alpha 2 agonist)	5–10 minutes	1.8–3 hours	None	1 µg/kg over 10 minutes	0.2–0.7 µg/kg/h	Bradycardia, hypotension, and hypertension with loading dose

site occurs commonly when propofol is administered through peripheral veins.

FURTHER READING

1. American Psychiatric Association. Diagnostic and statistical manual of mental disorders: DSM-5. American Psychiatric Association; 2013.
2. Barr J, Fraser GL, Puntillo K, Ely EW, Gélinas C, Dasta JF, et al; American College of Critical Care Medicine. Clinical practice guidelines for the management of pain, agitation, and delirium in adult patients in the intensive care unit. Crit Care Med. 2013;41:263-306.
3. Cascella M, Fiore M, Leone S, Carbone D, Di Napoli R. Current controversies and future perspectives on treatment of intensive care unit delirium in adults. World J Crit Care Med. 2019;8:18-27.
4. Collet MO, Caballero J, Sonneville R, Bozza FA, Nydahl P, Schandl A, et al; AID-ICU cohort study co-authors. Prevalence and risk factors related to haloperidol use for delirium in adult intensive care patients: the multinational AID-ICU inception cohort study. Intensive Care Med. 2018;44:1081-9.
5. Ely EW, Inouye SK, Bernard GR, Gordon S, Francis J, May L, et al. Delirium in mechanically ventilated patients: validity and reliability of the confusion assessment method for the intensive care unit (CAM-ICU). JAMA. 2001;286:2703-10.
6. Fraser GL, Devlin JW, Worby CP, Alhazzani W, Barr J, Dasta JF, et al. Benzodiazepine versus nonbenzodiazepine-based sedation for mechanically ventilated, critically ill adults: a systematic review and meta-analysis of randomised trials. Crit Care Med. 2013; 41(9 Suppl 1):S30-8.
7. Goldberg TE, Chen C, Wang Y, Jung E, Swanson A, Ing C, et al. Association of Delirium With Long-term Cognitive Decline: A Meta-analysis. JAMA Neurol. 2020;77: 1373-81.

8. Gusmao-Flores D, Salluh JI, Chalhub RA, Quarantini LC. The confusion assessment method for the intensive care unit (CAM-ICU) and intensive care delirium screening checklist (ICDSC) for the diagnosis of delirium: a systematic review and meta-analysis of clinical studies. Crit Care. 2012;16:R115.
9. Hayhurst CJ, Pandharipande PP, Hughes CG. Intensive Care Unit Delirium: A Review of Diagnosis, Prevention, and Treatment. Anesthesiology. 2016;125:1229-41.
10. Hughes CG, McGrane S, Pandharipande PP. Sedation in the intensive care setting. Clin Pharmacol. 2012;4:53-63.
11. Mitchell DA, Panchisin T, Seckel MA. Reducing Use of Restraints in Intensive Care Units: A Quality Improvement Project. Crit Care Nurse. 2018;38:e8-16.
12. Reade MC, Finfer S. Sedation and delirium in the intensive care unit. N Engl J Med. 2014;370:444-54.
13. Riker RR, Shehabi Y, Bokesch PM, Ceraso D, Wisemandle W, Koura F, et al; SEDCOM (Safety and Efficacy of Dexmedetomidine Compared With Midazolam) Study Group. Dexmedetomidine vs midazolam for sedation of critically ill patients: a randomised trial. JAMA. 2009;301:489-99.
14. Robinson TN, Raeburn CD, Tran ZV, Brenner LA, Moss M. Motor subtypes of postoperative delirium in older adults. Arch Surg. 2011;146:295-300.
15. Stollings JL, Kotfis K, Chanques G, Pun BT, Pandharipande PP, Ely EW. Delirium in critical illness: clinical manifestations, outcomes, and management. Intensive Care Med. 2021;47:1089-103.

CHAPTER

23 Bedsore and Pressure Injuries

Durgesh Satalkar

INTRODUCTION

Pressure injuries are localized skin and soft tissue injuries that develop due to prolonged pressure exerted over specific areas of the body, typically bony prominences. These injuries demand prompt treatment to prevent potential lethal complications. Pressure injuries, also termed "bedsores", "decubitus ulcers", or "pressure ulcers (PU)". Areas that are particularly prone to pressure sores are those that cover the boney areas such as occiput, trochanters, sacrum, malleoli, and heel. However, they can also occur in the scapula, elbow, heel, shoulder, and ear.

In 2016, the National Pressure Ulcer Advisory Panel (NPUAP) released new terminology guidelines, and the preferred name is now "pressured injury" to "better reflect all forms of tissue damage, including the stage before skin breakdown." The organization also publically announced the change from NPUAP to the National Pressure Injury Advisory Panel (NPIAP).

ETIOLOGY

The development of pressure injuries is complex and multifactorial. External and internal factors co-occur to form these ulcers. Externally, prolonged pressure, friction, shear force, and moisture can lead to tissue deformation and ischemia. Internal factors such as malnutrition, anemia, and endothelial dysfunction can speed up the process of tissue damage.

Decreased mobility, skin moisture, poor nutritional status, and loss of sensory perception are the most common risk factors. Other identified risk factor are older age, cognitive impairment, and comorbid conditions affecting tissue healing.

The dysfunction of nervous regulatory mechanisms responsible for regulating local blood flow is also somewhat culpable in forming these ulcers. The common sites of bedsore are shown in **Figure 1**.

PATHOPHYSIOLOGY

Most important factor that contributes to ulceration is tissue ischemia and necrosis. Tissues can sustain an abnormal amount of external pressure, but constant pressure exerted over a prolonged period is the main culprit. External pressure must exceed the arterial capillary pressure of 32 mm Hg to impede blood flow. The pressure must be greater than the venous capillary closing pressure of 8–12 mm Hg to impair venous blood return. Sustaining pressure above these values leads to tissue ischemia and necrosis.

Besides occluding the blood flow, tissue distortion also obstructs lymphatic flow which in turn leads to accumulation of metabolic waste products, proteins, and enzymes in the affected tissue. It can compound tissue damage.

To put it more simply, any individual, with or without a medical condition, who is incapable of avoiding prolonged periods of

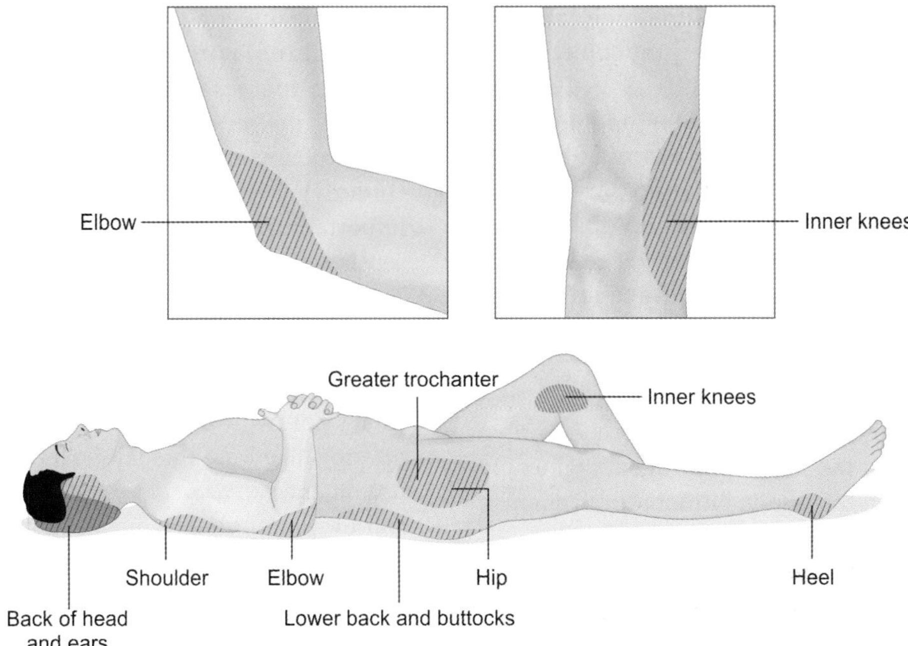

Fig. 1: Common sites of bedsore.

Flowchart 1: Cause of pressure ulcer.

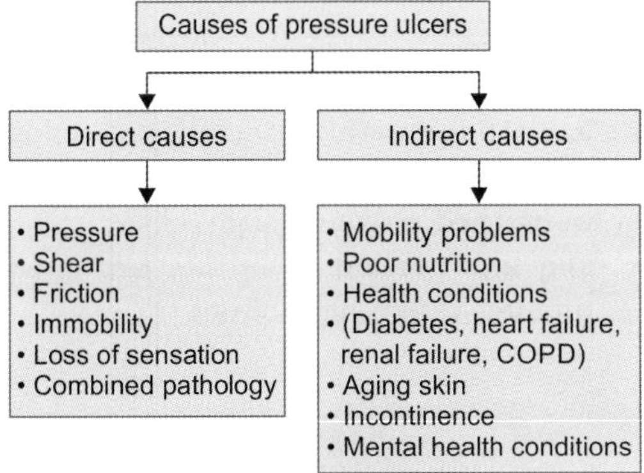

(COPD: chronic obstructive pulmonary disease)

an uninterrupted compression, is at a risk of PUs. The common causes of pressure sores are shown in **Flowchart 1**.

Failure of Reactive Hyperemia Cycle

It is a known fact that tissue distortion causes ischemia, that, in turn, stimulates protective movements to relieve pressure and circulatory activity to restore normal blood flow in the affected areas. Patients who fail to produce reactive hyperemia cannot recover from the pressure induced ischemic episodes resulting permanent damage to the tissues.

Clinically, this presents as white patches in pressure areas, which do not change color rapidly to the red of reactive hyperemia, as they would in a healthy person. Rather, the white patches remain for many minutes before slowly returning directly to a more normal skin color with little or no reactive hyperemia being observable.

INDIRECT CAUSES (ASSOCIATED FACTORS)

- *Age:* Advanced age contributes to the risk of PU development. Elderly individuals have less subcutaneous fat, decreased dermal thickness, and decreased sensory perception.
- *Delayed wound healing:* Conditions like diabetes mellitus (DM), peripheral

vascular diseases impair circulation, and will increase the probability of PU development.

- *Inadequate oxygenation:* Conditions that are associated with a hypoxia like heart failure, atrial fibrillation, myocardial infarction, and chronic obstructive pulmonary disease (COPD) can be major cause of PUs as oxygen is required for all stages of wound healing.
- *Contractures and spasticity:* It can contribute by repeatedly exposing tissues to pressure through flexion of a joint. Loss of sensations, the pain signal that would normally cause an immobile individual to change position is lost.
- Paralysis and insensibility may produce atrophy of skin leading to thinning of skin. Thus, skin becomes susceptible to frictional and shear forces when patients are being moved.
- Malnutrition, anemia, and hypoproteinemia can cause significant delays in wound healing.
- In trauma cases there is skin de-epithelialization happens and moisture causes maceration, adherence of the skin to clothing and any other supports in contact, resulting into further injury.
- Mental health conditions such as severe schizophrenia or severe depression have an increased risk of PUs due to neglect, malnutrition, and subsequent hypoproteinemia.
- Underlying disease severity is also an important factor for developing PU, e.g., sepsis and septic shock.

STAGING OF PRESSURE ULCERS

Stage I (Figs. 2A and B)

- Intact skin with nonblanchable redness of a localized area usually over a bony prominence.
- Darkly pigmented skin may not have visible blanching. Its color may differ from surrounding area.
- Discoloration of skin, warmth, edema, or pain may also be present.
- Involves only epidermal layer of skin.
- Indicate at risk person.

Stage II (Figs. 3A and B)

- Partial thickness loss of dermis presenting as a shallow open ulcer with a red/pink wound bed, *without* slough.
- May also present as an intact or open ruptured serum-filled blister.

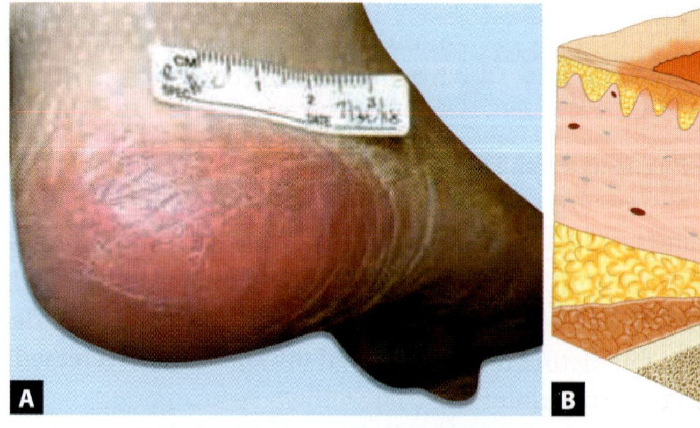

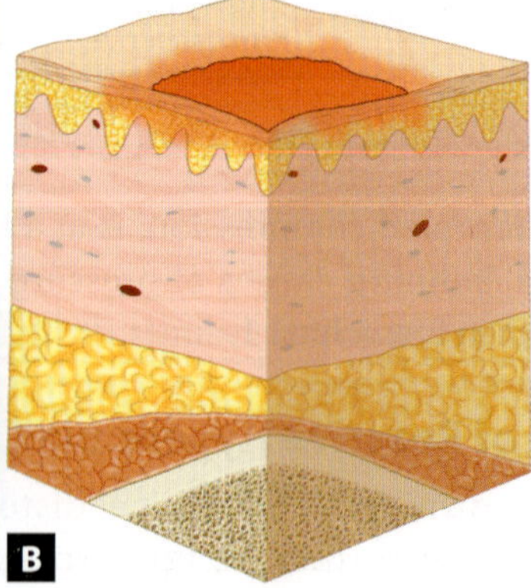

Figs. 2A and B: *Stages/classification of bedsores:* Stage I bedsore. The anatomical depth of involvement is shown in Figure 2B.

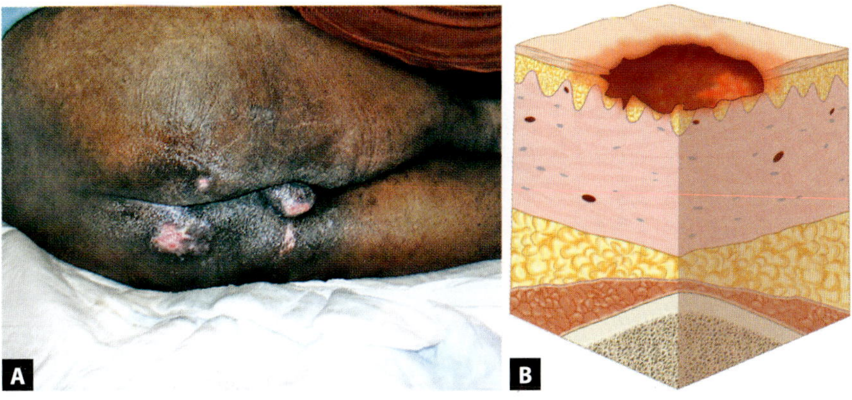

Figs. 3A and B: Stage II—pressure ulcer.

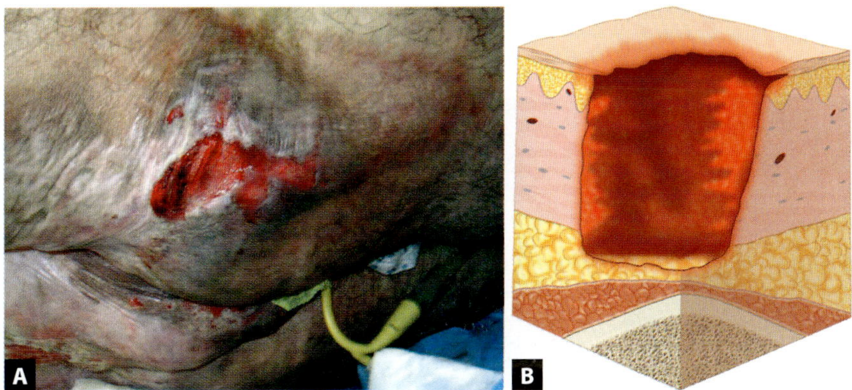

Figs. 4A and B: Stage III.

- Subcutaneous fat is not visible.
- Involves epidermis and dermis.

Stage III (Figs. 4A and B)

- Full thickness tissue loss. Subcutaneous fat may be visible, but bone, tendon, and/or muscle are not exposed.
- Slough may be present but does not obscure the depth of tissue loss. May include undermining and tunneling.
- Bone/tendon is not visible or directly palpable.

Stage IV (Figs. 5A and B)

- Full thickness tissue loss with exposed or directly palpable fascia, muscle, tendon, ligament, or bone
- Slough or eschar may be present on some parts of the wound bed. Often includes undermining and tunneling.

Unstageable (Figs. 6A and B)

- Full thickness tissue loss in which the base of the ulcer is covered by slough (yellow, tan, gray, green, or brown) and/or eschar in the wound bed.
- The wound bed is not visible.

Deep Tissue Injury (Figs. 7A and B)

- Localized and persistent nonblanchable purple or maroon discolored but intact skin or blood-filled blister.
- Due to damage of underlying tissue from prolonged pressure or shear at muscle bone interface.

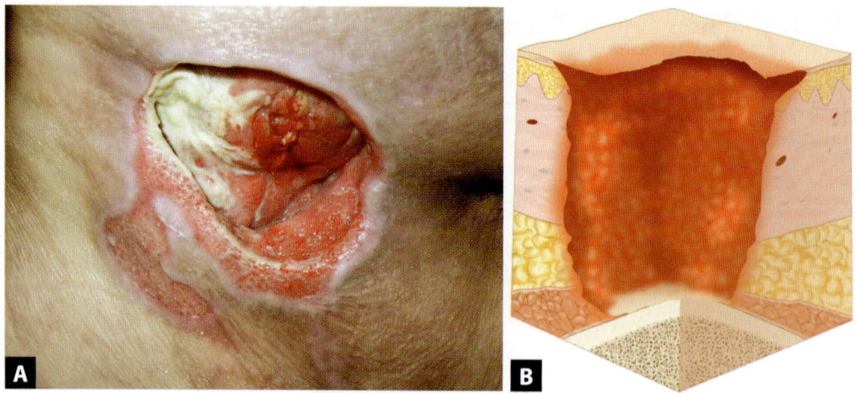

Figs. 5A and B: Stage IV.

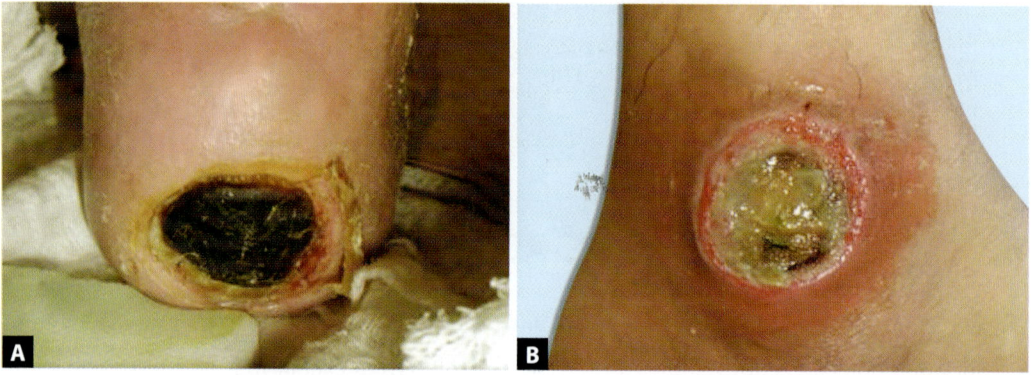

Figs. 6A and B: Unstageable—full thickness tissue loss.

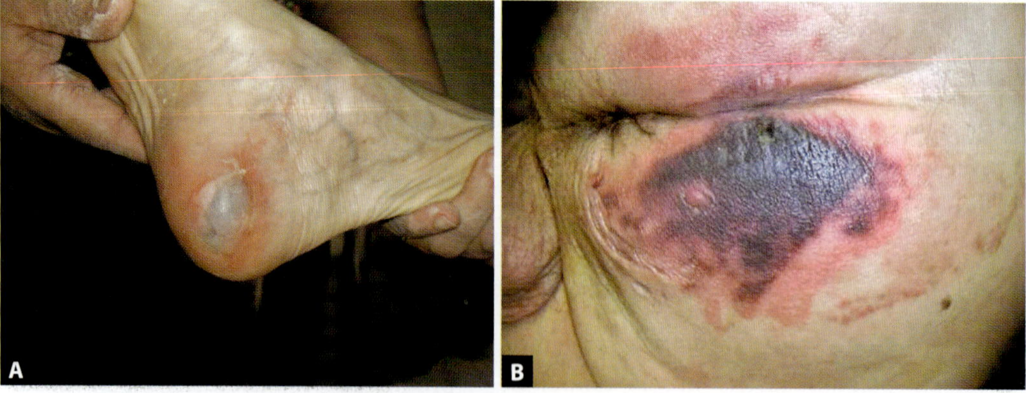

Figs. 7A and B: Deep tissue injury.

EVALUATION

Examine the following in a patient with a PU:

- Ulcer history, including etiology, duration, and previous treatment.
- Staging by thoroughly examining the depth of the wound, which this activity will cover in detail under "staging".
- Size of the affected area
- Sinus tracts, undermining, and tunneling
- The presence of drainage
- The presence of necrotic tissue

There are three risk assessment scales: (1) Waterlow, (2) Norton, and (3) Braden. *The Braden scale is the most common and accepted in the current literature.* It includes five sections worth 4 points and one section worth 3 points. Sum the points to provide a risk assessment score.

Braden Scale

- Sensory perception (1–4; completely limited, very limited, slightly limited, or no impairment).
- Mobility (1–4; completely immobile, very limited, slightly limited, or no limitations).
- Moisture (1–4; constantly moist, very moist, occasionally moist, and rarely moist).
- Nutrition (1–4; very poor, probably inadequate, adequate, and excellent).
- Activity (1–4; bedfast, chairfast, walks occasionally, and walks frequently).
- Friction and shear (1–3; problem, potential problem, and no apparent problem).

Scores

- Mild risk = 15–18
- Moderate risk = 13–14
- High risk = 10–12
- Very high risk = 9 or below.

MANAGEMENT

- Aim to reverse the factors that have originally caused the ulcer.
- Ulcers are often the result of combined pathology (like diabetes, pressure, and loss of sensation).
- In general, remove the possible causative factor (pressure, shear, and friction).

Always Emphasize Upon Prevention (Fig. 8)

Prevention consists of maintaining and improving tissue tolerance and appropriate offloading.

SKINCARE (FIG. 9)

- Skin condition should be inspected and documented daily for temperature, color, turgor, moisture status, and integrity.

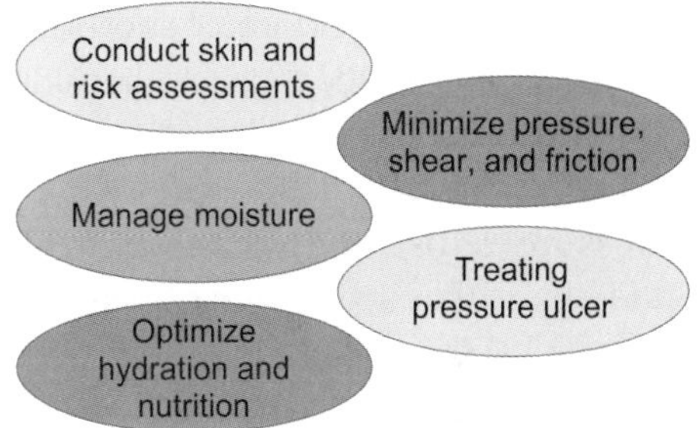

Fig. 8: Emphasis upon prevention.

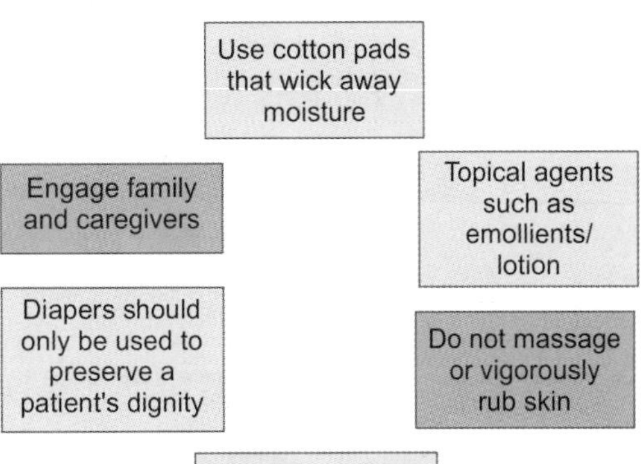

Fig. 9: Skincare.

- Avoid excessive dryness and scaling.
- Hot water to be avoided.
- Vigorous massage over bony prominence to be avoided.
- For incontinent patients protect skin from constant exposure to urine and feces.

Adequate Hydration/Nutrition (Fig. 10)

- Adequate nutrition helps to prevent ulcer formation and promote healing of early-stage ulcer.
- Ensure adequate nutrition. Target protein intake 1–1.5 g/kg/day unless contraindicated.

PROPER POSITIONING AND TURNING SCHEDULES

- Turning should be performed successively from back to one side then to other side to minimize interface pressure and maintain microcirculation at risk areas.
- Pressure redistribution through beds and chairs that avoid direct pressure on anatomical risk areas.
- Turning every 4 hours on a viscoelastic foam mattress/surface results in fewer PUs than turning every 2 hours on a standard mattress.
- Pillows or foam wedges should be placed between ankles and knees to avoid pressure at these sites when patients have no mobility at these areas.
- Keep pillows under lower legs to elevate hills and special heel protectors can be used.
- Patient should be placed at an angle of ≤30° when lying on their side to avoid direct pressure over greater trochanter or other bony prominences.
- Prevention of progression of a stage 1 pressure injury may require frequent positioning.

The salient features are summarized in **Figure 11**.

GENERAL CARE

- Appropriate local care which also includes debridement for patient with necrotic tissues.
- Consider adjunctive therapies such as negative pressure wound therapy.

Nutrition assessment:
- Weight status and weight loss
- Ability to eat independently
- Adequacy of intake

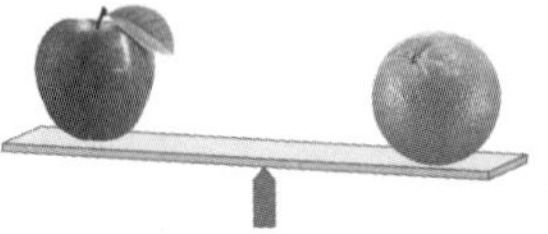

The three key food groups

Protein and energy and vitamin intake: Provide
- 1.25–1.5 g/kg body protein
- 30–35 kcal/kg body of energy
- Vitamin A and C contributes wound healing
- Enteral/parenteral supplement

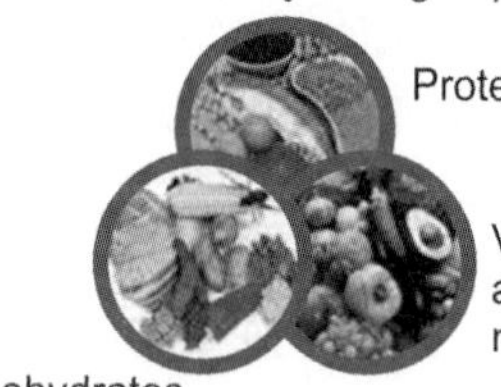

Hydration:
Monitor signs and symptoms of dehydration:
- Change in weight, skin turgor, urine output, and serum sodium
- Provide additional fluid

Fig. 10: Adequate hydration/nutrition assessment.

- Monitor document of patient's progress.
- Adequate analgesia using systemic and topical local anesthetics.

WOUND MANAGEMENT

- *Stage 1:* Skin injuries should be covered for protection.
- *Stage 2:* Generally, there is need of little debridement and requires dressing to maintain moist wound environment.
- *Stages 3 and 4:* Pressure or deeper injuries require debridement.
- Of necrotic tissue and possibly treatment of infection.
- After adequate wound bed preparation coverage involve skin grafting or other tissue transfer procedure.

The various measures to prevent pressure sores are shown in **Figures 11 to 13** and **Box 1**.

Minimize pressure shear and friction:

Off-load pressure over bony prominences:
- Position knees in slight flexion for offloading the heels
- If awake, ask about any complaints of pain
- Reposition patients at least every 2 hours in bed
- Every 15 minutes if chair bound
- Avoid positioning on existing pressure ulcer
- Use a 30-degree side-lying position (alternately, right side, back, and left side)

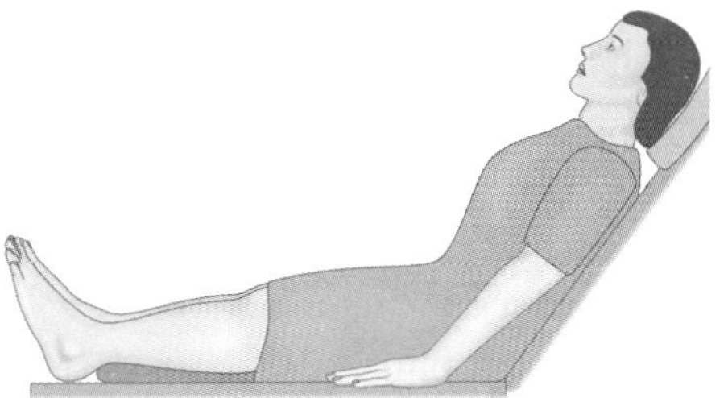

Fig. 11: Salient features of proper positioning and turning schedules.

Reduce friction and shearing forces:
- Wrinkle-free bed
- Proper seating alignment to reduce patient's tendency to slide down
- Do not drag/pull
- Use lift sheet while transferring patient

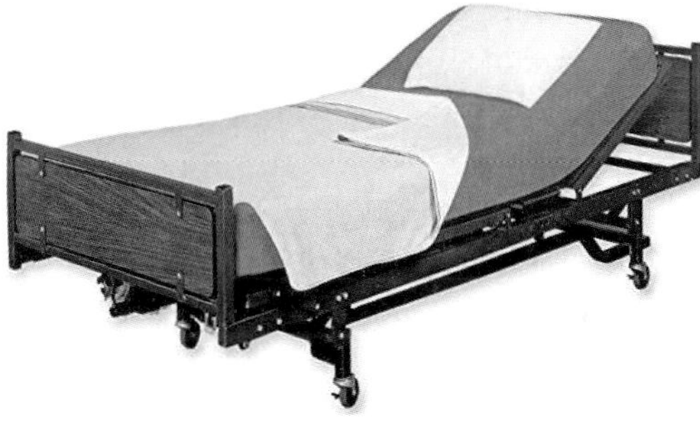

Fig. 12: Reducing friction and shearing forces.

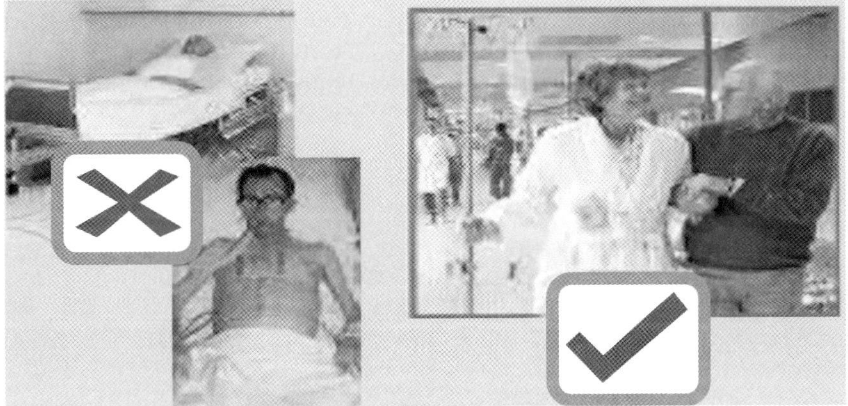

Fig. 13: Early mobilization.

BOX 1: Adequate support surfaces to redistribute pressure.

- Use pillows (only for limbs)
- Use special beds, mattresses, and foam wedges
- The following "devices" should not be used to elevate heels:
  - Synthetic sheepskin pads
  - Cutout ring, or donut-type devices
  - Intravenous fluid bags
  - Water-filled gloves

QUALITY INITIATIVES

- Education of staff on the best preventive practices.
- Standardize forms for documenting ulcer appearance and intervention.
- One or more nursing staff to be designated as skin champion.
- Instituting prompts for turning patient at regular intervals, e.g., music cues played over public address system at 2 hours interval.
- Availability of necessary supplies as special mattresses and overlay.
- Use of audit and feedback.

Uncertain Benefit for Adjunctive Therapies

Variety of adjunctive therapies have been investigated but their benefit remains uncertain:

- Hyperbaric oxygen therapy
- Topical oxygen
- Topical ultrasound
- Electrical stimulation

CONCLUSION

Pressure sore are a preventable complication in critical care. However, it requires training, awareness, and keen observation to assess them. Preventing pressure sores from happening and treating them when they occur both test the nursing standards of the unit.

FURTHER READING

1. Anders J, Heinemann A, Leffmann C, Leutenegger M, Pröfener F, von Renteln-Kruse W. Decubitus ulcers: pathophysiology and primary prevention. Dtsch Arztebl Int. 2010;107(21):371-81; quiz 382.
2. Bhattacharya S, Mishra RK. Pressure ulcers: Current understanding and newer modalities of treatment. Indian J Plast Surg. 2015;48(1):4-16.
3. Gefen A, Ousey K. COVID-19: pressure ulcers, pain and the cytokine storm. J Wound Care. 2020;29(10):540-2.
4. National Pressure Injury Advisory Panel. (2025). Prevention and Treatment of Pressure Ulcers/Injuries: Clinical Practice Guideline: The International Guideline. [online] Available from http://guidelinesales.com. [Last accessed February, 2025].
5. Zaidi SRH, Sharma S. Pressure Ulcer. In: Stat Pearls [Internet]. Treasure Island (FL): Stat Pearls Publishing; 2024.

CHAPTER

24 Physiotherapy and Mobilization

Parshotam Lal Gautam, Rubina Khullar Mahajan, Anoopjit Kaur

INTRODUCTION

Physiotherapy is a vital component in the management of patients admitted to the intensive care unit (ICU). Early mobilization plays a pivotal role to counteract the adverse physiological consequences of surgical stress and immobilization. This is one of the components of enhanced recovery after surgery (ERAS) pathways. There is a substantial evidence to support that it reduces the risk of postoperative complications. The role of physiotherapy conventionally has been limited to respiratory management, but rehabilitation and mobilization have equal priority for patients admitted to the ICU. Prolonged mechanical ventilation and immobilization can lead to muscle deconditioning and weakness, thus increasing morbidity, mortality, and physical impairment even after ICU discharge. Not only this, prolonged immobility has its effects on multiple systems of the body **(Fig. 1)**.

Despite the numerous reported benefits of physiotherapy in ICU, studies have shown

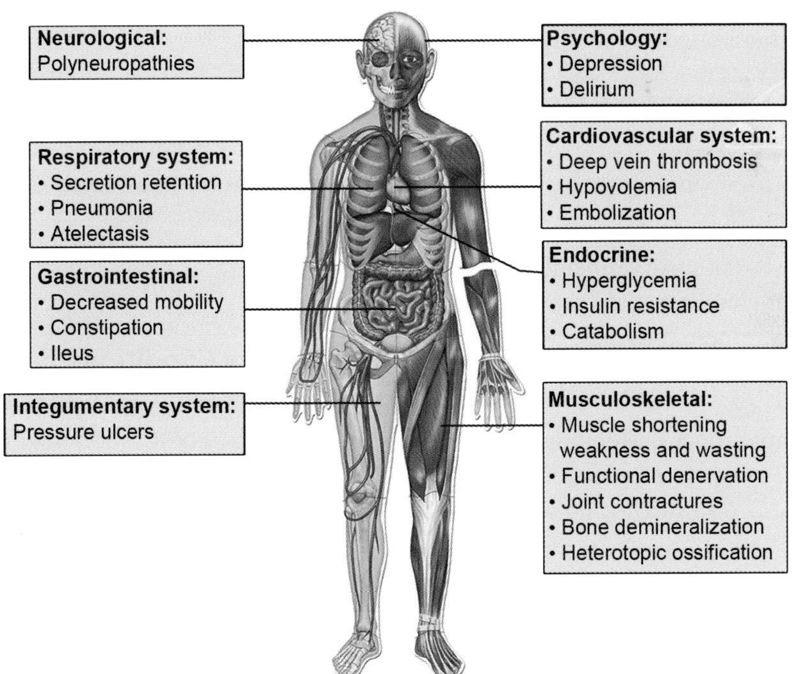

Fig. 1: Illustration of effects of prolonged immobility on various organ systems of the body.

TABLE 1: Barriers to physiotherapy in intensive care unit (ICU).

Patient related	*System related*	*Clinician related*	*Provider related*
• Lack of patient cooperation • Medical instability • Cognition level • Inadequate analgesia • Agitation • Excessive sedation	• Unavailability of a protocol • Lack of cost for protocol development • Lack of leadership management • Lack of environment, equipment, and resources • Interprofessional clinician staffing, workload, and time concerns • Interprofessional team coordination	• Lack of knowledge about protocol • Lack of confidence in protocol development • Patient's safety concerns • Safety concern regarding tubes and catheters • Perceived workload	• Limited staff • Poor communication • Inadequate training • Safety concerns • Perceived workload

that only 54% of all patients' days involved mobility and that too 95% of all patients on mechanical ventilation cannot be mobilized within first 72 hours. This inadequacy is probably because of lack of adequate manpower, safety concerns, and lack of availability of trained physiotherapists in the ICU. The various barriers to physiotherapy for ICU patients are listed in **Table 1**.

GOALS OF PHYSIOTHERAPY

Short-term Goals

- To maintain integrity of the respiratory system by reducing secretion retention, atelectasis, optimize ventilation perfusion ratio, oxygenation, improve respiratory muscle strength, minimize postoperative complications, and to reduce ventilator dependency.
- To prompt proper positioning throughout the ICU stay, thus protecting patient's joints and minimizing potential nerve damages and pressure sores and deconditioning related complications.
- To maintain the stability of musculoskeletal system by early ambulation
- Effective communication and emotional healing

Long-term Goals

- Reduce morbidity and mortality
- Reduce postintensive care weakness
- Rehabilitation of the patient and improve health-related quality of life.

ROLE OF PHYSIOTHERAPY IN INTENSIVE CARE UNIT

Physiotherapy plays a major role in three clinical areas in the ICU.

1. Respiratory conditions
2. Deconditioning and its related complications
3. Effective communication and emotional support in the ICU

Respiratory Conditions

Respiratory dysfunction is one of the most common causes of ICU admission. This may be related to the primary pathology of patient (pneumonias, acute respiratory distress syndrome, chest trauma, etc.) or be due to the prolonged immobility and ventilation (retention of secretions, atelectasis, etc.). Physiotherapy in respiratory dysfunction helps to clear secretions, improve lung ventilation and compliance, and to reduce

BOX 1: Techniques for optimization of cardiopulmonary function.

Techniques used in patients on mechanical ventilation:
- Lung hyperinflation techniques:
  - Manual hyperinflation
  - Ventilator hyperinflation
- Suction

Techniques which can be used in all patients:
- *Manual techniques:* Chest wall compression, chest shaking and vibrations, chest clapping/percussion
- Positioning/gravity-assisted positioning
- Mobility/rehabilitation
- Active cycle of breathing technique
- Intermittent positive pressure breathing
- Continuous positive airway pressure (CPAP)
- Oropharyngeal/nasopharyngeal suctioning
- Positive expiratory pressure (PEP) mask and flutter valve

Techniques which can be used only in spontaneously breathing patients (to help avoidance of intubation or facilitate weaning):
- Noninvasive ventilation (NIV) insufflator
- Incentive spirometry

airway resistance and work of breathing. The objective is to recruit areas of atelectasis and improve ventilation/perfusion (V/Q) matching, regional lung ventilation, lung compliance, and hence oxygenation. The various techniques for optimization of cardiopulmonary function are listed in **Box 1**.

- *Lung hyperinflation techniques:*
  - *Manual hyperinflation (MHI):* Using a manual resuscitator or an AMBU bag, tidal volumes (Vt) 100–150% more than the baseline Vt, with a slow inspiratory flow are delivered, to target a peak airway pressure of no >40 cmH_2O, followed by an inspiratory hold of 2–3 seconds and a fast expiratory flow which generates a whirlwind peak expiratory flow and mimics forced expiration. The dosage varies from two cycles of six breaths to six cycles of six breaths.
  - *Ventilator hyperinflation (VHI):* The settings of the ventilator are altered to achieve larger than baseline Vt. Advantages over MHI include maintenance of positive end-expiratory pressure (PEEP) and reproducibility of the technique. It can be performed in both spontaneous and controlled modes of ventilation.
    - *Advantages:* Increased Vt along with inspiratory hold allows alveolar recruitment, reduces atelectasis, and improves lung compliance. Increased expiratory flow helps to mobilize secretions.
    - *Disadvantages:* Hyperinflation of the lung can lead to marked hemodynamic instability due to raised intrathoracic pressure.
- *Suctioning:* Patients admitted to the ICU may have excessive secretions either due to placement of an artificial airway or poor cough reflex. Accumulation of secretions leads to airway obstruction and ineffective airflow. Mechanical aspiration of secretions by suctioning helps to keep the respiratory tract clear, ultimately improving the gas exchange.

  Indications:
  - Removal of secretions/blood from the respiratory tract and taking samples for diagnostic purposes (microbiological or histological)
  - To keep a clear field of vision with certain procedures like during fiberoptic bronchoscopy
  - To maintain the patency of artificial airways like endotracheal tube or tracheostomy tube

Personnel: Respiratory therapists, nurses, physicians, and even relatives can learn the procedure.

Equipment required (for suctioning of artificial airway):

- Oxygen source and vacuum with calibrated collection container
- Personal protective equipment (PPE) including (clean and sterile gloves, masks, and goggles)
- Sterile saline
- Manual resuscitator or Bains circuit for ventilation
- Monitoring equipment (stethoscope, pulse oximetry, and heart rate)
- A sterile suction catheter
- Medication for patient's comfort (if required)

Procedure: The patient should be explained about the procedure if awake. After proper preoxygenation, wearing PPE and ensuring adequate monitoring, airway is suctioned with appropriately sized suction catheter according to the size of the airway (i.e., 50% of the internal diameter of endotracheal tube). Suction pressure kept should be <200 mm Hg in adults and 80–120 mm Hg in neonates.

Complications: Hypoxemia, atelectasis mechanical trauma, bacterial contamination, cardiac arrhythmias, patient's distress, and anxiety.

- *Chest physical therapy (CPT):* It consists mainly of chest percussion, vibration, breathing exercises, coughing and cough stimulation techniques, postural drainage, suctioning, and patient's mobilization. The forced expiration technique, active cycle of breathing, intermittent positive pressure breathing, positive expiratory pressure, and use of a flutter valve are other techniques which help to keep the airway open in cooperative patients.

Indications:

- *Prophylactic use:*
    - Acute neurological diseases in which the innervation of intercostal, diaphragmatic, and abdominal muscles is involved.
    - Smoke inhalation
    - Acute brain injury
- *Therapeutic use:*
    - Retained secretions not amenable to removal by coughing, turning, and suctioning.
    - Radiological presence of acute atelectasis or infiltrate
    - Retained secretions causing decrease in arterial oxygenation (PaO_2) or oxygen saturation (SpO_2) **(Flowchart 1)**.
- *Incentive spirometry:* It reduces atelectasis and improves airway clearance.

Technique: Patient's cooperation is required. The patient holds the device and does a maneuver mimicking a yawn or a sigh, which increases the lung volume and opens up the collapsed areas of lung. After a normal expiration, the patient breathes in slowly and deeply for as long as possible and then holds his breath for a period of 5–10 seconds (maximizing distribution), followed by a normal expiration. The device gives feedback on performance from the gauge.

Deconditioning and its Related Complications

Because of the nature of critical illness, prolonged bed rest is unavoidable in ICU. The fear that the critically ill patients may not tolerate mobilization, and has been put to rest by the recent studies. It is now proven that early physical activity is safe after cardiorespiratory and neurological stabilization. Early mobilization, commenced within 2–5 days, is early application and intensification of physical rehabilitation in

Flowchart 1: Illustration of pathways and modalities for increasing airway clearance.

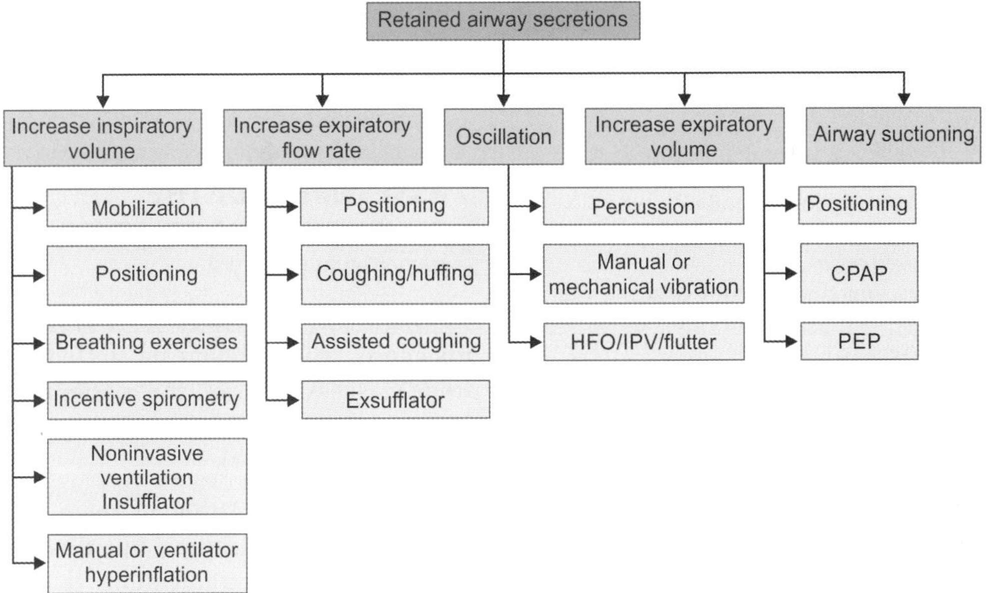

(CPAP: continuous positive airway pressure; HFO: high-frequency oscillation; IPV: intermittent percussive ventilation; PEP: positive expiratory pressure)

Source: Reproduced from the article "Physiotherapy for adult patients for critical illness: recommendations from the European Respiratory Society and European Society of Intensive Care Medicine Taskforce on Physiotherapy of Critically Ill Patients".

critically ill patients. Physical activity is not shown to have any adverse effects on the inflammatory status of ICU patients.

Once the patient stabilizes, the specific need for mobilization is determined and then form of mobilization or exercise in a dosage (intensity) that will match the patient's oxygen carrying capacity is decided. Monitoring is done by monitoring the oxygen transport and its indices, and patient's vitals. The mobilization is repeated as the patient tolerates and the intensity increased if patient's capacity permits and vitals are stable.

The treatment modalities to prevent physical deconditioning include:

- *Positioning:* Strategies include—
  - *Head tilt:* It increases gravitational stress and fluid shifts.
  - *Upright position:* It increases lung volumes and improves gas exchange. It also stimulates autonomic activity and reduces cardiac stress from compression.
- *Mobilization:* It is defined as physical activity sufficient enough to induce acute physiological effects which will improve ventilation, circulation, perfusion, muscle metabolism, alertness, and prevent venous stasis and hence deep vein thrombosis. The various strategies for mobilization are illustrated in **Box 2**. Apart from these, abdominal belts stabilize, and improve exercise capacity and vital capacity in spinal cord injury patients. Some patients (some neurological diseases, burns, and trauma) who are at hight risk for soft-tissue contractures may

BOX 2: Strategies for mobilization in the intensive care unit (ICU).

Strategies for mobilization:
- Passive and active range of motion
- Active side-to-side turning
- Bed sitting
- Exercising in the bed
- Use of cycling pedals in bed
- Continuous lateral rotational therapy with specialized beds
- Transfers from the bed to the chair and vice versa
- Chair exercises
- Standing aids (modified walking frames, and tilt tables)
- Walking
- Hoist therapy (allows the patient to move to vertical position and mobilize safely)
- Resistive muscle training
- Neuromuscular electrical stimulation
- Aerobic training and muscle strengthening (in chronic critical illness)

require splinting. Noninvasive ventilation (NIV) during mobilization may improve exercise tolerance.

Effective Communication and Emotional Support in Intensive Care Unit

Critically ill patients admitted in the ICU often feel lonely and anxious. Anxiety adversely affects their recovery, and many patients suffer from post-traumatic stress disorder. Physiotherapists play an important role in emotional well-being of the patient by:

- *Relaxation interventions:* Decrease anxiety and promote sleep.
- *Body positioning and repositioning:* May improve breathlessness and decrease anxiety.
- *Therapeutic touch:* Provides comfort and enhances sleep.
- *Massage:* Reduces pain, anxiety, and enhances relaxation.
- *Communication:* Promotes patient's satisfaction and provides emotional support. Informed consent provides patient's autonomy and makes them feel empowered.

ASSESSMENT OF THE PATIENT BEFORE STARTING PHYSIOTHERAPY

Although physiotherapy is a very safe procedure, still it should be started after proper assessment of the patient and ensuring safety through safety criteria checklist **(Flowchart 2)**.

Contraindications: Although there is no absolute contraindication, but there are some relative contraindications to avoid unintentional harm. These are as follows:

- Head injury with raised intracranial pressure
- Unstable cervical spine injury
- Hemodynamic instability
- Undrained pneumothorax
- Severe bronchospasm
- Positive end-expiratory pressure ventilation
- High frequency of oscillation ventilation
- Nitric oxide ventilation

Precautions have to be taken in patients who are on high PEEP as they may desaturate during the procedure.

ADVERSE EFFECTS

The frequency of adverse effects with early mobilization in the ICU is <4% and most of these are benign. Tachypnea, desaturation, heart rate elevation over 20%, postural hypotension, discomfort, agitation, unplanned extubation, device dislodgment, and falls have been reported.

Flowchart 2: Ensuring safety before mobilization of critically ill patients.

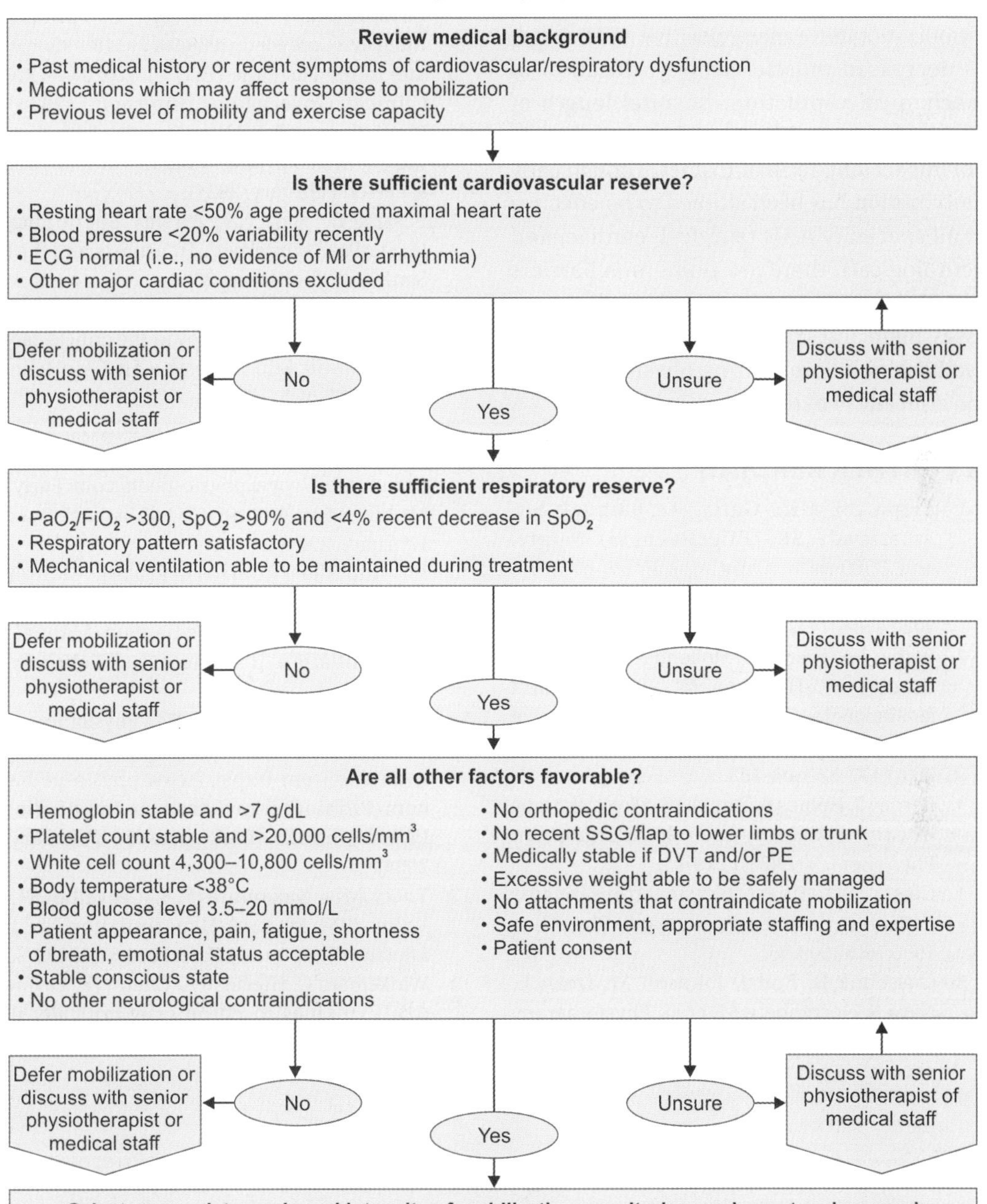

Source: Reproduced from the article "Physiotherapy for adult patients for critical illness: recommendations from the European Respiratory Society and European Society of Intensive Care Medicine Taskforce on Physiotherapy of Critically Ill Patients".

CONCLUSION

Respiratory physiotherapy and early mobilization have many positive effects such as decreased muscle atrophy, duration of mechanical ventilation, hospital length of stay, and increased functional capacity but do not impact long-term outcomes. Though early mobilization has been studied to be effective in all speciality ICUs (surgical, cardiac, and neurological), there are numerous barriers which need to be overcome, and proper assessment and safety of the patient has to be established before starting physiotherapy in the critically ill patients.

FURTHER READING

1. Alaparthi GK, Gatty A, Samuel SR, Amaravadi SK. Effectiveness, Safety, and Barriers to Early Mobilization in the Intensive Care Unit. Crit Care Res Pract. 2020; 2020:e7840743.
2. Barber EA, Everard T, Holland AE, Tipping C, Bradley SJ, Hodgson CL. Barriers and facilitators to early mobilisation in Intensive Care: a qualitative study. Aust Crit Care. 2015; 28(4):177-82; quiz 183.
3. Berney S, Haines K, Denehy L. Physiotherapy in Critical Care in Australia. Cardiopulm Phys Ther J. 2012;23(1):19-25.
4. Ciesla ND. Chest physical therapy for patients in the intensive care unit. Phys Ther. 1996;76(6):609-25.
5. Gosselink R, Bott J, Johnson M, Dean E, Nava S, Norrenberg M, et al. Physiotherapy for adult patients with critical illness: recommendations of the European Respiratory Society and European Society of Intensive Care Medicine Task Force on Physiotherapy for Critically Ill Patients. Intensive Care Med. 2008;34(7):1188-99.
6. Life in the FastLane (FITFL). (2020).—CCC Clinical Governance [Internet]. (2024). Physiotherapy in ICU. [online] Available from https://litfl.com/physiotherapy-in-icu/ [Last accessed February, 2024].
7. Pasrija D, Hall CA. Airway Suctioning. In: StatPearls [Internet]. Treasure Island (FL): StatPearls Publishing; 2024.
8. Pathmanathan N, Beaumont N, Gratrix A. Respiratory physiotherapy in the critical care unit. Contin Edu Anaesth Crit Care Pain. 2015;15(1):20-5.
9. Physiopedia [Internet]. (2024). Early Mobilization in the ICU. [online] Available from https://www.physio-pedia.com/Early_Mobilization_in_the_ICU [Last accessed February, 2024].
10. Physiopedia [Internet]. (2024). Manual Hyperinflation. [online] Available from https://www.physio-pedia.com/Manual_Hyperinflation [Last accessed February, 2024].
11. Physiopedia [Internet]. (2024). Physiotherapy Assessment of the Patient in ICU. [online] Available from https://www.physio-pedia.com/Physiotherapy_Assessment_of_the_Patient_in_ICU [Last accessed February, 2024].
12. Tucci MR, Nakamura MA, Carvalho NC, Volpe MS. Manual Hyperinflation: Is It Effective? Respiratory Care. 2019;64(7):870-3.
13. Winkelman C, Higgins PA, Chen YJK, Levine AD. Cytokines in chronically critically ill patients after activity and rest. Biol Res Nurs. 2007;8(4):261-71.

CHAPTER 25

Transferring a Critically Ill Patient

Manish Munjal, Bikram K Gupta, Preeti Singh

INTRODUCTION

Patient care transfer can be defined as moving a patient from one flat surface to another or to other definitive care units. Patient care transfer can also be defined as transferring patients within the same facility and between facilities.

Patient care transfers are an essential yet often neglected aspect of patient care. Patient care transfers are an indispensable aspect of patient care, requiring rigorous adherence to clinical guidelines. Proper transfers are based on the concept that focuses on maintaining continuity of care both during and after the transfer. Poorly organized patient's transfers can result in increased morbidity and mortality and should be performed with careful attention.

For trauma patients, if definitive care cannot be provided at a local hospital, transfer the patient to the closest appropriate hospital that has the resources and capabilities to care for the patient is required. Ideally, this facility should be a verified trauma center at a level that is appropriate to the patient's needs.

DETERMINING THE NEED FOR PATIENT'S TRANSFER

It is essential that clinicians assess their own capabilities and limitations, as well as those of their institution, to allow for early differentiation between patients who may be safely cared for in the local hospital and those who require transfer to specialty centers.

Decision to Transfer and Communication

- The decision to transfer the patient should be taken by a senior consultant level doctor after thorough discussion with patient's relatives about the benefits and risks involved.
- A written and informed consent of patient's relatives along with the reason to transfer is mandatory before the transfer.
- Dedicated critical care transfer groups should be established to coordinate and facilitate the patient's transfer.
- These groups also arrange appropriate facilities at the receiving hospital or facility. A direct communication between the transferring and receiving facility should be undertaken with sharing of complete information on patient's clinical condition, treatment being given, reasons for transfer, mode of transfer, and timeline of transfer in a written document.
- *Check for following before transfer:* Perform proper hand hygiene, check the patient's chart/room for any additional precautions, introduce the team to the patient and the patient's family, confirm the patient's identification, and ensure patient's privacy.
- The pretransfer stabilization and preparation checklist is shown in **Table 1**.

TABLE 1: Pretransfer stabilization and preparation.

Primary survey	*Findings*	*Interventions*	*Consider transfer?*
Airway	Airway compromise	Intubate, end-tidal CO_2, pulse oximeter, EKG, chest X-ray	Yes
	High risk for airway loss	Monitor EKG, pulse oximeter, and arterial blood gas	Yes
Breathing	Tension pneumothorax	Needle, finger, and chest tube	Yes
	Hemothorax Open pneumothorax	Chest X-ray and chest tube	Yes
	Hypoxia/hypoventilation	Intubate	Yes
Circulation	Hypotension	Reliable IV/IO access, warm IV fluids, control external hemorrhage using pressure, topical hemostatic, or tourniquets	Yes
	Pelvic fracture	Pelvic X-ray, pelvic binder, or sheet	Yes
	Vascular injury	Reliable IV/IO access, warm IV fluids, control external hemorrhage using pressure, topical hemostatic, or tourniquets	Yes
	Open fracture	Reduce and splint and dress	Yes
	Abdominal distention	Focused assessment with sonography in trauma (FAST)	Yes
Disability	GCS <13	Intubate if GCS is <8	Yes
	Intoxicated patient who cannot be evaluated	Sedate and intubate	Yes
	Evidence of paralysis	Restrict spinal motion	Yes
Exposure	Severe hypothermia	External warming	Yes

(GCS: Glasgow Coma Scale; IO: intraosseous IV: intravenous)

SAFE PATIENT'S TRANSFER TECHNIQUES

Safe patient's transfer techniques involve several steps, including assessing the patient's ability to participate in a transfer, preparing the environment for the transfer, and using the correct assistive devices. Before transferring a patient, caregivers should assess the patient's ability to bear weight, stability, and level of consciousness. The environment should be well-lit and free of obstacles.

TYPES OF TRANSFERS

There are several types of patient's transfer techniques, each tailored to accommodate the individual physical ability and specific needs of the patient. Healthcare professionals should consider factors such as mobility limitations, motor skills, and medical conditions to determine the most suitable transfer method for each individual patient.

- *Pivot transfer:* The patient moves from one surface to another with the aid of a pivot point, which are generally the patient's feet or buttocks. It is commonly used for wheelchair transfers and is particularly beneficial for individuals with limited mobility. This transfer helps to rotate the patient from one direction to the other. Patient's safety belts are often used in conjunction with pivot transfers.

- *Lift transfer:* This technique involves the use of a mechanical or electrical device designed to safely and efficiently lift and move the patient without the need for physical lifting. This is especially helpful for patients with no mobility, and can greatly reduce both the risk of injury and number of caregivers needed during the transfer. A sling is placed snugly around the patient and attached securely to the lift to prepare for a safe transfer.
- *Board transfer:* Different types of boards can be used to transfer patients either laterally for those with no mobility or in a seated position for those with limited mobility. To facilitate the process, the caregiver carefully places a board beneath the patient and provides assistance as the patient moves or is moved from one surface to another.
- *Air-assisted lateral transfer:* Air-assisted lateral transfer systems work similarly to air hockey tables, reducing friction by circulating low-pressure, high-volume air through 100s of microperforations. This creates a cushion of air to help smoothly, comfortably, and safely lift and glide patients from surface to surface, drastically reducing overall pull force and the risk of staff injuries compared to traditional transfer devices.

TRANSFER EQUIPMENT

Transfer equipment is used to facilitate safe and easy transfers for both patients and caregivers. Some of the most commonly used types of transfer equipment include grab bars, gait belts, transfer sheets, shifters, roll boards, lifts and slings, transfer boards, pivot disks, and air-assisted lateral transfer systems.

- *Grab bars:* Grab bars offer support for patients, enabling them to confidently and independently pull themselves up to a standing position or maintain their balance during transfers.
- *Gait belts:* Also called transfer belts or patient's safety belts, gait belts are commonly used in healthcare settings to provide additional support and stability to patients who may be unsteady on their feet or have weakened leg muscles. By securely fastening the transfer belt around the patient's waist, healthcare providers can ensure a higher level of safety and confidence during transfers, thus reducing the risk of falls or injuries.
- *Transfer sheets:* Slide sheets allow you to move a patient without lifting them. They come in various sizes and materials, ensuring flexibility and adaptability for different patients' needs.
- *Shifters:* Shifters are placed between two surfaces to safely bridge any gaps or height differences. Most models are made using materials that allow the patient to slide easily across the board for a smooth and easy transfer.
- *Roll boards:* The cover of a roll board rotates around the frame and moves with the patient, acting like a conveyer belt. This gently pushes the patient from one surface to another, helping to reduce the overall friction and force required.
- *Lifts and slings:* Mechanical or electric lifts eliminate the need for manual lifting, helping reduce the risk of injury for staff. The patient is placed securely into a sling, which is attached to the lift to facilitate a comfortable and safe transfer.

- *Transfer boards:* Transfer boards can be used with patients who have limited upper and/or lower body strength and are able to sit up while maintaining balance. These boards help to facilitate transfers between two-seated surfaces, such as a bed, chair, wheelchair, or toilet.
- *Pivot disks:* Pivot disks are designed for use during pivot transfers with patients who can stand but cannot readily move their legs. Patient's safety belts or slings are recommended for use with pivot disks to provide additional support.
- *Air-assisted lateral transfer systems:* These systems help to transfer patients up to 1,200 lbs. from surface to surface with only two caregivers needed. This method reduces overall pull force and decreases the risk of staff injuries.

Equipment required for monitoring **(Fig. 1)**

TRANSFER PROTOCOLS

- *Information from referring doctor:* The doctor who determines that patient's transfer is necessary should speak directly to the physician accepting the patient at the receiving hospital. The ABC-SBAR (airway, breathing, circulation followed by situation, background, assessment, and recommendation) can serve as a checklist for the telephone report between physicians and the verbal report to transporting personnel **(Table 2)**.
- *Information to transferring personnel:* Information regarding the patient's condition and needs during transfer should be communicated to the transporting personnel.
- *Documentation*: A written record of the problem, treatment given, and the patient's status at the time of transfer, as well as certain physical items.
- *Treatment during transport:* Trained personnel should transfer the patient, based on the patient's condition and potential problems. Treatment during transport typically includes: Monitoring vital signs and pulse oximetry, and

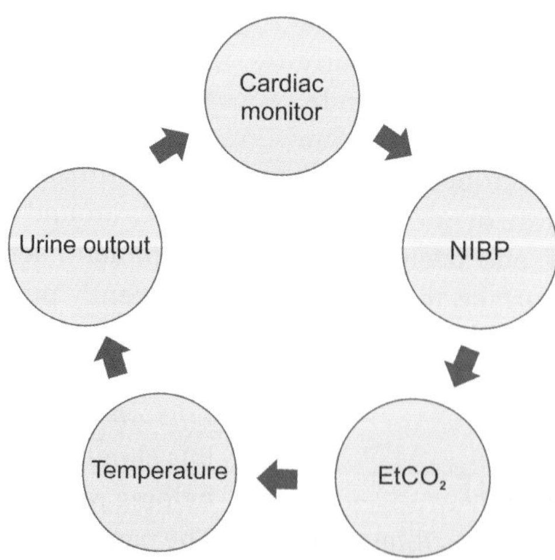

Fig. 1: Basic monitoring checklist during the patient's transfer. ($EtCO_2$: end-tidal carbon dioxide; NIBP: noninvasive blood pressure)

TABLE 2: Checklist for patient's transfer note and documentation.

ABC-SBAR—an acronym		
Acronym	***Meaning***	***Information to provide***
A *B* *C*	• Airway • Breathing • Circulation	All airway, breathing, and circulation problems identified and interventions performed
S	Situation	• Patient's name: ____ • Age: ____ • Referring facility: ____ • Referring physician's name: ____ • Reporting nurse's name: ____ • Indication for transfer: ____ • IV access site: ____ • IV fluid and rate: ____ • Other interventions completed: ____
B	Background	• Event history: ____ • AMPLE assessment: ____ • Blood products: ____ • Medications given (date and time): ____ • Imaging performed: ____ • Splinting: ____
A	Assessment	• Vital signs: ____ • Pertinent physical examination findings: ____ • Patient's response to treatment ____
R	Recommendation	• Vital signs: ____ • Transport mode: ____ • Level of transport care: ____ • Medication intervention during transport: ____ • Needed assessments and interventions: ____

(AMPLE: allergies, medications, past medical history, last meal time, events leading to presentation; IV: intravenous)

continuing support of cardiorespiratory system.

A typical documentation during patient's transfer is shown in **Table 2**.

CONCLUSION

Most of the critically ill patients are unstable. Their condition may deteriorate during any transfer. Set protocols, specialized instruments and a properly trained team are all necessary to make the process of transfer safer.

FURTHER READING

Book

1. ATLS INDIA, 10th edition.
2. Bergman R, De Jesus O. Patient Care Transfer Techniques. [Updated 2022 Oct 17]. In: StatPearls [Internet]. Treasure Island (FL): StatPearls Publishing; 2024.

3. Kulshrestha A, Singh J. Inter-hospital and intra-hospital patient transfer: Recent concepts. Indian J Anaesth. 2016;60(7):451-7.

Online

1. https://www.ncbi.nlm.nih.gov/books/NBK564305/
2. AliMed. (2023). Patient Transfer Techniques for Safe, Effective Transfers. [online] Available from https://www.alimed.com/patient-transfer-techniques-for-safe-effective-transfers-blog/ [Last accessed February, 2024].
3. Access Physiotherapy. (2014). Chapter 13: Patient Transfers and Mobility. [online] Available from https://accessphysiotherapy.mhmedical.com/content.aspx?bookid=1472§ionid=86198760 [Last accessed February, 2024].
4. BCcampus. (2015). 3.7 Patient Transfers. [online] Available from https://opentextbc.ca/clinicalskills/chapter/3-7-transfers-and-ambulation/ [Last accessed February, 2024].
5. Munjal M, Ahmed SM, Garg R, Das S, Chatterjee N, Mittal K, et al. The Transport Medicine Society Consensus Guidelines for the Transport of Suspected or Confirmed COVID-19 Patients. Indian J Crit Care Med. 2020;24(9):763-70. [online] Available from https://www.ncbi.nlm.nih.gov/pmc/articles/PMC7584832/ [Last accessed February, 2024].

CHAPTER

26 Nutrition

Sanjith Saseedharan Saroja

Until you get nutrition right nothing will change

—Anonymous

INTRODUCTION

Medical nutrition therapy includes the delivery of calories, amino acids, vitamins, electrolytes, minerals, and trace elements and fluid and encompasses the use of oral feeding, nutritional supplements, enteral tube feeding, and parenteral nutrition (PN) therapy.

Enteral nutrition (EN) refers to provision of nutrition by oral or tube feed into the stomach, duodenum, or jejunum. PN refers to provision of nutrition through parenteral route (intravenous lines). Generally, all patients admitted to the hospital need screening with a screening tool like the Subjective Global Assessment (SGA), Nutrition Risk Score 2002 (NRS 2002) or the NUTRIC (Nutrition Risk in the Critically Ill) Score, Global Leadership in Malnutrition (GLIM criteria) by the Clinical Nutrition Team. All patients admitted in the intensive care unit (ICU) for >48 hours should be considered candidates for medical nutrition therapy.

ASSESSMENT FOR NUTRITION

Assessment of nutrition should be made on the basis of history. This should contain the history of present illness as well as important past histories like diabetes mellitus, malignancies (and the therapies for them), chronic diseases like liver disease or kidney disease, etc. Clinical examination like general build, anemia, skinfold thickness, edema as well as basic laboratory reports may also throw some light on the nutrition status of the patient. Malnutrition is defined as the presence of any two or more of these entities: Insufficient energy, intake, weight loss, loss of muscle mass, loss of subcutaneous fat, localized or generalized fluid accumulation, or decreased functional status. Critically ill patients are at an increased risk for undernutrition, as they are often in a state of inflammation. This induces catabolic hormones and proinflammatory cytokines, which are also catabolic in nature. Moreover, these patients often lack in proper food intake.

NUTRIC score: The NUTRIC score is designed to quantify the risk of critically ill patients developing adverse events that may be modified by aggressive nutrition therapy. The score, of 1–10, is based on six variables that are explained below in **Table 1**. The scoring system is shown in **Tables 2 and 3**.

TYPES OF NUTRITION THERAPY

Enteral Nutrition

Enteral nutrition is preferred because it is more physiological, cost-effective, and safer. Enteral feeding also has beneficial effects on gut, it reduces infection rate, preserves

TABLE 1: Nutrition Risk in the Critically Ill (NUTRIC) score variables.

Variable	*Range*	*Points*
Age	<50	0
	50 to <75	1
	≥75	2
APACHE II	<15	0
	15 to <20	1
	20–28	2
	≥28	3
SOFA	<6	0
	6 to <10	1
	≥10	2
Number of comorbidities	0–1	0
	≥2	1
Days from hospital to ICU admission	0 to <1	0
	≥1	1
IL-6	0 to <400	0
	≥400	1

(ICU: intensive care unit; IL-6: interleukin 6; SOFA: Sequential Organ Failure Assessment)

TABLE 2: *Nutrition Risk in the Critically Ill (NUTRIC) score scoring system:* If IL-6 available.

Sum of points	*Category*	*Explanation*
6–10	High score	• Associated with worse clinical outcomes (mortality, ventilation) • These patients are the most likely to benefit from aggressive nutrition therapy
0–5	Low score	These patients have a low malnutrition risk

TABLE 3: *Nutrition Risk in the Critically Ill (NUTRIC) score scoring system:* If no IL-6 available.[†]

Sum of points	*Category*	*Explanation*
5–9	High score	• Associated with worse clinical outcomes (mortality, ventilation) • These patients are the most likely to benefit from aggressive nutrition therapy
0–4	Low score	These patients have a low malnutrition risk

[†]It is acceptable to not include IL-6 data when it is not routinely available. It was shown to contribute very little to the overall prediction of the NUTRIC score.[‡]

[‡]Rahman A, Hasan RM, Agarwala R, Martin C, Day AG, Heyland DK. Identifying critically-ill patients who will benefit most from nutritional therapy: Further validation of the "modified NUTRIC" nutritional risk assessment tool. Clin Nutr. 2016;35(1):158-62.

functional and structural gut integrity and supports immune function. Hence, it is important to start enteral feeding early and within 48 hours of ICU admission. There is no need to look for bowel sounds before starting the feeding. If patient is able to eat at least 70% of his daily needs by day 3, then oral diet is the preferred route of nutritional support. If this is not achieved, then it is advisable to pass an enteral feeding tube [nasogastric (NG) route] and feed through this route. This feeding can be intermittent feeding where the patient is fed with intermittent bolus of prepared feed via the enteral feeding tube using a gravity technique to flow in the feed or could be delivered continuously using a feeding pump. There is no evidence to say that intermittent bolus feeding is superior to continuous feeding or vice versa. However, it is important to remember that reconstituted feeds should not be hung for >6 hours during feeding.

During feeding, there is no need to perform an aspiration an monitor gastric residual volumes as there is no evidence indicating any benefit from doing so. However, if the unit protocol demands monitoring of gastric residual volume then feeds should not be reduced or suspended until the gastric residual volume is >500 mL.

Contraindications to enteral nutrition:
- Severe shock, requiring high dose of vasopressors
- Uncorrected severe hypoxemia/hypercapnia
- Active upper gastrointestinal bleed
- Over intestinal ischemia
- Large-volume fistula
- Abdominal compartment syndrome
- Gastric aspirate >500 mL in 6 hours

In the event that the patient has abdominal distension, abdominal pain, a gastric residual volume of >500 mL, or intractable vomiting, then it important to pass a nasojejunal tube also called as a post-pyloric route of feeding. At this time it will also help to use prokinetic drugs like metoclopramide and erythromycin (either oral or intravenous).

At times enteral tube feeding is done using a percutaneous endoscopic gastrostomy (PEG) tube, a surgically created gastrostomy tube, or a jejunostomy tube.

Post-pyloric feeding tube is inserted under radiographic guidance, endoscopically, percutaneous endoscopic, percutaneous radiological, or surgically. Tubes may have two ports; distal port is to deliver nutrition in jejunum or distal duodenum and proximal port to drain stomach. These tubes are especially useful in patients with gastric outlet obstruction, duodenal obstruction, intolerance to gastric feeding, and severe gastroesophageal reflex or gastric or duodenal fistula.

Some Special Orders

Sometimes the physician might order a clear liquid diet prior to an endoscopic procedure or just after a major surgery. Clear liquid diet is by definition transparent (can be colored for example grape juice). Such diets are high in sugars and works as a transition before proper diet can be commenced. It is impossible to provide the nutrient requirements while providing a clear diet.

A bland diet also called a soft diet or a low-residue diet may be prescribed for patients with acid peptic disease, sometimes post surgery, gastroenteritis, and when the patient complains of excessive gas formation. This usually consists of boiled vegetables, juices, low-fat yoghurt, eggs, broth, etc. Again a bland diet might not be able to match the nutritional requirements of a patient admitted to the ICU. Certain diets are disease-specific diets; for example, a salt-restricted diet for hypertensive patient, a low-sugar diet for diabetic patients, a high-protein diet for patients on hemodialysis, or a low-potassium diet for patients with kidney disease and hyperkalemia.

Parenteral Nutrition

When the entire nutritional requirements for the individual are delivered via parenteral route, it is called as total parenteral nutrition (TPN) and when PN is delivered partially, it is called as partial parenteral nutrition (PPN). PN may consist of bags that contain water, energy (carbohydrates and lipids), amino acids, vitamins, and trace elements, which are infused together and called as the "all-in-one admixtures" and also as "3-chamber bags". This is also available as "2-chamber bags" containing dextrose and amino acids with intravenous fat emulsions infused separately.

Parenteral nutrition can be delivered through central route (via short-term central venous catheter or a peripherally inserted central line) and peripheral route. PN delivered through the central route will be of high serum osmolarity (>900 mOsm/L) while that delivered via peripheral route has lower osmolarity (<900 mOsm/L). In order to decrease the risk of infection, it is advisable to use a dedicated single-lumen central venous catheter for PN. Alternatively one port of a multilumen central venous catheter can be exclusively dedicated for the infusion of PN. It is advisable to discard the infusion line and the remaining fluid in the TPN bag at the end of 24 hours, as it is known that beyond 24 hours the multiplication of microorganisms would increase and may lead to infection and septicemia.

PRESCRIPTION

The energy prescription should be based on a measured value of energy expenditure using the indirect calorimetry. In the absence of indirect calorimetry, we could use predictive equations like Harris-Benedict equation **(Box 1)**.

Even an universal simple calculation like 25–30 kcal/kg of energy as required calories to be delivered to the patient may be used. This calculation may be modified as per nutritional goals. For example, it can be increased to 30–35 kcal/kg if weight gain is a goal. It is important to deliver up to 70% of energy in the first 3 days of acute illness and reach 80–100% by day 7 of therapy. The protein requirement would range from 1.2 to 2 g/kg/day. Generally, the fluid requirement would be 30–35 mL/kg/day and would increase depending on the presence of fever, drains, etc.

The prescription per se would also be tailored to the condition of the patient. A fluid-restricted energy-dense formula would be used in patients who have fluid restriction orders. A mixed fiber-containing formula would be used for persistent diarrhea. If there is suspicion of malabsorption, a peptide-based formula may be used. An electrolyte-altered formula may be used in cases like renal impairment.

BOX 1: Harris–Benedict equation.

- *Male:* 13.75 × bodyweight + 5.00 × height – 6.75 × age + 66.47
- *Female:* 9.56 × bodyweight + 1.85 × height – 0.67 × age + 655.09

Enteral formula should be prepared for admission under strict aseptic precautions, preferably in a separate room, using sterile water with the intention to avoid contamination.

Enteral feeds:
- Usually, it is iso-osmolar (250–350 mOsm/L).
- Usually, the caloric concentration in 1 kcal/mL.
- Calorie-dense formulations may be used when fluid restriction is needed (like renal failure).
- Peptide-based low-fat formulations may be used in patients with pancreatitis.
- Low-sodium, low-potassium diets may be chosen as per situations.
- Low-calorie, high-fiber diets may be chosen for diabetic patients.

Feeding tubes:
- *For short duration:* Nasogastric or nasojejunal tubes
- *For long duration:* Percutaneous endoscopic gastrostomy (PEG) or feeding jejunostomy tubes

MONITORING

All tubes used for EN should be checked for proper placement. An NG tube can be checked by clinical methods like auscultation, X-ray, or ultrasonography. Also the fluid may be aspirated after a tube placement and checked visually or by the pH (<5.5). The oral cavity should be examined for coiling. An improperly placed NG tube may cause serious aspiration pneumonias, particularly if it is goes inside any bronchus.

Parenteral nutrition should preferably be delivered to through a dedicated venous access. Different nutrition formulas are available for delivery through central venous access or peripheral routes.

While feeding enterally it is important to watch out for intolerance, which is indicated by intractable vomiting, abdominal distension, pain, and intractable diarrhea. At such stages especially when there is abdominal pain and distension, monitoring of intra-abdominal pressure should be considered. It is important to ensure a head-end elevation of the patient during feeding and for at least 30 minutes after feeding. Before administering the next feed, it will help to verify the position of the tube by monitoring the mark at the nostril and look for the position of the tip in the X-ray (if done).

While on PN it is advisable to monitor liver function test at least twice in the week during the initial week and then at least weekly thereafter. Monitoring of sugar is of utmost importance as glucose contained in PN is known to cause hyperglycemia.

COMPLICATIONS

Complications of PN are classified into three groups, related to central venous access, metabolic effects, and bloodstream infections.

Complications Related to Central Venous Access

The immediate complication of the central venous access is related to the placement procedure, which would include bleeding, hematoma, pneumothorax, hemothorax, vascular injury, arrythmias, and venous air embolism. The late complications include thrombosis, infection, and port occlusion. The more the line remains in situ, the higher the chance of infection and related complications. Hence, it is important to daily inspect the line for infection in the proximity of the insertion site, thrombosis, and most importantly whether the line can be removed. Bacterial and fungal bloodstream infection are increased in patients receiving PN. These infections can be minimized by following proper hand hygiene, maximum barrier precaution during insertion of central venous catheter, which includes whole body draping of the patient, physician donning sterile gown, sterile gloves, mask and cap for insertion, using a jugular route in place of a femoral route especially in obese individuals, using strict aseptic precaution using an alcoholic chlorhexidine solution for skin preparation, and ensuring a daily inspection of the line and an assessment of whether this can be removed out.

Complication Related to Enteral Route Access

Placement of the NG tube may lead to discomfort, bleeding, and sometimes misplacement into the lungs, which may lead to catastrophic complications. All NG tubes should be verified using a chest X-ray before being used for feeding. Surgically placed tubes also have chances of misplacement, dislodgment, infection of the access site, and bleeding.

Metabolic effects: These include hyperglycemia, refeeding syndrome, Wernicke's encephalopathy, hepatic dysfunction, electrolyte disturbance, and macro- and micronutrient deficiency.

Hyperglycemia is very common in patients receiving PN. Hence, there is a need to monitor for glucose level and keep it between 140 and 180 mg/dL to decrease length of hospital stay, mortality, and infection.

Refeeding syndrome is seen after starting enteral or PN in malnourished patients characterized by severe electrolyte abnormalities (a decrease of serum phosphorus, potassium, and/or magnesium of >10%) occurring within 5 days of starting the feed.

Hypophosphatemia is the most common of the abnormalities, which can lead to cardiovascular collapse, arrythmias, respiratory failure, seizure, endocrine dysfunction, rhabdomyolysis, and neuromuscular dysfunction. Other manifestations of refeeding syndrome include hypokalemia, hypomagnesemia, and thiamine deficiency leading to Wernicke's encephalopathy.

Metabolic bone disease in the form of osteoporosis and osteomalacia can occur in patients with long-term home PN.

CONCLUSION

Nearly every patient who is in the ICU is at potential risk for malnutrition. Feeding these patients early and enterally is known to improve outcomes. A nutrition protocol will help in improving the conduct of nutrition in the ICU. Optimal, tailored, and personalized nutrition will help in improving outcomes and contribute in successful functional and physical rehabilitation for our critically ill patients.

FURTHER READING

1. da Silva JSV, Seres DS, Sabino K, Adams SC, Berdahl GJ, Citty SW, et al.; Parenteral Nutrition Safety and Clinical Practice Committees; American Society for Parenteral and Enteral Nutrition. ASPEN Consensus Recommendations for Refeeding Syndrome. Nutr Clin Pract. 2020;35(2):178-95. Erratum in: Nutr Clin Pract. 2020;35(3):584-5.
2. Fessler AG, Rejrat CE. Re-evaluating Safe Osmolarity for Peripheral Parenteral Nutrition in Neonatal Intensive Care Patients. J Pediatr Pharmacol Ther. 2021;26(6):632-7.
3. Jensen GL, Cederholm T, Correia MITD, Gonzalez MC, Fukushima R, Higashiguchi T, et al. GLIM Criteria for the Diagnosis of Malnutrition: A Consensus Report From the Global Clinical Nutrition Community. J Parenter Enteral Nutr. 2019;43(1):32-40.
4. Mehta Y, Sunavala JD, Zirpe K, Tyagi N, Garg S, Sinha S, et al. Practice guidelines for nutrition in critically ill patients: A relook for Indian scenario. Indian J Crit Care Med. 2018;22:263-73.
5. Saseedharan S. Comparison of Nutric Score, Nutritional Risk Screening (NRS) 2002 and Subjective Global Assessment (SGA) in the ICU: a Cohort Study. J Nutr Health Food Sci. 2019;7(4):1-4.
6. Singer P, Blaser AR, Berger MM, Calder PC, Casaer M, Hiesmayr M, et al. ESPEN practical and partially revised guideline: Clinical nutrition in the intensive care unit. Clin Nutr. 2023;42(9):1671-89.

CHAPTER 27

Defibrillation, Cardioversion, and Transcutaneous Pacing

Shyam Sunder Tipparaju, Shwetha Ram Chandankhede

INTRODUCTION

In critical cardiac emergencies involving abnormal rhythms, a defibrillator is employed to administer an electric shock to the heart, restoring its normal rhythm. This life-saving device, known as a *defibrillator*, serves three primary interventions: Defibrillation, cardioversion, and transcutaneous pacing (TCP). These swift interventions are crucial in preventing sudden cardiac death, significantly improving survival rates.

During a cardiac arrest lack of effective circulation can lead to severe oxygen deprivation to vital organs, including the brain, and can lead to potential complications including death. Early recognition and intervention often involving advanced cardiac life support (ACLS) measures including prompt defibrillation increase the chances of successful resuscitation.

Defibrillators are standard equipment in hospitals, while a more user-friendly variant, the automated external defibrillator (AED), is widely accessible in public spaces such as airports, bus and railway stations, shopping malls, and gated communities. The AED is designed for use by nonmedical individuals and paramedics during emergency situations in public settings, providing essential support in critical moments.

There are two primary types of defibrillators based on the flow of current: Monophasic and biphasic. Monophasic defibrillators deliver electrical current in a single direction, generating a singular waveform. Conversely, biphasic defibrillators employ a waveform that changes direction during the shock, resulting in a two-phase (positive and negative) current flow. In contemporary medical practice, biphasic defibrillators are predominantly favored due to their enhanced effectiveness and lower energy requirements, consequently reducing the potential risk of tissue damage. In the following chapter, we will delve into the specific applications of biphasic defibrillators.

TYPES OF EXTERNAL DEFIBRILLATOR

There are various types of external defibrillators for specific setups and user expertise.

Manual External Defibrillator (Fig. 1)

This is available in the hospitals and advanced life support settings for the use by trained healthcare professionals, such as doctors, nurses, and paramedics. This device gives a greater control over the defibrillation process, allowing it to analyze the rhythm manually and determines when to deliver the shock.

Automated External Defibrillator (Fig. 2)

It is a portable, user-friendly device designed for use by nonmedical individuals, including

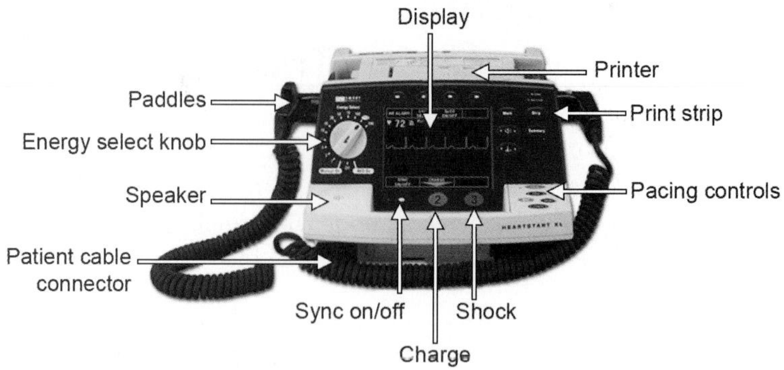

Fig. 1: Manual external defibrillator.

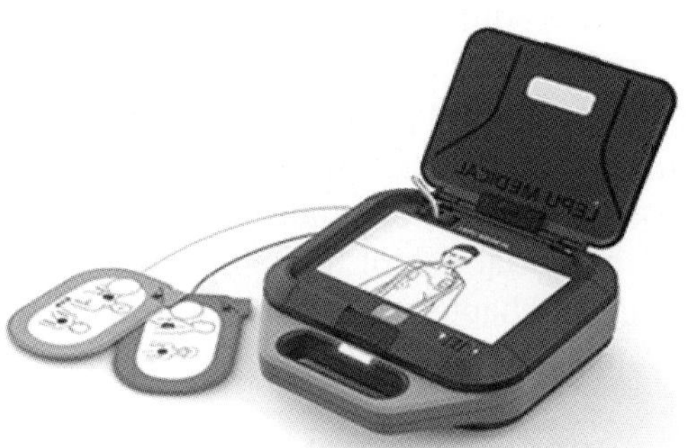

Fig. 2: Automated external defibrillator (AED) with adhesive pads.

nonexpert and first responders. AEDs provide audio and visual instructions to guide users through the defibrillation process. They analyze the heart rhythm and deliver an electric shock automatically.

Semiautomatic External Defibrillator

It is similar to AED. It guides the users through the process but require a manual trigger to administer the shock thus allowing the users to confirm the decision to shock.

PARTS OF DEFIBRILLATOR

A defibrillator is a sophisticated medical device equipped with essential components, including cables, controls, knobs, a display screen, alarms, and voice prompt. These features collectively contribute to the device's intricate functionality. Typically, defibrillators offer both manual and automatic modes, allowing users to select the appropriate mode based on their level of competence.

Power Supply

The defibrillator operates on a dual power system, utilizing both direct power and a battery backup. The duration of the battery backup varies depending on the specific make and model of the defibrillator. Ensuring the battery is adequately charged is paramount to prevent any malfunctions in the event of a power supply cutoff. This precautionary measure is crucial for maintaining the device's readiness and effectiveness during emergencies.

Energy Selection Knob

The energy select knob on a defibrillator serves the vital function of choosing the appropriate energy level for a shock, ranging from 2 to 200 joules. The selection is contingent on factors such as the specific cardiac rhythm and the patient's weight, particularly significant in pediatric cases.

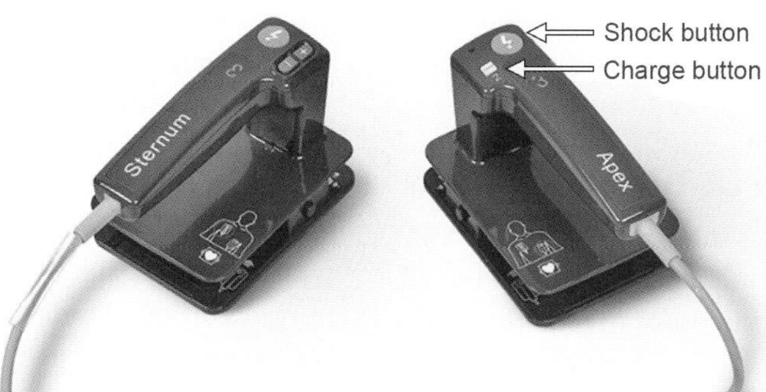

Fig. 3: Manual electrode pads with charge button, shock button, and marking for positioning.

Electrode Pads

Electrode pads come in two main types: Manual paddles and adhesive gel pads.

Manual Electrode Pads (Fig. 3)

- Manual electrode pads are strategically placed on the upper right and lower left chest of the patient after being charged.
- The shock is delivered by pressing the shock button, either located on the paddle itself or on the defibrillator unit.
- Noteworthy is their reusability; these pads can be cleaned and used again.
- The size of manual paddles varies between 8 and 13 cm for adults, with smaller paddles designed for pediatric patients.
- For ease of use in emergency, they are marked with labels, i.e., sternum and apex in most of the defibrillators.

Adhesive Gel Pads (see Fig. 2)

- Adhesive gel pads are affixed to the upper right and lower left chest of the patient.
- Primarily used for rhythm analysis and delivering the therapeutic shock.
- Unlike manual pads, adhesive pads are designed for single use and should be used for only one patient.

Sync On/Off Button

The defibrillator features a sync on/off button, offering versatility in its applications. With sync set to *off*, the device is primed for defibrillation purposes. Conversely, when sync is set to *on*, the same device becomes apt for cardioversion.

Pacing Control

The device is equipped with a pacing control feature, enabling its utilization for TCP when the pacing mode is activated.

Display

The defibrillator is equipped with a comprehensive display window that presents real-time information on the heart's rhythm and rate. This visual data is derived from inputs received either through electrocardiogram (ECG) cables or the connected paddles/pads. The display serves as a critical tool, facilitating the analysis of cardiac rhythm, providing essential insights for informed decision-making in planning appropriate interventions.

Printer

The defibrillator is equipped with an integrated printer that generates a printed copy of the rhythm strip. This functionality allows for the tangible documentation of the cardiac rhythm, providing a physical record for medical documentation and analysis.

DEFINITION OF DEFIBRILLATION

Defibrillation is a medical procedure that involves delivering a controlled electric shock to the heart in order to restore normal heart rhythm during life-threatening cardiac arrhythmias.

Indication

Indications for defibrillation include:

- *Ventricular fibrillation (VF)* ***(Fig. 4)****:* This is a serious and life-threatening cardiac arrhythmia characterized by chaotic and rapid contractions ventricles. In VF, the electrical signals in the heart become disorganized, leading to a quivering or fibrillating motion of the ventricles. This chaotic activity results in the heart's inability to effectively pump blood.
- *Ventricular tachycardia (VT) without pulse* ***(Fig. 5)****:* Pulseless VT is a serious and life-threatening cardiac arrhythmia characterized by a rapid and sustained rhythm originating in the ventricles. In this condition, the heart beats at a dangerously fast rate, but the contractions are uncoordinated and ineffective in pumping blood. Despite the rapid ventricular contractions, there is little to no forward blood flow, resulting in the absence of a palpable pulse.

Note: During a cardiac arrest, four distinct abnormal heart rhythms may occur: Asystole, pulseless electrical activity, VF, and pulseless VT. It is essential to note that defibrillation is not effective in treating asystole and pulseless electrical activity. Defibrillation is only applicable and beneficial in addressing the two shockable rhythms—VF and pulseless VT.

Procedure

Defibrillation is a time-sensitive emergency procedure crucial for enhancing outcomes during cardiac arrest. Following ACLS guidelines, in the case of a cardiac arrest with pulseless VT or VF, immediate defibrillation is prioritized when a defibrillator is already attached. It is recommended to deliver the shock before initiating chest compressions.

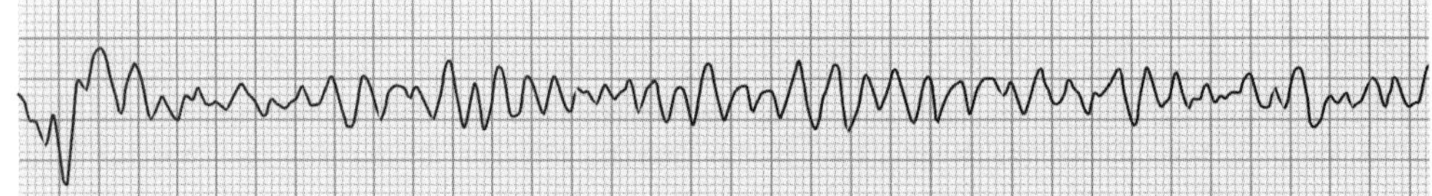

Fig. 4: Ventricular fibrillation.

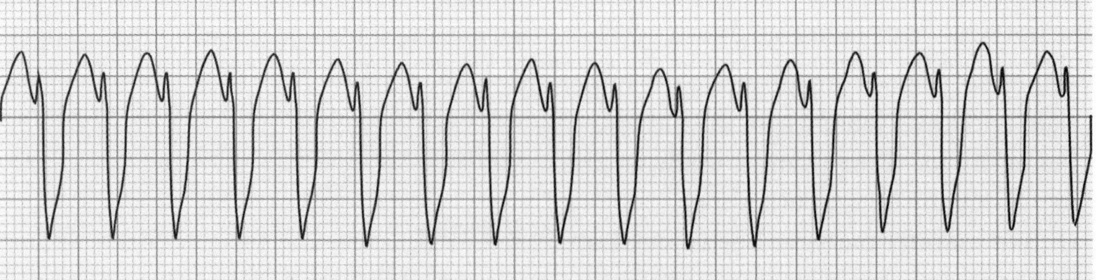

Fig. 5: Ventricular tachycardia.

After the shock is administered, prompt commencement of cardiopulmonary resuscitation (CPR) is essential, accompanied by regular rhythm assessments at intervals to guide further interventions.

The following procedure should be carried out during cardiac arrest:

- *Scene assessment:* Assess for scene safety, call for help and defibrillator.
- *Confirmation of cardiac arrest:* Cardiac arrest is identified based on the absence of a pulse, unresponsiveness, and abnormal or absent breathing.
- *Defibrillator setup:* When employing a manual defibrillator, the initial shock for VF or pulseless VT is typically chosen within the range of 120–200 joules. Subsequent shocks, if required, may be administered at the same or higher energy levels. In contrast, AEDs, commonly utilized in public settings by laypersons, are typically configured to deliver a standardized energy level, often ranging from 120 to 200 joules.

  Note: For pediatric defibrillation, the initial shock may fall within the range of 2–4 joules per kilogram.
- *Electrode placement:* External defibrillator paddles, or electrode pads, are typically placed on specific locations on the patient's chest. There are two main pad placements commonly used:
  1. *Anterior-lateral placement* **(Fig. 6)**: One pad is placed on the upper right side of the chest lateral to the right border of the sternum, just below the right clavicle. The second pad is positioned on the left side of the chest, at the apex of the heart (below the nipple) in the anterior or midaxillary line.
  2. *Anterior-posterior placement* **(Fig. 7)**: One pad is placed left side of the chest below the nipple, in the anterior or midaxillary while the second pad is placed on the left side of the back below the scapula.
- *Rhythm analysis:* Analyze whether the rhythm is shockable or nonshockable.

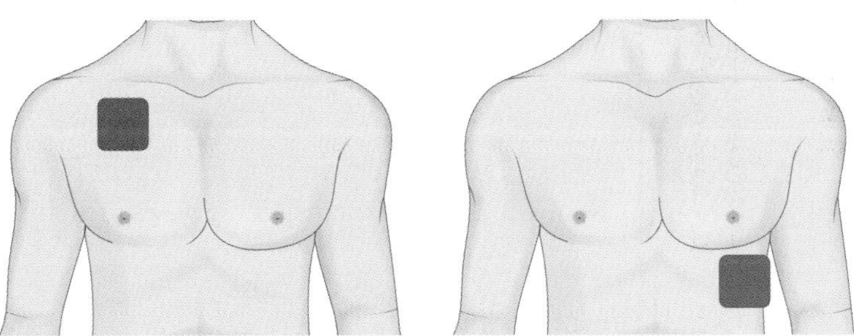

Fig. 6: Anterolateral placement of paddles.

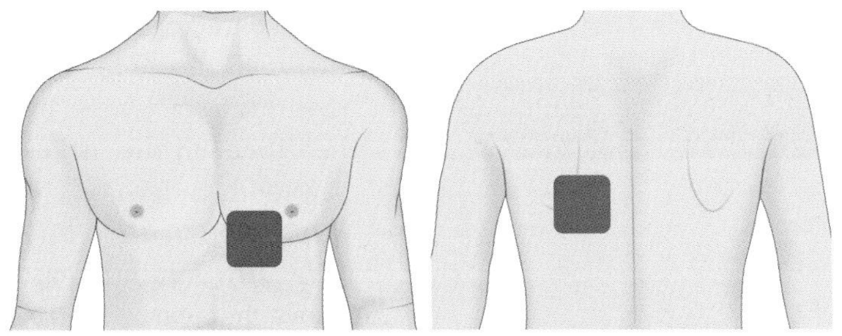

Fig. 7: Anteroposterior placement of the paddles.

- *Clear the patient:* Before administering a shock, it is imperative for all personnel to ensure a clear space around the patient. No one should be in physical contact with the patient or the immediate surroundings during the delivery of the shock. The team leader assumes the responsibility of verifying that the area is free from any contact, thereby minimizing the risk of harm to both the patient and those involved in the resuscitation effort.
- *Shock delivery and CPR:* Upon confirmation of a shockable rhythm, the defibrillator is promptly charged, and the paddles are coated with a conductive gel for optimal contact with the skin. Placing the paddles in the appropriate position on the chest is crucial to ensure effective delivery of the shock. The shock is administered by pressing the button on the paddle or the defibrillator device. Throughout the entire preparation process, the uninterrupted continuation of CPR is paramount. The only interruption occurs during the actual shock delivery. Following the shock, CPR is resumed promptly, ensuring a minimal delay of no >10 seconds. Chest compressions and rescue breaths are continued until the next rhythm analysis.

Note: Defibrillation is a live-saving procedure but it is associated with few complications **(Box 1)**.

BOX 1: Complications of defibrillation and cardioversion.

- Skin burns
- Pain or discomfort
- New arrhythmias
- Myocardial injury
- Hemodynamic instability
- Thromboembolism

USE OF AUTOMATED EXTERNAL DEFIBRILLATOR FOR DEFIBRILLATION

The process of defibrillation with an AED closely mirrors manual defibrillation, with the primary distinction being the AED's automated rhythm analysis. If a shockable rhythm is identified, the AED issues clear and audible prompts instructing rescuers to stand clear and press the shock button. Immediately after the shock, CPR is resumed following the AED's voice or visual prompts. Chest compressions and rescue breaths are continued until the next rhythm analysis.

DEFINITION OF CARDIOVERSION

Cardioversion is a medical procedure designed to address abnormal heart rhythms associated with a pulse, leading to hemodynamic instability. This involves delivering a precisely timed electric shock to the heart with the primary aim of restoring a normal heart rhythm. Unlike defibrillation, which is typically an unplanned and emergency intervention used during cardiac arrest, cardioversion is often a scheduled and elective or semi-urgent procedure intended to treat specific types of arrhythmias.

Indications

- *Atrial fibrillation (AF)* ***(Fig. 8)****:* A rapid and irregular heartbeat originating in the atria characterized by absent "P" waves.
- *Atrial flutter* ***(Fig. 9)****:* Abnormal heart rhythm characterized by a regular but fast heartbeat in the atria characterized by saw tooth pattern.
- *Supraventricular tachycardia (SVT)* ***(Fig. 10)****:* A rapid heart rate originating above the heart's ventricles characterized by regular, narrow QRS complexes with hidden "P" waves.

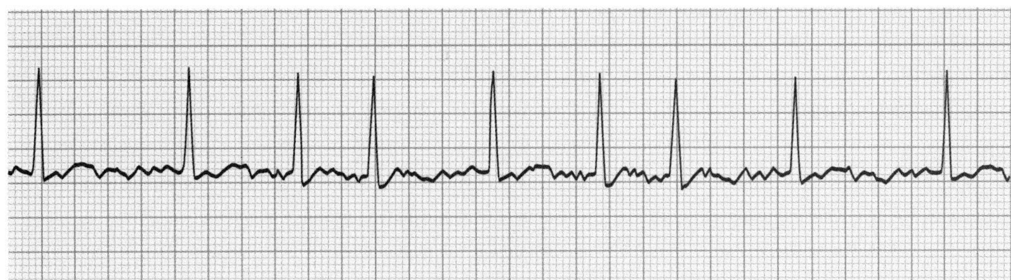

Fig. 8: Atrial fibrillation.

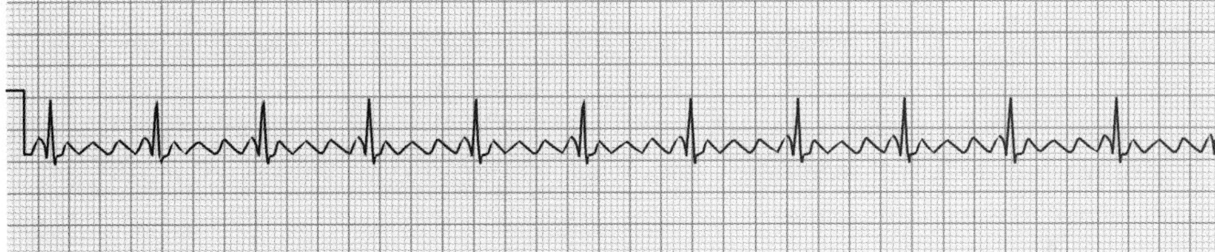

Fig. 9: Atrial flutter.

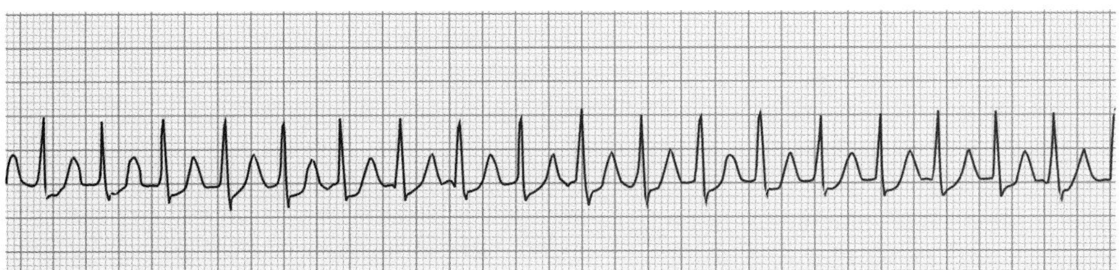

Fig. 10: Supraventricular tachycardia.

- *VT with pulse:* A potentially life-threatening rapid heartbeat originating in the ventricles.
  Note: Defibrillation is done for pulseless VT whereas cardioversion is done for VT with pulse.
- *Wolff-Parkinson-White syndrome **(Fig. 11)**:* A condition where an extra electrical pathway in the heart leads to episodes of rapid heart rate. It is characterized by a wide QRS complex with delta waves which gives the QRS complex a slurred or notched appearance.

The procedure of cardioversion and defibrillation are almost same with few striking differences **(Table 1)**.

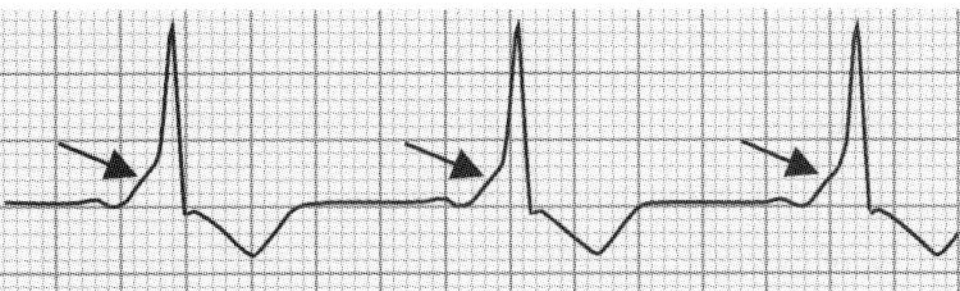

Fig. 11: Wolff–Parkinson–White syndrome.

Procedure

- The patient's medical history, current medications, blood tests, imaging studies, and an ECG are assessed.
- Informed consent is obtained procedure, its purpose, potential risks, and benefits.
- If cardioversion is planned, patients are instructed to fast for 6–8 hours before the procedure to reduce the risk of

TABLE 1: Difference between defibrillation and cardioversion.

Defibrillation	*Cardioversion*
Emergency procedure	Elective, semi urgent, or emergency procedure
Asynchronized	Synchronized
Indications: • Pulseless ventricular tachycardia (VT) • Ventricular fibrillation (VF)	*Indications:* • Supraventricular tachycardia • Atrial fibrillation • Atrial flutter • Ventricular tachycardia with pulse
No need of sedation	Needs sedation
Shock energy is higher than cardioversion	Shock energy may be lower than defibrillation

aspiration if sedation is used. If it is a semi urgent procedure, cardioversion is done irrespective of the fasting status.

- *Airway, breathing and circulation (ABC) management*: ABC assessment is performed and prompt intervention is done if any abnormality is detected.
- Heart rate, blood pressure, ECG, and oxygen saturation are monitored periprocedure.
- Electrode paddles placement is similar to defibrillation procedure.
- Sedation is given for the comfort of the patient.
- The energy level for cardioversion is tailored to the specific type and rate of the arrhythmia **(Table 2)**. Typically, the selected energy is lower than that used for defibrillation. In the event that the initial shock fails to restore the rhythm to a normal rate and pattern, subsequent shocks may be administered with higher energy levels. According to the guidelines set forth by the American College of Cardiology (ACC) and the American Heart Association (AHA), the following are the recommended initial energy selection levels for various arrhythmias.
- Synchronization during cardioversion refers to the timing of the delivery of an electric shock during the R-wave of the QRS complex on the ECG. Synchronization minimizes the risk of inducing VF during the delivery of the shock.

TABLE 2: Energy level selection for various arrhythmias.

Rhythm	*Energy in joules*
Atrial fibrillation	120–200
Atrial flutter	120–200
Supraventricular tachycardia	50–100
Ventricular tachycardia (VT) with pulse	100

- Shock is delivered by pressing the button on the paddles or the device. After shock delivery, the response is monitored on ECG. If the initial cardioversion is not successful, additional attempts may be made with adjustments to energy levels.
- Cardioversion is associated with a few complications **(*see* Box 1)**.

Check list for elective cardioversion is provided in **Box 2**.

DIFFERENCE BETWEEN DEFIBRILLATION AND CARDIOVERSION

While defibrillation and cardioversion share several procedural similarities, distinct

BOX 2: Check list for elective cardioversion.

- Empty stomach for 6–8 hours
- 48 hours off digitalis
- Hypo- and hyperkalemia should be corrected
- Crash trolley ready
- Intravenous access to be secured
- Oxygen and intubation set to be ready
- Electrocardiogram (ECG) monitor with recorder/printer to be attached (if the defibrillator does not have it)
- Informed consent is preferable
- Sedation

differences exist in their indications and the energy levels applied during the intervention (*see* **Table 1**).

TRANSCUTANEOUS PACING

Transcutaneous pacing is a medical procedure used to temporarily manage and correct life-threatening bradycardias or heart block by delivering external electrical stimuli through electrodes placed on the skin.

Indication

- Symptomatic bradycardia unresponsive to medication
- Heart block (third degree or complete)
- As a bridge to permanent pacemaker
- When pacing is required for small duration

Paddle placement for TCP involves positioning adhesive electrode pads on the patient's chest. Normally the negative electrode is placed on the anterior chest wall at the V3 position and the positive electrode is placed on the back, exactly opposite to the negative electrode. In case the patient cannot be turned, the positive electrode cane be placed at the V1 position. The external pulse generator delivers controlled electrical stimuli through the skin to pace the heart and maintain an adequate heart rate. The pacing rate, current amplitude, and other parameters can be adjusted based on the patient's response with continuous monitoring of the patient's heart rhythm, blood pressure, and clinical status. The rate is kept above the patient's intrinsic rate. The output is started from a lower level, say 10 mA and then increased by 5–10 mA, step by step till there is capture. The output is kept 10 mA higher than the capture threshold. In case the patient is in arrest, the initial output is kept at 200 mA to ensure capture and then slowly reduced to identify the threshold. Most patients can be successfully paced with an output between 20 and 140 mA.

CONCLUSION

Defibrillation, cardioversion, and TCP are vital interventions used in the management of cardiac arrhythmias, each serving distinct purposes based on the clinical scenario. These interventions are integral components of ACLS, contributing to improved outcomes in patients experiencing cardiac emergencies. Every healthcare worker should possess a thorough understanding of cardioversion, defibrillation, and TCP. Team collaboration is essential to ensure effective and timely application of these life-saving techniques. Maintenance of optimal device functionality is crucial to prevent failures that could compromise patient outcomes. Additionally, public awareness regarding the use of AEDs in public spaces during emergency situations is of paramount importance. Widespread knowledge empowers the public to take swift and appropriate action, potentially saving lives in critical situations.

FURTHER READING

1. Adams A, Adams C. Transcutaneous Pacing: An Emergency Nurse's Guide. J Emerg Nurs. 2021;47(2):326-30.

2. Goyal A, Chhabra L, Sciammarella JC, Cooper JS. Defibrillation. Treasure Island (FL): StatPearls Publishing; 2024.
3. Panchal AR, Bartos JA, Cabañas JG, Donnino MW, Drennan IR, Hirsch KG, et al; Adult Basic and Advanced Life Support Writing Group. Part 3: Adult Basic and Advanced Life Support: 2020 American Heart Association Guidelines for Cardiopulmonary Resuscitation and Emergency Cardiovascular Care. Circulation. 2020;142(16_suppl_2):S366-468.
4. Philips. Philips HeartStart XL Defibrillator Manual. [online] Available from https://www.aedsuperstore.com/pdf/philips-heartstart-xl-defibrillator-manual.pdf. [Last accessed February, 2025].

CHAPTER

28 Injections and Infusions

Rohit Kumar Patnaik, Nupur Karan, Tapas Kumar Sahoo

INTRODUCTION

In the realm of critical care nursing, injections and infusions are fundamental techniques used to administer medications, fluids, and other therapeutic agents directly into the body. These methods offer precise delivery, allowing for rapid absorption and targeted action. Injections involve the introduction of a substance into the body using a syringe and needle, typically into veins (intravenous), muscles (intramuscular), or beneath the skin (subcutaneous). On the other hand, infusions involve the slow, controlled administration of fluids or medications into the bloodstream through a catheter or intravenous line. Both injections and infusions play crucial roles in critical care nursing, providing efficient and often life-saving interventions across a wide spectrum of conditions and settings **(Boxes 1 and 2)**. Understanding the principles and techniques of injections and infusions is essential for healthcare professionals (HCPs) to ensure safe and effective patient's care.[1]

BOX 1: Common routes of injections and infusions in critical care.

- Intravenous
- Subcutaneous
- Intramuscular
- Epidural
- Intradermal
- Intrathecal
- Intraosseous
- Intra-articular

The topic of critical care injections and infusions can be categorized into the following sections:

- Patient's safety and quality
- Infection prevention and control
- Injections and infusions equipment
- Site and device selection and placement
- Site care and maintenance
- Specific devices
- Infusion therapies
- Infusion-related complications
- Education and training
- Infusion therapy teams

PATIENT'S SAFETY AND QUALITY

The objective is to ensure patient's identification through the use of a patient's ID tag, while upholding the patient's rights, autonomy, and dignity. The venous access procedure, all administered injections and infusions, and any observed adverse medication reactions should be recorded. Essential information regarding vascular access devices (VADs) should encompass the following: informed consent, precise date and time of insertion, rationale for insertion, specific site of insertion, number and location

BOX 2: Common infusions in critical care.

- Medications (fluids, vasopressors, insulin, sedatives, antibiotics, and heparin)
- Enteral and parenteral nutrition
- Chemotherapeutic agents

of insertion occurrences, type of VAD (such as peripheral or central line, and number of lumens in central line), exact length of the inserted catheter, and the appearance of the catheter site. Details regarding care and maintenance of VAD—presence of phlebitis (if observed), specifics of flushing solution (type, volume, and frequency), date of dressing change, length of catheter insertion (to detect migration). Information regarding injections and infusions includes the specific drug, dosage, route of administration, rate of administration, timing, and technique of administration, as well as the patient's tolerance and response to therapy, any adverse drug reactions, and potential problems **(Fig. 1)**.

Vascular access devices removal information includes the rationale for removal, the specific date and time of removal, the condition of the VAD's integrity, the appearance of the site after VAD removal, the kind of dressing placed following removal, any difficulties encountered during the removal process, and the discontinuance of infusion. The expiry date of the injection/infusion should be noted. Labeling should include the brand name and generic name of the drug, as well as its strength, total volume, mode of administration, and any relevant warnings **(Fig. 1)**. For epidural infusion sets, it is important to clearly mark them as "For Epidural Use Only". Any faults in injection/infusion products, bad responses to drugs, complications, and adverse reactions to blood/blood components should be reported.

Pt's Full Name: XYZ	**MRN:** 12345
Fluid Name: NS	**Drug added:** FENTANYL
Rate: 500 µg in 50 mL	**Started Date/Time:** 24-01-24 10 AM
Ended Date/Time: –	**Started by:** ABC

Fig. 1: Labeled drug infusion.

INFECTION PREVENTION AND CONTROL

For all infusion-related treatments, it is necessary to employ an aseptic technique, adhere to standard precautions including hand hygiene and full aseptic technique. Especially central venous catheter insertions need the adoption of maximal sterile barrier precautions.

Sharp objects utilized for injections should be discarded in designated sharp disposal containers. Once sharp containers are filled up to the designated fill line, they must be securely sealed and emptied. The department should also monitor the rate of catheter-related bloodstream infections (CRBSI):

(CRBSI rate = Number of IV device related infections/Total number of catheter days × 1,000)

Else the department can also look out for catheter-linked bloodstream infections (CLABSI).

INJECTION AND INFUSION EQUIPMENT

- *Administration sets* ***(Fig. 2)****:* Administration sets for continuous infusion should be replaced every 96 hours, or sooner if they become detached or if there is any compromise in the integrity of the product or the system **(Fig. 2)**. Administration sets for continuous infusion of blood and blood products should be changed at least every 12 hours or upon completion of the transfusion. Platelet transfusion should be administered using separate administration sets, distinct from those used for other blood components. Blood administration sets should be equipped with an integrated mesh filter with a pore size of 170–200 µ. Blood administration

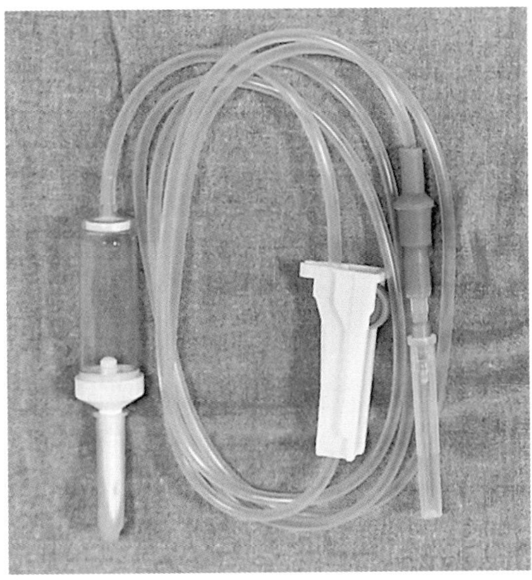

Fig. 2: Intravenous infusion set.

sets are not interchangeable with solution administration sets. Administration sets for continuous infusion of parenteral nutrition should be replaced every 24 hours. Infusion sets must have date and time markings affixed to them in order to ensure compliance with the correct time intervals for replacing them. It is preferable to change add-on devices such as stop cocks or filters at the same time as changing administration sets. Administration sets must be changed using aseptic method and standard precautions.

- *Flow control devices:* Manual flow control devices such as slides, roller clamps, and drop controls assist in regulating the rate of infusions.

  Central venous access device infusions are best administered with electronic flow control devices, such as volumetric infusion pumps and powered syringe pumps **(Fig. 3)**. The electronic infusion pumps come with safety features such as electrical safety, audible alarms, battery life and operation indicators, anti-free flow protection,

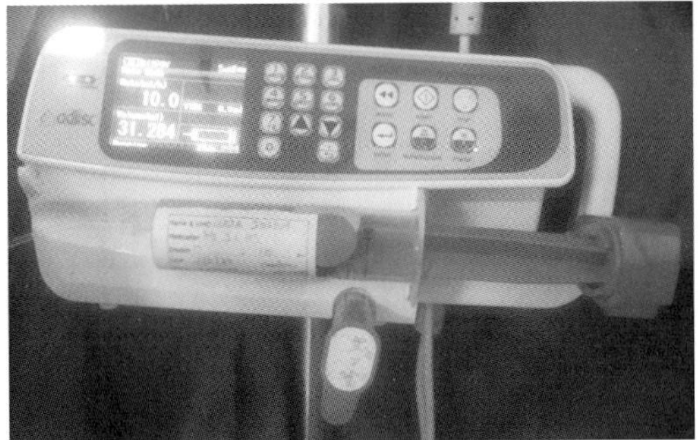

Fig. 3: Electronic flow control device.

  adjustable occlusion pressure levels, in-line pressure monitoring, etc. They should be periodically checked at regular intervals. The nursing staff should be well trained about these instruments.

- *Add-on devices:* The add-on devices include of three-way taps/stopcocks, extension sets, blind hub caps, needleless systems, and filters. All add-on devices must be designed with a closed Luer-Lok™ mechanism. The add-on devices should be checked for compatibility. As the norm standard aseptic procedures should be followed.
- *Injection and access devices:* Injection and access devices encompass caps, needle-free caps, catheter hubs, and ports. It is necessary to disinfect all injection and access sites using a solution consisting of 2% chlorhexidine and 70% alcohol. The solution should be applied with friction and given sufficient time to dry both before and after usage. Devices should always be kept with their caps securely closed and protected **(Figs. 4A and B)**.
- *Blood/fluid warmers **(Fig. 5)**:* Blood and blood components should be heated to a temperature of 37°C using blood/fluid warmers. Other techniques, such as using a microwave oven, radiator, or immersing the pack in hot water, should not be used to warm it. Prior to being authorized to use blood/fluid warmer devices, all healthcare

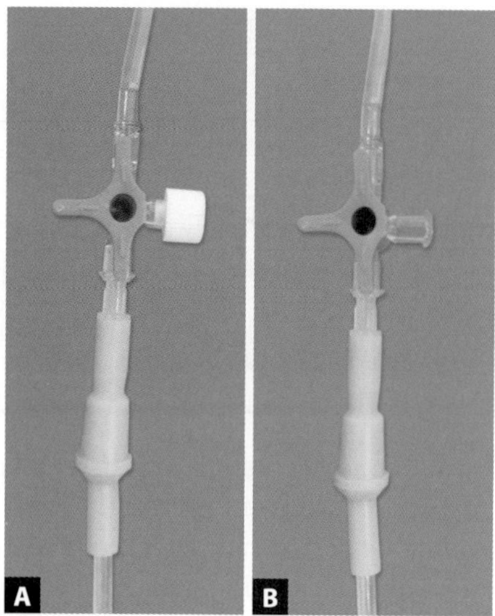

Figs. 4A and B: Three-way stop cock. (A) Capped and (B) uncapped.

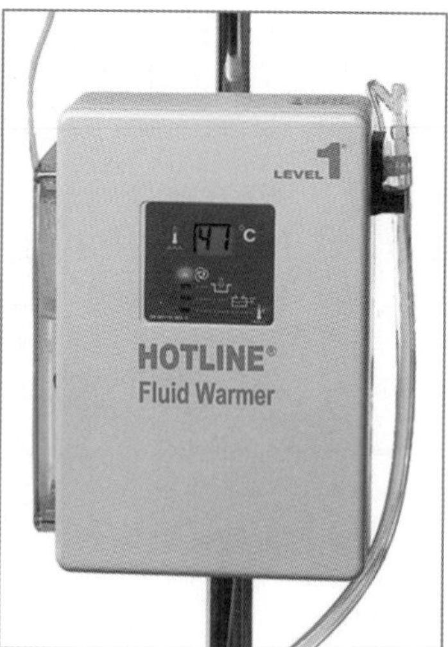

Fig. 5: Fluid warmer.

staff must complete competency-based training.

- *Filters:* Filters should be bacteria/particulate-retentive and air-eliminating. For clear solutions, it is recommended to use a 15-μ filter. For lipid infusions or whole nutrition preparations, a 1.2-μ filter is recommended. For blood components, it is recommended to use an integrated mesh filter with a pore size of 170–200 μ.
- *Tourniquets:* It is important to avoid using a tourniquet for >60 seconds in order to prevent the occurrence of "hemoconcentration" at the site of venepuncture, which can lead to inaccurate blood chemistry readings. The tourniquet should be applied with sufficient tightness to encourage distention of the veins, while yet allowing normal blood flow via the arteries.

SITE AND DEVICE SELECTION AND PLACEMENT

- *Peripheral devices:* Peripheral cannulae are usually used to get a venous access for injections or infusions **(Fig. 6)**. Initially, the most distal regions of the upper extremities are cannulated, followed by the cannulation of more proximal areas if necessary **(Fig. 7)**. The preferred site for cannulation should be the nondominant arm, avoiding places that are prone to flexion. It is advisable to refrain from using blood pressure cuffs on the limb that has been cannulated. To mitigate the risk of lymphedema formation, it is advisable to avoid cannulation on the same side for patients who have received axillary lymph node dissection or radiotherapy. Medications with an osmolarity over 900 Osm/L should not be administered through a peripheral cannula. Peripheral access devices require the application of a sterile clear film dressing. Aseptic procedure is necessary for every dressing change.
- *Central venous access devices* ***(Fig. 7):*** With the exception of hemodialysis catheters, the subclavian vein is the preferred choice over the internal jugular vein. Whenever feasible, it is advisable to avoid using the femoral vein due to its

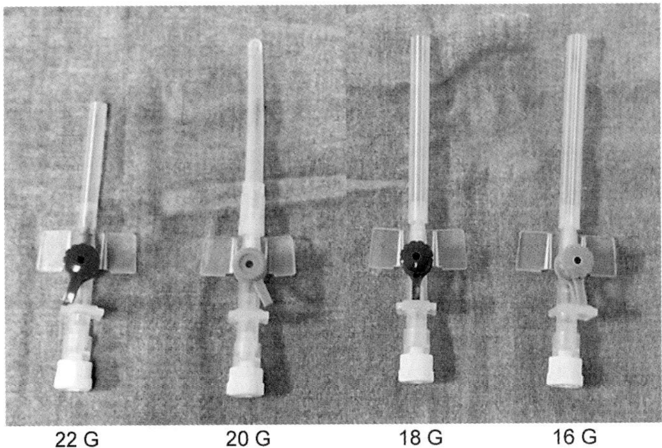

Fig. 6: Peripheral cannulae in various sizes.

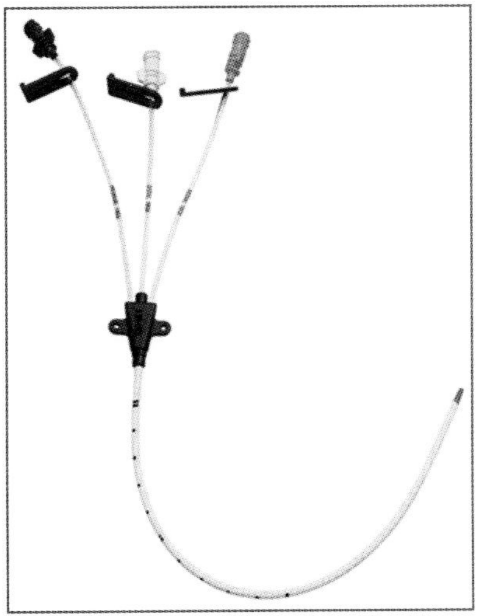

Fig. 7: Triple-lumen central venous catheter.

elevated susceptibility to infection. The cephalic, basilic, or medial cubital veins in the arm are suitable for the insertion of a peripherally inserted central catheter (PICC). Central venous access devices require the application of a sterile transparent film dressing. It is necessary to employ an aseptic method for every dressing change.

- Sterile gauze dressings are necessary in some situations, such as when a patient experiences excessive perspiration or when the insertion site is leaking. Nevertheless, it is imperative to promptly substitute it with a sterile, transparent film dressing when possible. Sterile clear film dressings should be replaced every 7 days or earlier if there is any damage to their integrity.

SITE CARE AND MAINTENANCE

It is necessary to follow aseptic technique and standard precautions when taking care of the vascular access site.

Periodic pulsatile flush using 0.9% normal saline aid in preserving the patency of the VAD. When central venous access devices are aspirated, blood should be observed returning. If not, then it is necessary to make an attempt to flush the device. Nevertheless, in the event of encountering resistance, it is advisable not to employ force. Routine use of systemic anticoagulants for maintaining patency is not recommended. When removing either peripheral or central vascular access, it is important to inspect the tip for integrity. It is important to take precautions to prevent air-embolism when removing central venous access catheters. After removal, digital pressure should be administered until hemostasis is achieved.

INFUSION THERAPIES

- *Medication and solution administration:* It is essential to use aseptic technique along with standard precautions while administering injectable drugs and solutions. Before administering, the HCP should adhere to the safety measures outlined in **Box 3**. It is essential to record the patient's identity and allergy status accurately. A separate inventory of "high-risk injectable drugs" must be created and a dedicated storage area should be provided in the ICU for their safekeeping. All medications present in the patient area must be either administered or disposed of within a 24-hour timeframe. An extravasation procedure is necessary for the administration of chemotherapeutic medicines. Do not use the affected limb for future placement of the VAD.

  Table 1 provides a comprehensive list of commonly used injections and infusions, along with their respective dilutions and dosages.
- *Transfusion therapy:* It is essential to verify and validate the correct blood (component, group, and type), as well as the correct patient, correct time (including volume and rate of transfusion), and correct location for the blood transfusion. The blood component administration set must include a built-in mesh filter with a pore size ranging from 170 to 200 μ **(Fig. 8)**. Blood warmers are necessary for warming the administered blood component to a temperature of 37°C. The patient's vital signs should be documented before initiating the blood component transfusion and at 15-minute intervals during the duration of the transfusion. It is necessary to document all adverse responses associated with blood transfusions, including the specific blood component and administration set used, and send them to the blood bank for analysis. Red blood cell transfusions must be administered within 4 hours after being taken out of a controlled temperature environment. Once thawed, fresh frozen plasma (FFP) cannot be refrozen. It should be transfused over a period of roughly 30 minutes. Platelets are transfused within a time frame of 30–60 minutes. Nevertheless, it is imperative to avoid transfusing it via sets that have been previously utilized for other blood components. It is important to avoid administering dextrose solution (5%) and blood component therapy through the same infusion line, since the dextrose solution can lead to the destruction of red blood cells (hemolysis).
- Epidural analgesia injections and infusion HCPs should receive proper training in the correct usage of epidural catheter. A readily accessible acute pain service team should be present to provide guidance and assistance on epidural infusions. The patient must have a venous access device in place during epidural infusions. Epidural analgesic catheters should be color-coded, devoid of injection sites,

BOX 3: List of safety features to be ensured before medication administration.

- Appropriately label containers, vials, and syringes
- Identify patient
- Correct date and time
- Verify contents, dose, rate, and route
- Verify expiration date and integrity of medications or solution being used

TABLE 1: Common injections and infusions dilutions and doses.

Drug	*Preparation*	*Concentration*	*Dosing/Infusion rate*	*Route*
Amiodarone	• 150 mg in 100 mL of 5% dextrose • 900 mg in 500 mL of 5% dextrose	• 1.5 mg/mL • 1.8 mg/mL	• Bolus over 10 minutes • 33.3 mL/hour in first 6 hours, then 17 mL/hour in next 18 hours	IV (P and C)
Cisatracurium	• 100 mg in 50 mL of 0.9% saline • (2 mg/mL)	2 mg/mL	5–10 mL/hour	IV (P and C)
Dexmedetomidine	200 µg in 50 mL of 0.9% saline	4 µg/mL	1–10 mL/hour	IV (P and C)
Dobutamine	250 mg in 50 mL of 5% dextrose	5 mg/mL	1–10 mL/hour	IV (C)
Epinephrine	6 mg in 50 mL of 5% dextrose	120 µg/mL	1–20 mL/hour	IV (C)
Fentanyl	500 µg in 50 mL 0.9% saline	10 µg/mL	5–10 mL/hour	IV (P and C)
Heparin	500 IU in 50 mL of 0.9% saline	10 IU/mL	1–10 mL/hour	IV (P and C)
Insulin (Human actrapid)	20 IU in 20 mL 0.9% saline	1 IU/mL	1–5 mL	IV (P and C)
Labetalol	250 mg in 50 mL of 5% dextrose	5 mg/mL	1–20 mL/hour	IV (P and C)
Morphine	50 mg in 50 mL of 0.9% saline	1 mg/mL	1–5 mL/hour	IV (P and C)
Midazolam	50 mg in 50 mL 0.9% saline	1 mg/mL	1–5 mL/hour	IV (P and C)
Nitroglycerin	50 mg in 50 mL of 5% dextrose	1 mg/mL	1–5 mL/hour	IV (P and C)
Norepinephrine	6 mg in 50 mL of 5% dextrose	120 µg/mL	1–20 mL/hour	IV (C)
Propofol	Neat 100 mg in 10 mL (no dilution needed)	10 mg/mL	1–5 mL/hour	IV (P and C)
Vasopressin	20 mg in 20 mL of 5% dextrose	1 mg/mL	0.5–2.4 mL/hour	IV (C)
Vecuronium	20 mg in 20 mL of 0.9% saline	1 mg/mL	2–5 mL/hour	IV (P and C)

Note: All infusion rates mentioned have been approximated. Final infusion rate to be decided based on titration to affect.
(C: central venous access; P: peripheral venous access)

and equipped with an antibacterial filter at all times **(Fig. 9)**. The catheter should be fixed in place with regular monitoring of the insertion site. The documentation should explicitly specify the concentration of the medicine and the rate at which it is being infused. Competency-based training is mandatory for all HCPs who

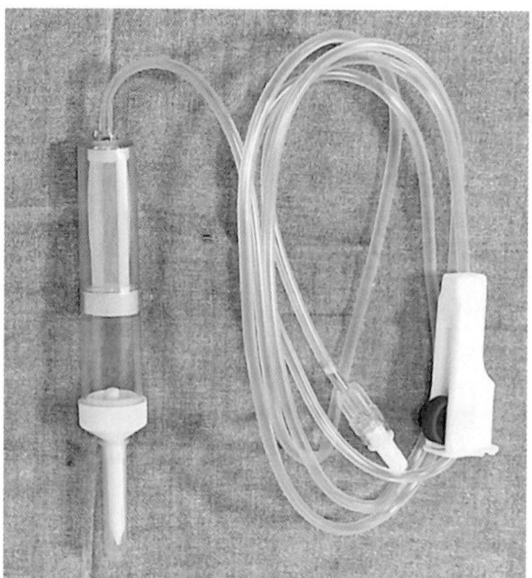

Fig. 8: Blood component administration set.

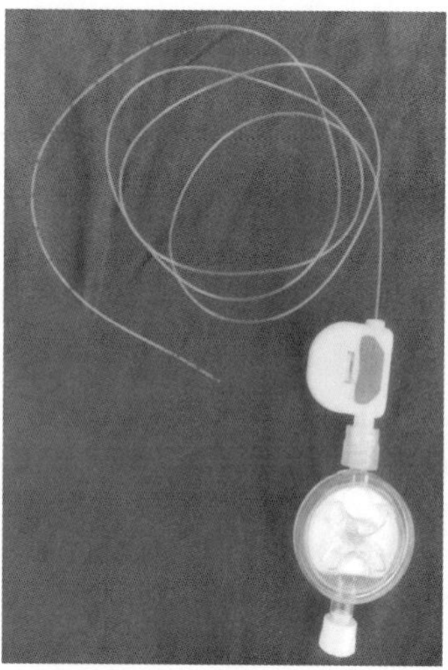

Fig. 9: Epidural catheter infusion set.

utilize epidural devices before they are authorized to use these devices.

- *Subcutaneous injections and infusions:* The subcutaneous injection location should be chosen carefully, ensuring that the skin is undamaged and positioned away from places with prominent bones, joints, inflammatory or fractured skin, previously irradiated areas, or limbs affected by lymphedema. Subcutaneously administered medications should be as isotonic as possible. Aseptic technique with standard precautions must be adhered to in administration of subcutaneous medications and solutions.
- *Intraosseous (IO) injections:* To be used in urgent situations or when it is challenging or impossible to establish vascular access. Aseptic technique with standard precautions must be adhered to in administration of IO medications and solutions. It is advisable to refrain from accessing the IO route in cases of broken bones, traumatized limbs, or areas affected by infection or cellulitis. The possible locations for IO access include the proximal humerus, proximal or distal tibia, and sternum. The location of IO placement can be verified by flushing with 5–10 mL of 0.9% normal saline. If problems such as extravasation/infiltration, compartment syndrome, skin necrosis, or infection are noted, IO access should be promptly discontinued.
- *Arteriovenous (AV) fistula, grafts, and hemodialysis catheters:* Arteriovenous fistula, grafts, and hemodialysis catheters are not suitable for routine administration of parenteral medications/solutions. Aseptic technique with standard precautions must be adhered to in usage of these devices. Hemodynamic monitoring and venepuncture should be avoided on the extremities with an AV fistula or graft, unless it is an emergency situation. The internal jugular veins are the preferred site for the placement of hemodialysis catheters **(Fig. 10)**. It is advisable to avoid using the subclavian and femoral veins for hemodialysis catheters due to the significant risk of stenosis. It is important to take precautions to prevent air embolism when removing hemodialysis

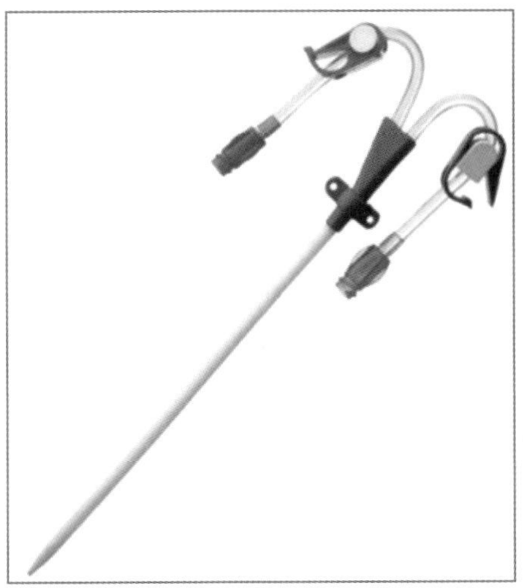

Fig. 10: Double-lumen hemodialysis catheter.

catheters. Applying digital pressure after removal until hemostasis is achieved can help to prevent this complication.

COMPLICATIONS RELATED TO INJECTION AND INFUSION

- *Phlebitis:* Regular monitoring of peripheral vascular catheter insertion sites for indications of phlebitis is essential during each shift. This can be done using a visual infusion phlebitis (VIP) scale, as indicated in **Table 2**. The cannula should be replaced once Stage 2 of the VIP score is attained.
- *Air embolus:* Air-in-line detectors are necessary for monitoring the presence

TABLE 2: Visual infusion phlebitis scale.

Appearance	***Score***	***Stage***
IV site appears healthy *Action:* Observe cannula	0	No signs of phlebitis
One of the following signs is evident: • Slight pain near IV site, or • Slight redness near IV site *Action:* Observe cannula	1	Possibly first signs of phlebitis
Two of the following are evident: • Pain at IV site • Redness • Swelling *Action:* Resite cannula	2	Early stage of phlebitis
All of the following signs are evident: • Pain along path of cannula • Redness around site • Swelling *Action:* Resite cannula and consider treatment.	3	Medium stage of phlebitis
All of the following signs are evident and extensive: • Pain along path of cannula • Redness around site • Swelling • Palpable venous cord *Action:* Resite cannula and consider treatment	4	Advanced stage of phlebitis or start of thrombophlebitis
All of the following signs are evident and extensive: • Pain along path of cannula • Redness around site and swelling • Palpable venous cord • Pyrexia *Action:* Initiate treatment/resite cannula	5	Advanced stage thrombophlebitis

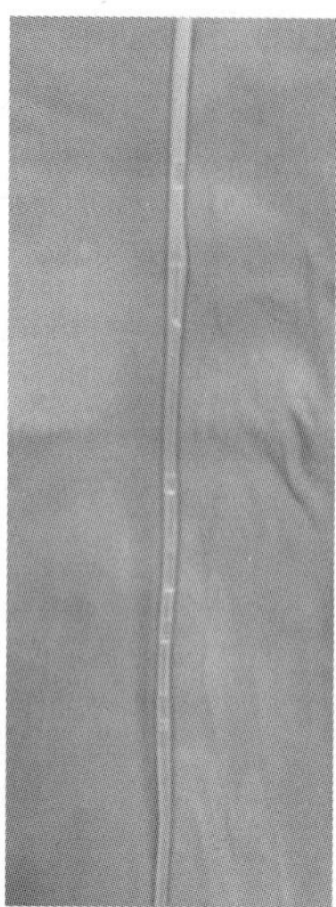

Fig. 11: Air bubble in intravenous administration set.

BOX 4: Ten rights of safe injections and infusions medication administration.

1. Right patient
2. Right drug
3. Right dose
4. Right route
5. Right time and frequency
6. Right to refuse
7. Right reason
8. Right documentation
9. Right response and outcomes
10. Right education and information

of air bubbles in administration sets during delivery using electronic infusion devices. It is necessary to remove air from administration sets and extension tubes before attaching them **(Fig. 11)**. The use of luer-locking connections aids in the prevention of air embolisms.

- *Other complications:* Other risks associated with injections and infusions include infiltration, extravasation, infection, thrombosis, hematoma, hemorrhage, speed shock, and fluid overload.

INFUSION THERAPY TEAMS

Enhancing the proficiency of HCPs in administering injections and infusions safely is facilitated by the implementation of specialized infusion therapy teams, hence promoting quality improvement. The 10 rights of safe administration of medications are listed in **Box 4**.

CONCLUSION

The meticulous understanding and application of injection and infusion methods by HCPs ensure not only the efficacy of treatment but also the safety and comfort of patients.

FURTHER READING

1. Dolan SA, Arias KM, Felizardo G, Barnes S, Kraska S, Patrick M, et al. APIC position paper: Safe injection, infusion, and medication vial practices in health care. Am J Infect Control. 2016;44:750-7.
2. Gallant P, Schultz AA. Evaluation of a visual infusion phlebitis scale for determining appropriate discontinuation of peripheral intravenous catheters. J Infus Nurs. 2006;29:338-45.
3. Gorski LA, Hadaway L, Hagle ME, Broadhurst D, Clare S, Kleidon T, et al. Infusion Therapy Standards of Practice, 8th Edition. J Infus Nurs. 2021;44:S1-S224.
4. Gorski LA. A look at 2021 infusion therapy standards of practice. Home Healthcare Now. 2021;39:62-71.
5. Kruer RM, Jarrell AS, Latif A. Reducing medication errors in critical care: a multimodal approach. Clin Pharmacol Advan Appl. 2014;1:117-26.
6. Loveday HP, Wilson JA, Pratt RJ, Golsorkhi M, Tingle A, Bak A, et al. epic3: national evidence-based guidelines for preventing healthcare-associated infections in NHS hospitals in England. J Hospital Infect. 2014;86:S1-70.

CHAPTER

29 Transfusion Medicine

Chandrashish Chakravarty

INTRODUCTION

Blood and blood product transfusion in any hospital comprises strict protocols and process flow to ensure safety, reduce wastage of blood products, and avoid medicolegal consequences. Just like physicians, who mostly decide on need for transfusion and manage complications, nurses play a key role in carrying out the bedside check of blood products, spiking and transfusing the products, reporting any complication, and documentation of the details.

BLOOD AND BLOOD PRODUCTS

It is rare to use whole blood transfusion in civilian hospitals now. Component transfusion is preferred. These components are:

- Packed red cells (PRBC)
- Platelet concentrate (random donor or single donor)
- Fresh frozen plasma (FFP)
- Cryoprecipitate
- Platelet-rich plasma
- Granulocyte concentrate

Packed Red Cells

Usual indications are acute hemorrhage with hemodynamic changes or end-organ injury and hemoglobin <7 g/dL in the intensive care unit (ICU). Hemoglobin targets may be higher in acute ongoing ischemia of the heart (8–9 g/dL).Symptomatic chronic anemia may need transfusion after blood investigations are sent for workup.

Storage: 4–6°C (±2°); expiry 35 days.

Transfusion should be started within 30 minutes of arrival from blood bank and the process completed within 4 hours.

Transport: Whole blood and PRBC are transported in cold box maintaining 4–6°C. It may be warmed to not >37°C before transfusion.

Platelet

Unlike PRBC, platelets, platelet-rich plasma, and granulocytes are issued from blood bank in an insulated carrier maintaining a temperature of 22° ± 2°C. Platelets should never be refrigerated. They are best kept on a slow rocking surface if there is delay in transfusion, so that they do not clump. Best transfused immediately and within 30 minutes of arrival from blood bank.

Usual indications are prophylactic transfusion in very low platelet count. The absolute numbers vary between 5,000 and 20,000/μL. Above 20,000 and below 50,000/μL transfusion of platelet is restricted to obvious bleeding or perioperative situations. Rarely platelet transfusion may be necessary above 50,000/μL in neurosurgical patients or ocular surgery where the target is 10^5/μL. Recent data suggest to transfuse platelet before central line placement if <50,000/μL. This decreases significant bleeding.

Target platelet count for:

- *Diagnostic endoscopy or bronchoscopy:* 20–30,000
- *Therapeutic endoscopy or bronchoscopy:* 50,000
- *Lumbar puncture:* 50,000 (in hematological malignancy may be lower up to 20–30,000)
- *Epidural anesthesia:* 80,000
- *Peripheral line, central line removal, and bone marrow biopsy:* No prophylactic transfusion

Platelet transfusion has high risk of transfusion-related acute lung injury (TRALI) like FFP transfusion.

Platelet transfusion is better to be ABO matched but not mandatory if short supply (platelets have short shelf life of 5–7 days). For immune thrombocytopenia or single donor platelet (SDP) transfusion, ABO compatible platelet should be given.

The administration set should be fresh or primed with normal saline.

Fresh Frozen Plasma

Usual indications of FFP are coumarin-induced bleeding, bleeding in liver failure, etc. FFP is also used in thrombotic thrombocytopenic purpura (TTP) and plasmapheresis. FFP transfusion to improve low albumin states is condemned.

Fresh frozen plasma and cryoprecipitate, like PRBC, are transported in cold box at 4–6°C, but unlike PRBC should be transfused immediately and finished within 20 minutes. Risk of TRALI and infection is high.

Group O is commonly referred to as the universal red cell donor. Similarly, Group AB individuals have neither anti-A nor anti-B antibodies in their plasma and can therefore be given to patients of any ABO blood group. AB is therefore universal plasma donor.

Dosage of FFP is usually 15 mL/kg. In case of massive hemorrhage, a PRBC:FFP ratio of 1:1 to 2:1 may be used.

Cryoprecipitate

Cryo is rich in fibrinogen and used to replace low fibrinogen states like trauma. Usually 5–10 packets are required in a single transfusion. Now, fibrinogen concentrate is available in vials and can reduce cryo transfusion. Cryoprecipitate like FFP needs to be ABO compatible.

PRETRANSFUSION CHECKING AND MONITORING

The requisition should be made for the blood products and sample collected from the recipient's blood. The samples collected are one clotted blood and one with EDTA (ethylenediaminetetraacetic acid) anticoagulation. A hemolyzed sample is not acceptable.

The appropriate requisition form must be sent to blood bank mentioning patients full name, age gender, bed number, and hospital identification number, types and units of blood products required, ABO and Rh group (if known), and indication of transfusion. Special instructions if any should also be mentioned. The compatibility of various blood groups is shown in **Table 1**.

Before transfusion, the bag of blood or blood product and the form sent with it

TABLE 1: Compatibility of blood products.

Patients group	*Compatible RBC*	*Compatible plasma*
O	O	O, A, B, AB
A	A, O	A, AB
B	B, O	B, AB
AB	AB, A, B, AB	AB

(RBC: red blood cell)

must be matched with the patient details before transfusion to ensure ABO-Rh compatibility, expiry date of the blood, and date of compatibility testing. Once checked, it can be transfused. *The documentation of pretransfusion check is of paramount medicolegal importance.* Also, it is important to give a follow-up note after 15 minutes and at the end of the transfusion for uneventful transfusion without any obvious transfusion reaction or discomfort.

The nurse has to check the bag for any damage or leak and do the bedside identity check just before transfusion.

Watch for following transfusion reactions:

- Tachycardia
- Chest discomfort or dyspnea
- Red urine
- Hypotension or bleeding from access sites
- Chills, rigor, fever, and heat sensation

In case of such an event:

- Stop transfusion
- Inform doctor
- Send blood samples to blood bank for testing along with the bag of blood being transfused
- Medications as per consultant physician

Physician responsibilities:

- Informed consent for transfusion (consent valid for 30 days)
- Documenting indication of transfusion
- Signing the pretransfusion check and monitoring thereafter
- Rate of transfusion
- Explaining any transfusion reaction and reassuring the patient

Infection control and quality: All blood administration sets are disposable and must be changed 12 hourly. Sterile blood administration sets with 170 micron filter is to be used for whole blood, red cell, granulocyte, plasma, and cryoprecipitate transfusion.

COMPLICATIONS OF TRANSFUSION

- *Febrile nonhemolytic transfusion reaction (FNHTR):* Fever within 4 hours up to 48 hours with mild discomfort or nausea. Mostly from antibodies in donor plasma and biological response modifier (BRM) released during storage. It can be reduced by leukoreduction and replacing residual plasma in platelet.
- *Allergic/anaphylaxis:* Severe reaction can happen in immunoglobulin A (IgA) deficiency. This can be prevented by giving washed platelet. It is rare but an emergency.
- *Transfusion-associated graft versus host disease (TAGVHD):* It is rare but fatal. Mostly occurs in immunocompromised host, congenital T-cell defect, homozygous human leukocyte antigen (HLA) between donor and recipient, and first-degree relative donor. It involves skin, liver, intestine, and bone marrow. Irradiated platelets should be used for prevention. It occurs after 1–6 months of transfusion when donor lymphocytes invade into host tissue by engraftment and proliferation.
- *TRALI:* Mostly reversible hypoxia starts within 6 hours of transfusion. It may need ventilation.
- *Post-transfusion purpura:* Self-limiting drop in platelet within 21 days from autoantibody.
- *Transfusion-related immunomodulation (TRIM):* It may predispose to infection. Leukodepletion of blood product is protective.
- *Platelet refractoriness:* Multiple immune and nonimmune factors can cause

inadequate increase in platelet after transfusion. Antigen-matched platelet should be transfused.
- *Transfusion-associated circulatory overload (TACO):* Volume overload responds to diuresis.
- Physical injury
- Sepsis and viral infection transmission
- *Hypotensive reaction:* Angiotensin-converting enzyme (ACE) inhibitor may cause hypotension after transfusing leukodepleted blood products.

WHO CAN BE A DONOR?

Healthy donors with hemoglobin of 12.5 g/dL can donate 8–9 mL/kg of blood every 12 weeks. Patient should have normal vitals, afebrile, and 18–60 years age.

Where should donation be deferred?
- *Minor surgery:* 3 months
- *Major surgery:* 6 months
- *Tuberculosis:* 5 years
- *Exposure to hepatitis by tattoo, body piercing:* 12 months
- *Received blood product transfusion:* 12 months
- *Malaria:* 3 months after treatment
- *Coronary artery bypass graft (CABG), coronary artery disease (CAD), or chronic kidney disease (CKD):* Usually not accepted as donor
- *History of vaccination for smallpox, oral polio vaccine (OPV), measles, mumps, and rabies:* Defer by 2 weeks
- *Dental surgery under anesthesia:* 1 month
- *Tooth extraction:* 3 days

CONCLUSION

This chapter outlines the protocols and information that a nurse should be aware of if working in an environment where he/she is required to handle blood transfusion. This is particularly true for emergency wards, trauma units, operation theaters, intensive care units, etc. It is also important for the nursing team to pick-up transfusion reactions early and seek help. This will reduce damage and prevent death.

FURTHER READING

1. Blood transfusion protocol. Accessed at HYPERLINK "http://www.NSCCM.ORG.NP" www.NSCCM.ORG.NP on March 11, 2025.
2. Sibinga CT. Clinical Use of Blood: A Different Approach. Springer Nature; 2024.
3. Tolich DJ, Blackmur S, Stahorsky K, Wabeke D. Blood management: Best-practice transfusion strategies. Nursing. 2013;43(1): 40-7.
4. Transfusion complications monitoring. Centers for Disease Control and Prevention. September 20, 2022. Accessed at www.cdc.gov/ncbddd/hemoglobinopathies/blood-transfusions.html on May 4, 2023.
5. What happens to donated blood. American Red Cross. Accessed at www.redcrossblood.org/learn-about-blood/what-happens-donated-blood/blood-testing on May 4, 2023.
6. World Health Organization. Educational modules on clinical use of blood. InEducational modules on clinical use of blood 2021.

CHAPTER 30

Intravenous Fluid Therapy in Intensive Care Nursing

Anand Vinaykumar Joshi

INTRODUCTION

Use of intravenous (IV) fluid is universal in intensive care unit (ICU). Fluid management is challenging in ICU due to deranged physiology of the patients, altered fluid distribution, and unpredictable fluid loss. The situation gets complicated due to dynamic nature of critical illness and frequent and rapidly changing fluid requirements. Optimal fluid management requires critical care nurses to know and understand the fluid homeostasis, composition of fluid, and impact on hemodynamics.

INDICATIONS FOR INTRAVENOUS FLUID THERAPY (FLOWCHART 1)

In intensive care fluid management strategy, one-size-fits-all approach cannot be implemented. Critically-ill patients require individualization in terms of type of fluid, amount or volume to be infused, rate and duration of infusion, and when to stop. Indication for IV fluid therapy in intensive care can be broadly classified as follows:

- *Resuscitation:* Target of resuscitation is to restore intravascular volume when there is life threatening intravascular fluid depletion and compromised end organ perfusion. Typically, clinical goals of this type of infusion include mean arterial pressure (MAP) >65 mm Hg, urine output >0.5 mL/kg/h or normalization of lactate in septic shock. So far, superiority of any particular type of IV fluid has not been established for resuscitation. Surviving sepsis guidelines recommend an initial resuscitation fluid of 30 mL/kg ideal body weight.
- *Maintenance:* Routine maintenance fluids are required for patients who are otherwise euvolemic, hemodynamically stable but are unable to maintain their regular fluid intake orally. This happens when patient is nil per oral or has no nasogastric tube as in dysphagia patient or gastrointestinal obstruction. Here, clinical goal is to supplement daily fluid need and not correct ongoing major loss or correct electrolytes or supplement nutrition **(Table 1)**.
- *Replacement*: Replacement fluids are administered in a hemodynamically stable patient to replace the ongoing fluid loss, as in vomiting, diarrhea, high fever, excess of diuresis, etc., and replacement of electrolytes. The main purpose is to avoid decompensation needing resuscitation, maintain homeostasis and maintain tissue perfusion.
- *Supplementing redistribution:* Certain situations such as sepsis, low albumin, congestive cardiac failure, renal failure, causing fluid shifts leading to intravascular depletion and increased fluid in third space. Clinical signs are unreliable as patient may appear fluid

Flowchart 1: Algorithm for intravenous fluid therapy in adult.

NICE National Institute for Health and Care Excellence

Algorithm 1: Assessment

Using an ABCDE (Airway, Breathing, Circulation, Disability, Exposure) approach, assess whether the patient is hypovolemic and needs fluid resuscitation
Assess volume status taking into account clinical examination, trends and context, indicators that a patient may need fluid resuscitation include: Systolic BP <100 mm Hg; heart rate >90 bpm; capillary refill >2 s or peripheries cold to touch; respiratory rate 20 breaths per min; NEWS ≥5: 45° passive leg raising suggests fluid responsiveness.

Yes → **Algorithm 2: Fluid resuscitation**

Initiate treatment:
- Identify causes of deficit and respond
- Give a fluid bolus of 500 mL of crystalloid (containing sodium in the range of 130–154 mmol/L) over less than 15 minutes

- Reassess the patient using the ABCDE approach
- Does the patient still need fluid resuscitation? Seek expert help if unsure

Yes → >2,000 mL given?
- Yes → Seek expert help
- No → Give a further fluid bolus of 250–500 mL of crystalloid → (back to Reassess the patient)

No → Does the patient have signs of shock?
- Yes → Seek expert help
- No → Assess the patient's likely fluid and electrolyte needs

No → **Assess the patient's likely fluid and electrolyte needs**
- History: Previous limited intake, thirst, abnormal losses, comorbidities
- Clinical examination: Pulse, BP, capillary refill, JVP, edema (peripheral/pulmonary), postural hypotension
- Clinical monitoring: NEWS, fluid balance charts, weight
- Laboratory assessments: FBC, urea, creatinine and electrolytes

Can the patient meet their fluid and/or electrolyte needs orally or enterally?

Yes → **Ensure nutrition and fluid needs are met**
Also see Nutrition support in adults (NICE clinical guideline 32)

No → **Does the patient have complex fluid or electrolyte replacement or abnormal distribution issues?**
Look for existing deficits or excesses, ongoing abnormal losses, abnormal distribution or other complex issues.

No → **Algorithm 3: Routine maintenance**

Give maintenance IV fluids
Normal daily fluid and electrolyte requirements:
- 25–30 mL/kg/d water
- 1 mmol/kg/day sodium, potassium*, chloride
- 50–100 g/day glucose (e.g., glucose 5% contains 5 g/100 mL)

Reassess and monitor the patient
- Stop IV fluids when no longer needed
- Nasogastric fluids or enternal feeding are preferable when maintenance needs are more than 3 days

Yes → **Algorithm 4: Replacement and redistribution**

Existing fluid or electrolyte deficits or excesses
Check for:
- Dehydration
- Fluid overload
- Hyperkalemia/hypokalemia

Estimate deficits or excesses

Ongoing abnormal fluid or electrolyte losses
Check ongoing losses and estimate amounts. Check for:
- Vomiting and NG tube loss
- Biliary drainage loss
- High/low volume ileal stoma loss
- Diarrhea/excess colostomy loss
- Ongoing blood loss, e.g., melena
- Sweating/fever dehydration
- Pancreatic/jejunal fistula/stoma loss
- Urinary loss, e.g., post-AKI polyuria

Redistribution and other complex issues
Check for:
- Gross edema
- Severe sepsis
- Hypermatremia/hyponatremia
- Renal, liver and/or cardiac impairment
- Postoperative fluid retention and redistribution
- Malnourished and refeeding issues

Seek expert help if necessary and estimate requirements

Prescribe by adding to or subtracting from routine maintenance, adjusting for all other sources of fluid and electrolytes (oral, enteral and drug prescriptions)

Monitor and reassess fluid and biochemical status by clinical and laboratory monitoring

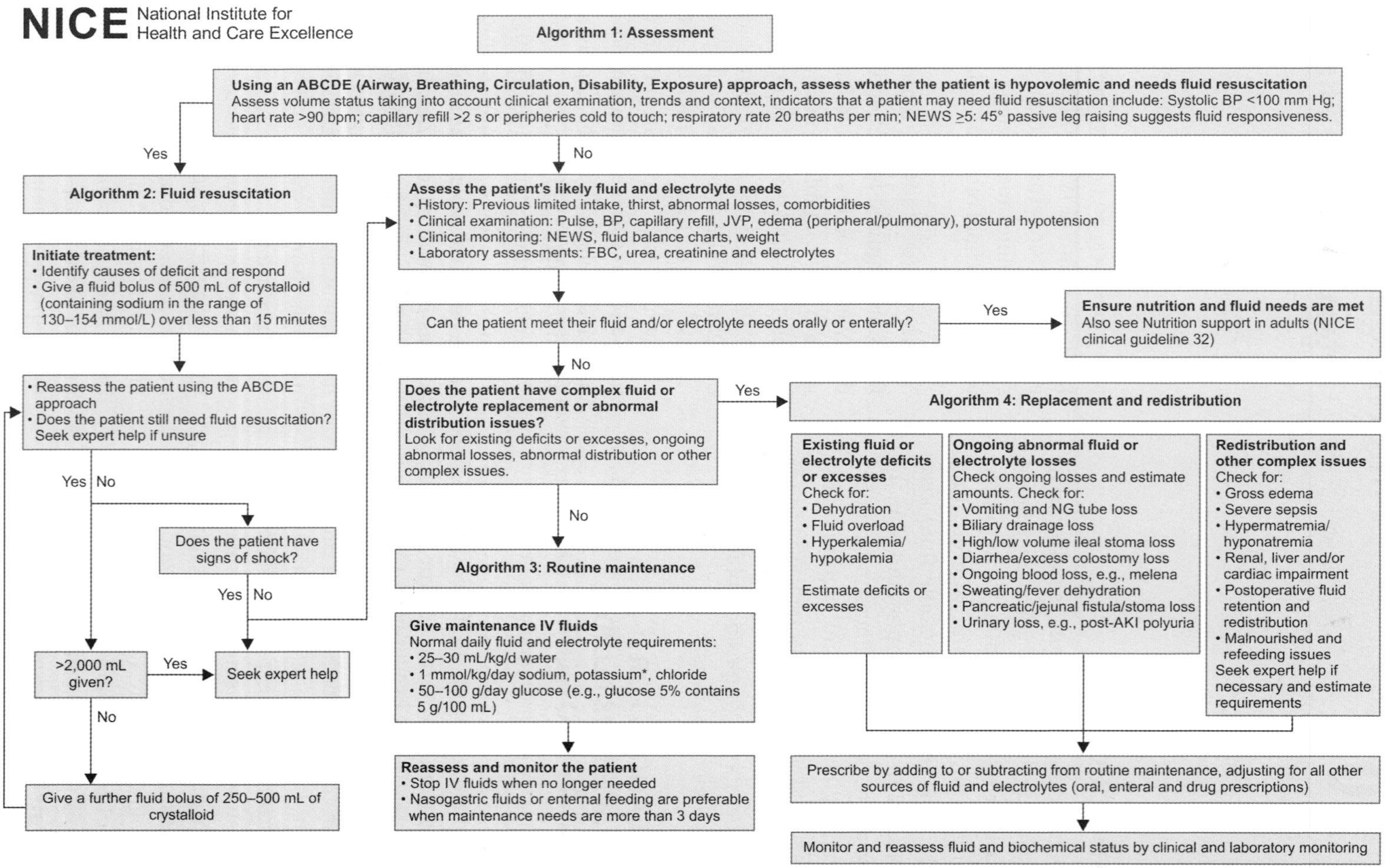

*Weight-based potassium prescriptions should be rounded to the nearest common fluids available (for example, a 67 kg person should have fluids containing 20 mmol and 40 mmol of potassium in a 24-hour period). Potassium should not be added to intravenous fluid bags as this is dangerous.
"Intravenous fluid therapy in adults in hospital", NICE clinical guideline 174 (December 2013. Last update December 2016)

TABLE 1: Relative concentration of electrolytes in various fluids compared to human plasma.

Fluid	*Sodium mmol/L*	*Potassium mmol/L*	*Chloride mmol/L*	*Calcium mmol/L*	*Lactate mmol/L*	*Glucose mmol/L*	*Osmolality mOsm/L*
Human plasma	135–145	3.5–4.5	98–105	2.2–2.7			280–300
5% dextrose						50	278
10% dextrose						100	556
50% dextrose						500	2,778
0.9% saline	154		154				308
0.45% saline	77		77				154
3% saline	513		513				1,026
0.9% saline + 5% dextrose	154		154			50	585
Plasmalyte 148	140	5	98				298
Hartmann's	131	5	111	2	29		278
Ringer's	130	4	109	2.7	28		273
5% albumin	145 ± 15		128				260
20% albumin	145 ± 15						130
Haemaccel (Polygeline)	154		120				274

Note: This table does not represent all the ingredients of each fluid.

over loaded with peripheral edema, but intravascularly they are depleted. IV fluids will be required to maintain intravascular volume to avoid organ hypoperfusion. Volume optimization in these patients requires delicate balance between replacing intravascular volume and minimizing accumulation. The type of fluid preferred in this situation are usually colloids.

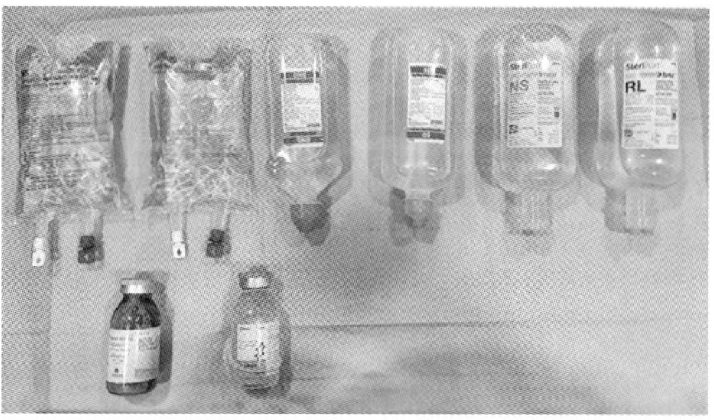

Fig. 1: Types of intravenous fluid infusion containers.

AVAILABILITY OF INTRAVENOUS FLUIDS (FIG. 1)

Intravenous fluids are available in bottle containers or collapsible fluid bag. Depending on containers they are classified as follows.

- *Open system*: Historically, IV fluids were available in a glass bottle with rubber cork and a vent. As fluid left the glass bottle, room air would enter via a tube vent, subjecting potential contamination and air embolism. Incidence of sepsis were reported time to time. Additionally, they were heavy, fragile, difficult to store, and expensive. With advent of polyvinyl chloride (PVC) bottles, use of these bottles is rarely seen now.

- *Close system:* The new generation containers for IV fluids are available as PVC bottles and more recently as collapsible PVC bags. These containers collapse as the fluid leaves and hence does not need any vent. This makes it as a close system. These containers are flexible, clear, and unbreakable. Being closed system, sterility is preserved, and chances of air embolism is minimal. PVC has less contamination as compared to glass. It is compatible with wide spectrum of drugs and other biologics. The newer generation bags are hangable and allows universal spike insertion and removal.

TYPES OF INTRAVENOUS FLUIDS

Based on their property to remain intravascular versus rapid distribution, two types of fluids are available: crystalloids and colloids **(Fig. 2)**.

Crystalloids (Figs. 3A to D)

Crystalloids are solutions of electrolytes and/or dextrose in water. They resemble mineral content of blood. They are the most common of fluids used in intensive care. They quickly diffuse out of blood vessels in to interstitium. They are further classified based on its tonicity, measured as mOsm/L, and compared to blood plasma tonicity. Normal range of tonicity of blood plasma is approximately 275–295 mOsm/L.

Isotonic Solutions

These are the crystalloids which has tonicity near around that of blood. It ranges from 250 to 375 mOsm/L. As they are isotonic, osmotic pressure inside and outside the cells remains the same, hence cells neither shrink nor swells with fluid movement. They freely distribute in body in same proportion as total body water. They get distributed as one-third intravascular and interstitium, while two-thirds get intracellularly. This makes them fluid of choice for resuscitation and maintenance.

Classic example of isotonic solution is normal saline. It is also called 0.9% saline and has sodium and chloride (154 mEq/L of each). Since the electrolytes are far from what we have in plasma, the term "Normal" is a misnomer. It also lacks any acid buffer and has no other electrolytes as we have in blood plasma. Hence, this crystalloid is called "Unbalanced" crystalloid solution.

"Balanced crystalloid solution" examples are Ringer lactate, Hartmann solution, PlasmaLyte solutions were designed to

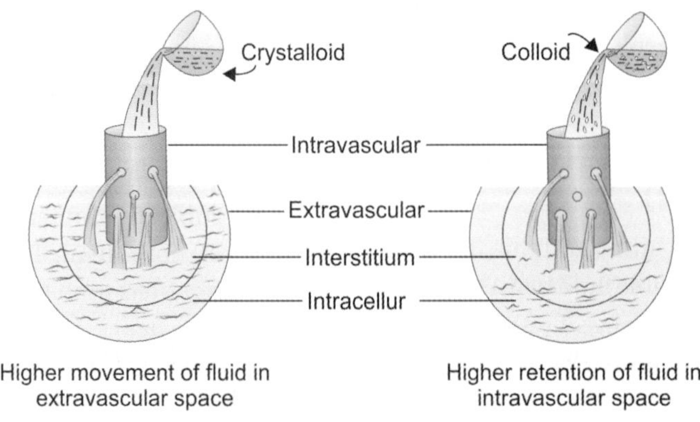

Fig. 2: Behavior of crystalloids versus colloids in body compartment.

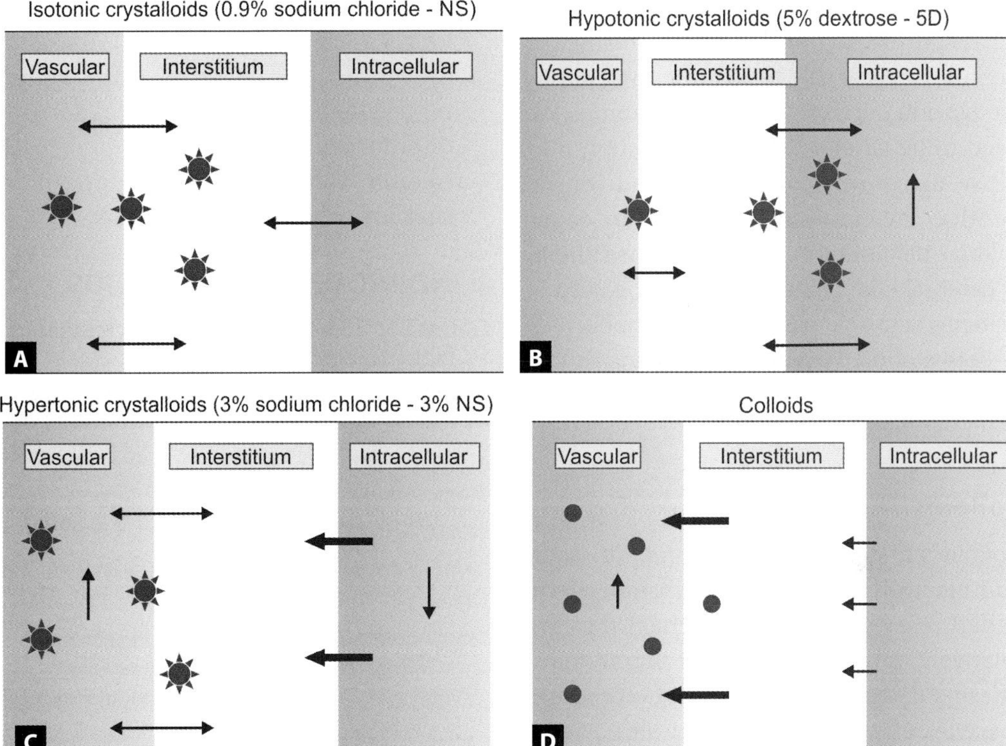

Figs. 3A to D: Crystalloid and colloid movement in body compartments crystalloids and colloids; (A) Isotonic fluid; (B) Hypotonic fluid; (C) Hypertonic fluid; (D) Colloids.

complement blood plasma. They have become preferred for replacement fluids as in burns, trauma, surgery, gastrointestinal loss, etc.

Hypotonic Solutions

These are crystalloids with tonicity of <250 mOsm/L. It contains dextrose in water or half percentage of 0.9% sodium chloride (0.45% sodium chloride). Because it is hypotonic, it rapidly goes out of intravascular compartment, and distributes in interstitium and more intracellularly. Hence, it cannot be used in resuscitation or hypovolemia where intravascular volume is required. Additionally, in central nervous system it can cause cerebral edema and increased intracranial pressure. Large volume of hypotonic fluids can cause hyponatremia. Hence, hypotonic solutions are avoided in patients with traumatic brain injury or central nervous system disorder.

Hypertonic Solutions

Hypertonic crystalloids have tonicity of >375 mOsm/L, much higher than blood plasma. Commonly, it contains high amount of sodium, as in 3% saline or 7% saline. It not only tends to remain intravascularly, but because of high oncotic pressure developed, it draws fluids from extravascular compartments (interstitium and intra-cellular). Small volumes, will draw fluid from extravascular space, hence they are also called as plasma expanders. (*Note:* Plasma expansion is also property of colloids, see in the following text). Hypertonic (3%) saline are used in correction of hyponatremia. We need to be careful as rapid correction may cause dangerous condition called central pontine myelinolysis. Since it can cause cellular dehydration, it is used in treatment of cerebral edema but should not be used in diabetes keto acidosis or hyper osmolar state or dehydration. Hypertonic solutions should not be infused via peripheral cannula and requires a dedicated central line.

Colloids

Colloids are solutions where along with water and electrolytes, insoluble substances are added (e.g., proteins or starches) that are relatively impermeable to cell membranes. These substances add to oncotic pressure intravascularly, causing fluid shifts from extravascular space (interstitium and intracellular) to intravascular space. Hence, they are also included as plasma expanders. These substances gives plasma expansion for around 12-24 hours, compared to 3-4 hours in crystalloids.

Common colloids substances used are:

- *Albumin:* It is most commonly used colloid. It is produced endogenously by liver. Commercially available albumin is prepared from pooled human plasma. It is available as 5%, 20%, and 25% concentrations.
- *Starches and dextran:* Amylopectin extracted from maize or sorghum (starches) and dextran, glucose products from leuconostoc bacteria, are carbohydrate based products used to form colloid. They provide unpredictable period of volume expansion. Examples are hetastarch and dextran. They are no longer recommended in ICU due to its proven adverse effect of acute kidney injury, hepatotoxicity, and coagulation disorder, and bone marrow failure.
- *Gelatin:* Hexigel has gelatin as colloid substances.

INDIVIDUAL CRYSTALLOIDS

Tables 2 to 13 lists the individual crystalloids.

TABLE 2: Glucose 5%.

Available	Dextrose 5%, D5W, G5W
Composition	50 g of glucose/L of water, 200 kcal/L, pH 3.5–6.5, isotonic
Administration	Suitable for central and peripheral line
Uses	Replacement fluid without electrolyte requirements. Some calories and isotonic hydration
Caution	Hyperglycemia, hyponatremia, increased 3rd space edema, worsening of cerebral edema

TABLE 3: Glucose 10%.

Available	Dextrose 10%, D10W, G10W
Composition	100 g of glucose/L of water, 400 kcal/L, pH 3.5–6.5, hypertonic
Administration	Suitable for central and peripheral line
Uses	• Provides some calories and hydration in maintenance fluids • Prevention and treatment of hypoglycemia • Treatment of hyperkalemia (Insulin-dextrose drip)
Caution	Hyperglycemia, hyponatremia, increased 3rd space edema, worsening of cerebral edema, water intoxication

TABLE 4: Glucose 25%.

Available	Dextrose 25%, D25W, G25W
Composition	250 g of glucose/L of water, 998 kcal/L, pH 3.5–6.5, highly hypertonic
Administration	Central line is preferred as it can cause severe thrombophlebitis
Uses	• Treatment of hypoglycemia • Source of calories in parental nutrition • Treatment of hyperkalemia (Insulin-dextrose drip)
Caution	Severe hyperglycemia, large volume infusion will cause electrolyte disturbances and water intoxication

TABLE 5: Glucose 50%.

Available	Dextrose 50%, D50W, G50W
Composition	500 g of glucose/L of water, 1996 kcal/L, pH 3.5–6.5, very highly hypertonic
Administration	Suitable for infusion through central line only. Bolus doses can be given via peripheral line, but can cause severe thrombophlebitis
Uses	• Treatment of hypoglycemia • Source of calories in parental nutrition • Treatment of hyperkalemia (Insulin-dextrose drip)
Caution	Severe hyperglycemia, large volume infusion will cause electrolyte disturbances and water intoxication

TABLE 6: Compound sodium lactate (Hartmann's).

Available	Hartmann's
Composition	• Isotonic (278 mOsm/L), pH 5–7 • Sodium 131 mmol/L • Potassium 5 mmol/L • Calcium 2 mmol/L • Chloride 111 mmol/L • Bicarbonate as lactate 29 mmol/L • Composition of electrolytes may varies slightly with different brands
Administration	• Suitable for central or peripheral line • Do not give simultaneously with blood products
Uses	Fluid maintenance and replacement. Provides hydration. Source of bicarbonate in mild-to-moderate metabolic acidosis
Caution	Fluid and electrolyte overload. Use with caution in patients with lactic acidosis, congestive cardiac failure, or renal failure

TABLE 7: Ringer's solution.

Available	Lactated Ringer's injection, USP
Composition	• Isotonic (273 mOsm/L), pH 6–7.5 • Sodium 130 mmol/L • Potassium 4 mmol/L • Calcium 2.7 mmol/L • Chloride 109 mmol/L • Lactate 28 mmol/L • Composition of electrolytes may varies slightly with different brands.
Administration	• Suitable for central or peripheral line • Do not give simultaneously with blood products
Uses	Fluid maintenance and replacement. Provides hydration. Source of bicarbonate in mild to moderate metabolic acidosis
Caution	Fluid and electrolyte overload. Use with caution in patients with lactic acidosis, congestive cardiac failure, or renal failure

TABLE 8: Sodium chloride 0.9%.

Available	NS, normal saline
Composition	• Isotonic (308 mOsm/L) • pH 4–7 • Sodium 154 mmol/L • Chloride 154 mmol/L
Administration	• Suitable for central or peripheral line • Can be given simultaneously with blood products as it will not cause hemolysis of blood cells
Uses	• Fluid resuscitation, maintenance, and replacement. Provides hydration • Compatible with most of drugs
Caution	Hypernatremia, hyperchloremic acidosis

TABLE 9: Sodium chloride 0.45%.

Available	1/2 (half) NS, 1/2 (half) normal saline
Composition	• Hypotonic (154 mOsm/L) • pH 4–7 • Sodium 77 mmol/L • Chloride 77 mmol/L
Administration	Central line is preferred. May be given with caution via peripheral vein but may cause cell swelling and edema
Uses	Hypotonic hydration, with minimal replacement of sodium compared to water. Dehydration with hypernatremia
Caution	If too much is mixed with bloods cells during transfusions hemolysis can occur. Hyponatremia especially in children and elderly patients, postoperative patients

TABLE 10: Sodium chloride 3%.

Available	Hypertonic 3% saline
Composition	• Hypertonic (1,026 mOsm/L) • pH 4–7 • Sodium 513 mmol/L • Chloride 513 mmol/L
Administration	Preferred central line, but can be given with caution via peripheral line
Uses	• Severe hyponatremia • Lower intracranial pressure in traumatic brain injury
Caution	• Rapid infusion for correction of sodium may cause central pontine myelinolysis • Hypernatremia

TABLE 11: Sodium chloride 0.9% and glucose 5%.

Available	Dextrose normal saline
Composition	• Hypertonic (308 mOsm/L) • pH 4–7 • Sodium 154 mmol/L • Chloride 154 mmol/L
Administration	• Suitable for central or peripheral line • Can be given simultaneously with blood products as it will not cause hemolysis of blood cells
Uses	• Fluid resuscitation, maintenance, and replacement. Provides hydration • Compatible with most of drugs
Caution	Hypernatremia, hyperchloremic acidosis

TABLE 12: Plasmalyte–148.

Available	Plasmalyte 148, Kabilyte
Composition	• Isotonic (298 mOsm/L) • pH 7.4 (6.5–8) • Sodium 140 mmol/L • Chloride 98 mmol/L • Potassium 5 mmol/L • Magnesium 1.5 mmol/L • Acetate 27 mmol/L • Gluconate 23 mmol/L
Administration	• Suitable for central or peripheral line • Can be given simultaneously with blood products as it will not cause hemolysis of blood cells
Uses	Fluid resuscitation, maintenance, and replacement. Provides hydration
Caution	Use with caution in patients with hypochloremic hypokalemia alkalosis, severe metabolic acidosis, congestive cardiac failure, or severe renal impairment

TABLE 13: Water for injection.

Available	Small ampoules of water for injection
Composition	• Hypotonic • No electrolytes present
Administration	Should not be used for infusion, centrally or peripherally as it will cause hemolysis
Uses	Reconstituting medicines that are formulated as a powder or diluting medicines before injection only
Caution	Should never be used for direct infusion in large quantity in veins or arteries as it will cause hemolysis of red blood cells

TABLE 14: Albumin 5%.

Available	5% albumin, USP (100 mL and 250 mL), glass bottle or collapsible PVC bag
Composition	• Contains 5 g albumin in 100 mL, or 12.5 g albumin in 250 mL • Total sodium is between 130 and 160 mmol/L • Sodium is in form of chloride salt, sodium acetyltryptophanate and sodium caprylate • pH: 6.7–7.3
Preparation	• Albumin is a blood product. Strict guidelines need to be followed in handling, storage. If refrigerated allow to reach room temperature before infusion. Use immediately after opening • Do not freeze albumin • Ideal store 2–8°C temperature. Keep temperature below 30°C • Protect from light
Administration	• No intramuscular, no subcutaneous, no IV bolus • Infuse through a standard IV set. The glass bottle must be vented during use. Slow infusion to avoid pulmonary edema • Allergic reaction may occur • Anaphylaxis may occur • Should be infused with vitals monitoring
Compatibility	Compatible with 5% and 10% dextrose, dextrose saline, Hartmann's, Ringer's and normal saline
Noncompatibility	• Amino acid solutions, fat emulsions, solutions containing alcohol, water for injection • Drugs that bind to albumin—phenytoin, diazepam, ceftolozane-tazobactam, fosfomycin, isavuconazole, labetalol, micafungin, midazolam, piperacillin-tazobactam (EDTA free), vancomycin, verapamil

INDIVIDUAL COLLOIDS

Tables 14 to 18 lists the individual colloids.

TABLE 15: Albumin 20% and 25%.

Available	20% albumin, IP (100 mL), and 25% albumin, IP (100 mL) glass vial or collapsible PVC bag
Composition	• 20% albumin contains 20 g albumin in 100 mL and 25% albumin contains 25 g albumin in 100 mL • Total sodium is between 130 and 160 mmol/L • Sodium is in form of chloride salt, sodium acetyltryptophanate and sodium caprylate • pH: 6.7–7.3
Preparation	• Albumin is a blood product. Strict guidelines need to be followed in handling, storage. If refrigerated allow to reach room temperature before infusion. Use immediately after opening • Do not freeze albumin • Ideal store 2–8°C temperature. Keep temperature below 30°C • Protect from light
Administration	• NO intramuscular, NO subcutaneous, NO IV bolus • Infuse through a standard IV set. The glass bottle must be vented during use. PVC pouch comes with vent port. Slow infusion to avoid pulmonary edema • Allergic reaction may occur • Anaphylaxis may occur • Should be infused with vitals monitoring
Compatibility	Compatible with 5% and 10% dextrose, dextrose saline, Hartmann's, Ringer's, and normal saline
Noncompatibility	• Amino acid solutions, fat emulsions, solutions containing alcohol, water for injection • Drugs that bind to albumin—phenytoin, diazepam, ceftolozane-tazobactam, fosfomycin, isavuconazole, labetalol, micafungin, midazolam, piperacillin-tazobactam (EDTA free), vancomycin, verapamil

TABLE 16: Hydroxyethyl starch.

Available	Voluven 6%, Volulyte 6%, Hestar 6%, Expavon, Tetra Hes, Tetraspan, Pentaplasam, Nirhes
Composition	• Each bag contains 60 g/L of hydroethyl starch 130/0.4 • Also contains 0.9% sodium chloride • Other small amount of electrolytes may vary with brand • pH: 4–6.5
Preparation	• Ready to use bag • Store below 25°C • Do not freeze
Administration	• No intramuscular, no subcutaneous, no IV bolus • Infuse through a standard intravenous (IV) set • Slow infusion to avoid pulmonary edema • Allergic reaction may occur • Anaphylaxis may occur • Should be infused with vitals monitoring
Compatibility	Do not mix with other medicines
Noncompatibility	No information available yet
Caution	• Use in critically-ill patients is associated with an increased risk of death and/or need for renal replacement therapy due to renal failure • Coagulopathy issues have been reported with large volume transfusion

TABLE 17: Haemaccel.

Available	Haemaccel PVC bottle
Composition	• Contains 35 g/L of polygeline gelatine (MW 3,000 Dalton) • Sodium 145 mmol/L • Potassium 5.1 mmol/L • Chloride 145 mmol/L • Calcium ionized 0.25 mmol/L • pH: 7.3, isotonic solution
Preparation	• Ready to use • Store below 25°C • Do not freeze • Use immediately after opening bottle
Administration	• Should be infused with vitals monitoring • Allergic reaction may occur
Compatibility	No information regarding compatibility issue
Noncompatibility	Should not be mixed with citrated blood as calcium in haemaccel will cause clotting of blood
Caution	Coagulopathy issues have been reported with large volume transfusion

TABLE 18: Dextran.

Available	Microspan, Rallidex In, Nitran
Composition	• Contains 100 g/L of dextran 40 (10%) • Available in various combination of sodium chloride salt and dextrose • Please see individual product brochure for detail content • pH: 3.5–7.0
Preparation	• Ready to use • Store below 25°C • Do not freeze • Use immediately after opening bottle • The solution may crystallize after storage for long periods • Dextran crystals can be dissolved by heating the solution in water bath at 100° C until it becomes clear or by autoclaving at 110°C for 15 minutes
Administration	• No Intramuscular, no subcutaneous, no intravenous bolus • Should be infused with vitals monitoring • Infuse 10–20 mL slowly and watch for hypersensitivity reaction • Allergic reaction may occur
Compatibility	Nimodipine, tramadol, tranexamic acid, vecuronium via Y site
Noncompatibility	Amoxicillin, ampicillin, cephalothin, promethazine
Caution	Coagulopathy issues have been reported with large volume transfusion

CONCLUSION

Intravenous fluids are needed in treating most of the patients. There are variety of intravenous fluids with different compositions which are used for different indications. One should be aware of the compositions and their indications of use and contraindications.

FURTHER READING

1. Australian injectable drug handbook. Product Information. [online] Available from www.tga.gov.au [Last accessed February, 2025].
2. Barlow A, Barlow B, Tang N, Shah BM, King AE. Intravenous fluid management in critically ill adults: A review. Crit Care Nurse. 2020;40(6):e17-27.
3. Brown rm, Semler MW. Fluid Management in sepsis. J Intensive Care Med. 2019;34(5):364-73.
4. NICE. Intravenous fluid therapy in adults in hospital. London: National Institute for Health and Care Excellence (NICE); 2017.
5. Wesley JR. Intravenous containers and solution packaging. Nutrition. 2000;16(7-8):597-8.

CHAPTER

31 Setting Up Trays

Sananda Chakraborty, Sudipta Mukherjee

INTRODUCTION

Invasive and semi-invasive procedures are an integral part of critical care management. Critically ill patients while admitted in intensive care unit (ICU) may need the procedure as planned intervention; but sometimes there may be an urgent need for an intervention like vascular access in a near arrest scenario or temporary pacing while receiving a patient with complete heart block. Being an emergent procedure, time pressure is very high on healthcare professionals such as doctors, nurses, and ICU technicians. At the same time, maintaining sterility during the procedure is of paramount importance. Some of the procedures need absolute sterility like central vascular cannulation (CVC); but for some interventions like nasogastric tube, clean technique is adequate. A protocolized approach is desirable to perform all the ICU interventions in an appropriate manner to have reasonable success rate. All the standard ICUs have written protocol for the invasive procedures performed on regular basis.

Nursing is the cornerstone of any ICU services and active interventions are needed from nursing team for all ICU procedures. Some of the procedures are done by trained nursing personnel themselves like urinary catheter; in some procedures like CVC, active assistance by a nurse is required during the process. It is desirable that nurse should know the procedural steps so that he/she can help the doctor appropriately and also can guide him/her during any wrong step. **Box 1** shows the list of procedures done in ICU on a regular basis.

BOX 1: List of ICU procedures.

- Peripheral venous cannulation
- Urinary catheterization
- Insertion of central venous access device (CVAD)/dialysis line/arterial catheters
- Fiberoptic bronchoscopy
- Bone marrow aspiration/lumbar puncture
- Percutaneous tracheostomy
- Insertion of intercostal/intra-abdominal drainage catheter
- Nasogastric tube insertion

PREPARATION OF TRAY

Preparation of procedural tray is an important component of ICU facility management. Some of the procedural trays are disposable and come as preprepared form. For rest, they need to be assembled at certain area of the hospital. It can be "clean" tray or "sterile" tray depending on the procedure. It should be simple in design, should contain at least items for skin preparation, dressing draping, supplies to give local anesthetics and supplies to close procedural site, and the kits or instruments specific to the procedure. The purpose of the tray is to keep all the necessary equipment, instruments, and consumables related to the procedure in the same place. It helps in smooth functioning of the procedure. Some components are common and should be present in most of the trays. It is advisable to have back up of all the parts separately in busy clinical area so that if extra volume is needed, that can be provided. The tray utilization and use of different components should be reviewed annually for better cost-effectiveness. The basic steps of the procedures and necessary components have been tabulated in **Table 1**. Some of the components are reusable and need thorough sterilization before incorporation in the next tray. All the trays are prepared at Central Sterile Supply Department (CSSD). This needs to be done accurately and consistently. A "reference" material is used by CSSD to standardize the sterility technique. A basic understanding of different kinds of sterilization technique needed for varied equipment is necessary for the nursing team.

TABLE 1: Different ICU procedures and necessary equipment required.

Sl. No	*Name of the procedure*	*Articles required*	*Steps*	*Remarks*
1.	Peripherally inserted venous cannula (PIVC)	1. *Sterile tray containing:* – 2% chlorohexidine solution and sterile gauze – Sterile gloves – Transparent sterile dressing 2. Peripheral IV cannula 3. Tourniquet 4. 10 mL 0.9% normal saline (NS)	• For skin antisepsis • Aseptic insertion of cannula • To secure the line and prevent infection at insertion site • Tie to constrict the blood flow proximal to the PIVC site • To flush the PIVC	Check for return at the hub of the puncture needle for successful attempt
2.	Urinary catheterization	1. *Sterile tray containing:* – Sterile gallipots: 2 – Sterile sponge holding forceps: 1 – Sterile dissecting forceps: 1 – Sterile kidney dish – Sterile gauze pieces 2. Betadine 3. Sterile water 30 mL 4. Appropriate-sized rubber/silicon urinary catheter 5. Sterile lithotomy sheet 6. Sterile gloves, gown, and mask 7. 20 cc syringe 8. K-Y jelly 9. Fixative tape	• To keep betadine and sterile water • For skin antisepsis • Skin antisepsis • To inflate the catheter balloon • Strict asepsis and sterile field • Catheter lubrication	• Insert the full catheter till the hub is at the urethral meatus • Do not inflate water till urine is coming from the catheter hub • Local anesthesia is strongly recommended even in an unconscious patient • Give adequate time for antiseptic to act—wait till dryness

Contd...

Contd...

Sl. No	*Name of the procedure*	*Articles required*	*Steps*	*Remarks*
3.	Central venous access device (CVAD)/arterial cannula/dialysis catheter/ temporary pacemaker insertion	1. *Sterile tray containing:* – Sterile gallipots: 2 – Sterile sponge holding forceps: 1 – Sterile dissecting forceps: 1 – Sterile needle holder: 1 – Sterile gauze pieces 2. Sterile triple lumen CVAD/ arterial cannula/leader catheter/temporary pacing sheath and pacemaker box 3. 2% chlorhexidine solution 4. 100 mL 0.9% NS 5. 3.0 suture 6. 11 size sterile blade 7. Syringe: 5 cc—1, 10 cc—1 8. 2% lox injection 9. Sterile q-site/needleless connectors 10. Transducer set, 500 mL saline pouch bag 11. Sterile lithotomy sheet, gown, gloves, face shield, cap, and mask 12. Sterile probe cover	• Site preparation • Skin antisepsis • To transduce the arterial line • USG-guided insertion	• Ensure position of the guidewire within the vein before dilatation • Watch for local hematoma/need for compression dressing
4.	Fiberoptic bronchoscopy	1. Sterile fiberoptic bronchoscope 2. Suction tube, Y-connector, sterile kidney dish, and 20 cc syringe 3. Mucous extractor 4. Sterile gown, gloves, eye shield, apron, and lithotomy sheet 5. Normal saline	• Sample collection • To flush the scope	• Ensure adequate oxygenation before and during the procedure • Monitor saturation closely during the procedure
5.	Bone marrow aspiration/ lumbar puncture	1. *Sterile tray containing:* – Gallipots: 2 – Small kidney tray: 1 – Sponge holders: 1 – Gauze pieces and cotton balls		Local analgesia is strongly recommended

Contd...

Contd…

Sl. No	Name of the procedure	Articles required	Steps	Remarks
		2. Lumbar puncture needle/bone marrow aspiration needle of appropriate size 3. 2% lignocaine injection 4. 5 cc syringe and 10 cc syringe 5. Sterile cutsheet, gown, gloves, cap, and mask 6. Vacutainers, slides and slide tray, and white paper		
6.	Bedside percutaneous tracheostomy	1. *A large sterile tray containing:* – Sponge holding forceps: 2 – Towel clips: 4 – Straight Kocher forceps: 2 – Curved mosquito forceps: 4 – St. artery forceps: 2 – Curved artery forceps: 2 – Sharp hook: 1 – Allis forceps: 2 – Needle holder: 1 – Straight Mayo's scissors: 1 – Curved Mayo's scissors: 1 – Curved Metz scissors: 1 – Kocher-Langenbeck (LB) retractor: 4 – Cat's paw retractor: 2 – BP handle no 3 and no 4: 2 each, 2 sharp hook -2 – Tracheal dilator: 1 – Tracheal retractor: 1 – Debark forceps: 1 – Dissecting forceps: - Nontoothed: 1 - Toothed: 2 – Small bowl: 1 – Big kidney tray: 1 – Adson forceps: 1 – Mayo clip: 1 – Gauze pieces and cotton balls 2. Sterile lithotomy sheet, gown, gloves, cap, and mask 3. 2% lignocaine injection 4. 5 cc and 10 cc syringes 5. Required size tracheostomy tube 6. Tracheostomy tie, suture: 2.0 Mersilk	Local anesthesia administration	• Keep airway card ready at hand for emergency endotracheal intubation or change of tube • Monitor saturation closely

Contd…

Contd...

Sl. No	*Name of the procedure*	*Articles required*	*Steps*	*Remarks*
7.	Insertion of intercostal/ intra-abdominal drainage catheter	1. *A sterile tray containing:* – Sponge holding forceps: 1 – Gallipot: 1 – BP handle: 1 – Dunhill forceps: 6 – Needle holder: 1 – Mayo's scissors: 1 – Needle holder CVD: 1 – Sterile gauze pieces and cotton balls – Sterile blade size 15 2. Appropriate sizes ICD with or without trocar/ intra-abdominal drainage catheter and drainage bag 3. Injection lignocaine 2% 4. 2% chlorhexidine solution 5. Sterile cutsheet, gown, gloves, cap, and mask 6. Pressure dressing 7. Tincture benzene 8. Triple way connector: 1 9. 0.9% NS 100 mL		
8.	Nasogastric tube insertion	*A clean tray containing:* • Appropriate size nasogastric tube • K-Y jelly • Small butterfly tape • Magill's forceps • 50 cc syringe, stethoscope	• Lubrication • Fixation • Ensure position	Confirm tube position by chest X-ray anteroposterior (AP) view before staring feeding

The common ICU procedures and the trays needed for them are summarized in **Table 1**.

Usually, flat trays are used for most of the procedures lined with surgical towel. The equipment should be placed in its sequence of utilization—from left to right by convention. It is for the ease of usage—for example, from left to right, it would be items for skin preparation, items for local anesthetics, items for the procedure, followed by closure items. Any "gallipot" or "paint cup", that is used to receive betadine and chlorhexidine solution, should be kept facing upright. One end of long equipment (e.g., swab forceps) should be inside pouch formed by sterile sheet and other end (e.g., user side) should be open. While opening the tray, the outer clean part of the cover will be opened by nursing staff and the sterile inner cover will be opened by doctor doing the procedure. The trays have to be wrapped in that way.

CONCLUSION

Setting procedural trays properly can help ICU intervention to a great extent. It ensures availability of all items at the same place and during the procedure itself. Some of the items cannot be put inside sterile trays, but they are equally important components and required for the procedure. It needs to keep in mind while setting things in order for an intervention. Knowledge of the steps of intervention can help the attending staff to understand the sequence of items needed in the procedure. Properly functional CSSD will ensure proper sterilization and conglomeration of items while preparing the "procedural trays".

FURTHER READING

1. Infection Control Today. (2003). The Proper Processing of Procedure Trays. [online] Available from https://www.infectioncontroltoday.com/view/proper-processing-procedure-trays [Last accessed February, 2025].
2. Life in the First Lane. (2020). General Preparation for Procedures. [online] Available from https://litfl.com/general-preparation-for-procedures/ [Last accessed February, 2025].
3. Medline. Minor Procedure Trays. [online] Available from https://www.medline.eu/uk/minor-procedure-trays [Last accessed February, 2025].
4. Scribd. Procedure Trays. [online] Available from https://www.scribd.com/doc/258516821/Procedure-Trays [Last accessed February, 2025].
5. The Operating Room Global (TROG). Preparation for Surgery: How to Set Surgical Trays. [online] Available from https://www.operatingroomissues.org/preparation-for-surgery-how-to-set-surgical-trays/ [Last accessed February, 2025].

CHAPTER 32

Alarm Fatigue and Burn Out

Susruta Bandyopadhyay, Diptanjan Ray

INTRODUCTION

The word "Alarm" originated from the Latin word "ad arma" or the French word "a l'arme" which means "to your weapons". In other words, it indicates a call for immediate action for attack or defense. "The Joint commission" (TJC: an accreditation organization) defines a clinical alarm as "any alarm" that is intended to protect the individuals receiving care or alert the staff that the individual is at an increased risk and needs immediate assistance. In medical devices, clinical alarms are designed to draw attention of the medical staffs when a patient's vital parameters go beyond proper range or when a medical device cannot able to function properly, in order to ensure patient safety. In 2002, a sentinel event was published by TJC, in respect to the injury or death of patients receiving mechanical ventilation, where 65% of these events were linked with alarm dysfunction or inappropriate alarm setting. In 2012, alarm hazard was reported to be the most common cause among all medical technology-related death in US.

Alarms can be mostly visual or auditory. Interestingly, it has been shown that a healthcare person takes 1 second to respond to an auditory alarm but about 6 seconds to respond to a visual alarm. The auditory alarms are mostly abstract sounds. Again to differentiate between two alarms, temporal patterns (like rate or rhythm) fare better than other patterns (like change in tone or pitch).

GOALS OF CLINICAL ALARMS

- Detection of life-threatening situations, e.g., ventricular tachycardia, asystole, hypotension, and oxygen desaturation.
- Detection of imminent danger, e.g., low blood pressure trends, bradycardia, and ECG changes
- Diagnostic alarm, e.g., diagnosing a new onset arrhythmia like atrial fibrillation (AF)
- Detection of life-threatening device malfunction, e.g., ECG lead off alarm, ventilator circuit disconnection alarm, disconnection from power, gas or water supply alarm, and machine failure
- Detection of imminent device malfunction, e.g., low battery warning

Over the past decade, all the medical technology companies along with quality control bodies increasingly followed a principle of "better safe than sorry," which resulted in more number of alarms and lower thresholds for setting off those alarms. There has been simultaneously a significant increase in medical devices in the critical care. Another reason for excessive alarms has been lack of coordination between various instruments. Each instrument maker wants their instrument to be safe. Hence, the alarm for a syringe pump warning the end of a certain infusion raises an alarm of same priority as the alarm of a ventricular tachycardia. The biomedical incorporations have recognized this but the progress to a solution has been slow. This has resulted in a manyfold increase in the number of alarms in the ICUs. It is estimated that an ICU may have several hundred alarm incidences per day. One hospital recorded 100–120 alarms per nurse per 8 hours shift or 1 alarm in every 4 minutes per nurse. It has also been observed that a nurse can at most differentiate between 9 and 14 different types of alarms Not only this makes it difficult for the nurses to differentiate between the critical and noncritical alarms but also raises the noise level in the ICU. The ICU noise level may reach 80 dB because of the alarms (as loud as running a drilling machine in the ICU). This causes loss of concentration and loss of efficiency among the nurses and also makes it uncomfortable for the patient.

The various alarms can be technically correct or incorrect (i.e., it may actually detect the aberration or pick up an artifact) as well as clinically relevant or irrelevant. The unnecessary alarms may be classified as:

- *False alarm:* It is an alarm which is detected by the monitoring devices as a significant physiological event when there is no actual event, e.g., interference with pulse oximetry caused by ambient light or a disconnected ECG lead leading to an asystole alarm.
- *Nuisance alarm:* It is a clinically non-actionable alarm. It may also be defined as technically correct but clinically irrelevant alarm, e.g., in a patient of chronic AF, frequent alarm notifying AF with controlled ventricular rate is considered to be nuisance alarm as it has got minimal clinical implication and does not require any action.
- *Technical alarm:* When the monitor/equipment in concern, requires attention, e.g., ECG lead off alarm. Some technical alarms are considered to be low priority and are major cause of desensitization among nursing personnel. However, there are many which have significant clinical implications. For example, during an ECG lead off situation, the patient remains unmonitored and there is possibility of missing critical cardiac rhythm-related events which may lead to complications, even death.

Increased number of false and nuisance alarms in the clinical setting creates distrust on the alarm safety system. The nurses often start treating these alarms as "plain white noise" or resort to blanket disabling the alarms. These lead to a "cry wolf" situation where clinically significant alarms are ignored by the attending nursing personnel. This ultimately gives rise to patient safety-related issues.

Alarm fatigue is the condition where the medical staffs including nurses and technologists become overwhelmed by the increased number of alarms in the clinical setting, this in turn causes desensitization of the medical personnel, making them ignore alarms, respond late or inappropriately disable the alarms. Medical staffs over-exposed to clinical alarms may lead to loss of concentration leading to misjudgment and make them feel stressed. Over the last few decades, several studies have recognized that excessive clinical alarms may lead to alarm hazards which include improper application of alarm system, alarm fatigue.

EFFECTS OF ALARM FATIGUE

- *Patient safety-related issue:* Delayed/missed response against significant clinical alarm requiring medical attention leading to potentially hazardous patient condition.

- *Burn-out syndrome in healthcare providers*: Noisy environment in ICU may lead to burn-out syndromes (a syndrome resulting from chronic workplace stress causing a state of emotional, mental, and physical exhaustion) in nursing personnel.

STRATEGIES TO REDUCE THE ALARM FATIGUE

On the basis of various studies in the past, in 2010, standardized measures have been put forth in order to reduce alarm fatigue among staffs. There are various strategies suggested in different literatures for improving alarm management, as well as reducing false, nuisance, and technical alarms, intending to minimize alarm fatigue. In general, these processes are called "alarm management".

- *Creating awareness:* The nurses should understand the various types of non-actionable alarms and the phenomenon of alarm fatigue. There should be efforts to reduce them.
- *Technical approaches:* There are three technical approaches to minimize the false alarms, thus reducing the alarm fatigue:
  1. *Maintaining a situational awareness*:
     i. The alarm settings should be realistic consistent with a patient's clinical situation rather than conventional and conservative. The threshold for ventilator alarms for high respiratory rate should be different for a postoperative stable patient on ventilator and a patient in acute respiratory distress syndrome (ARDS).
     ii. *Phase-specific setting*: It is especially relevant in different stages of surgical procedures where different patterns of alarms specific for that condition (introduction of anesthesia, maintenance, and emergence) reduce the frequency of false alarms. There are several studies where different patterns of alarms and alarm responses have been identified in different phases of anesthesia.
  2. *Composite system of validation (cross-checking)*: Integration of different parameters in detection of a clinically significant event reduces the frequency of false alarm, e.g., a ventricular tachycardia alarm can be assumed to be false alarm, if the plethysmograph or arterial blood pressure waveform shows normal graph morphology.
  3. *Individualize alarm priority on the basis of patient status*: Changing the alarm setting according to patient's preexisting condition the incidence of false/nuisance alarms, e.g., in a patient of chronic AF, deactivating the rhythm alert may reduce the incidence of nuisance alarm or in a patient whose baseline HR is <60 beats/min or >100 beats/min, setting the lower/upper limit of the alarm setting a little beyond the normal range may help to reduce the incidence of false alarm.
- *Statistical approaches to improve signal extraction*: Several statistical models have been incorporated in the monitors/devices for improvement in signal extraction and it was proven to be effective in reducing false alarms caused by artifacts.
- Artificial intelligence and automation
- Keeping the monitors in standby mode when the patients are not connected.

All these will require a collaboration between medical personnel, biomedical engineers, organizations looking after accreditations or standards, and the authorities.

CONCLUSION

Alarms are a necessity in the ICUs. They draw attention to various events and various dangers. They have also been shown to save lives. However, if not used properly they may also proved to be a nuisance. Nurses should be aware of this and be able to set their alarms to their advantage.

FURTHER READING

1. Baillargeon E. Alarm Fatigue: A Risk Assessment. Master Sci Nurs. 2018;(23):1-43.
2. Cho OM, Kim H, Lee YW, Cho I. Clinical alarms in intensive care units: Perceived obstacles of alarm management and alarm fatigue in nurses. Healthc Inform Res. 2016;22(1):46-53.
3. Funk M, Clark JT, Bauld TJ, Ott JC, Coss P. Attitudes and practices related to clinical alarms. Am J Crit Care. 2014;23(3):e9-e18.
4. Johnson KR, Hagadorn JI, Sink DW. Alarm Safety and Alarm Fatigue. Clin Perinatol. 2017;44(3):713-28.
5. Koomen E, Webster CS, Konrad D, van der Hoeven JG, Best T, Kesecioglu J, et al. Reducing medical device alarms by an order of magnitude: A human factors approach. Anaesth Intensive Care. 2021;49(1):52-61.
6. McKinnell JA, Dwyer JP, Talbot GH, Connolly LE, Friedland I, Smith A, et al. Plazomicin for infections caused by carbapenem-resistant Enterobacteriaceae. N Engl J Med. 2019;380(8):791-3.

CHAPTER 33

Sample Collection

Kanwalpreet Sodhi, Manender Kumar

INTRODUCTION

Phlebotomy, the collection of blood samples for laboratory testing, is a routine bedside procedure. Blood sampling carries risks both for the patients and health workers, thereby, the procedure needs to be done meticulously. Patients may have pain, get bruised or there may occur needle-stick injuries to the healthcare workers, which can lead to infections with blood-borne organisms such as human immunodeficiency virus (HIV), hepatitis B, syphilis, or malaria. Each step of sample collection and handling can affect the quality of the specimen and the diagnosis. A contaminated specimen can lead to a misdiagnosis and even the clerical errors occurring with wrong labeling or errors during transport can prove fatal. The World Health Organization (WHO) has recommended guidelines for safe phlebotomy including drawing, collecting blood, and transporting blood to laboratories/blood banks, which reiterate quality and should be brought into clinical practice. **Table 1** depicts the standard quality elements required for safe blood sampling.

Sampling is considered a procedure and should be duly approved by the institutional authority and the persons who can do the procedure should be designated. Consideration should be given to regular training by competent authority for the procedure including strict asepsis, sample taking procedure, sample labeling, handling, and transport. The recommended standard operating procedures (SOPs) for sampling are mentioned in **Box 1**.

TABLE 1: Safe phlebotomy.

Procedures	Nurses should be trained about sampling procedures
Training	Training for all staff carrying out phlebotomy is mandatory which should include an understanding of anatomy, procedure details, awareness of the risks from blood exposure, and the consequences of poor infection control
Correct patient identification	Identification should be through the patient ID number matching to the laboratory request form
Condition of sample	Condition of the sample should be satisfactory to match the quality of the results: no clotting/hemolysis
Safe transport	Appropriate transport criteria as per the specimen should be part of best practices which will improve the quality of results from laboratory testing
Incident reporting system	*A system for reporting all adverse events should be there:* A logbook or register should be maintained with accurate details of the incident, possible causes, and management

Blood collection methods include:

- *Venipuncture,* i.e., penetrating a vein with a needle with an evacuated tube system, syringe method, or butterfly infusion set; and
- *Capillary blood system* whereby the skin puncture is done with the use of a lancet.

Sampling in ICUs should follow a *defined protocol* with defined elements including:

Practical considerations:

- Look for the physician orders
- Preplan the procedure to:
  - Arrange proper and labeled collection tubes
  - Arrange necessary equipment for processing the samples, e.g., tube roller/mixer or centrifuges etc. or for transport of sample, e.g., icepacks
  - Ensure sufficient staff resource is available to assist with the sampling procedure and for transport
  - Talk to the patient before performing sampling, explain the procedure to him. Be empathetic.
  - Use restrains, if needed

  The method and volume of blood to be collected will depend on many factors, including:
    - The specimen requirements for the specific laboratory test
    - The volume of sample required for a particular test
    - Patient's age (e.g., infant versus adult)
    - Available equipment for obtaining the specimens
    - Accessibility of proper specimen processing and storage facilities

BOX 1: Safe phlebotomy standards.

- Quality control
- Appropriate training of staff in phlebotomy
- Availability of appropriate supplies of protective equipment
- Avoidance of contaminated phlebotomy equipment
- Availability of postexposure prophylaxis (PEP)
- Cooperation on the part of patients
- Appropriate equipment for transport of specimens
- Quality of laboratory services

The various types of blood samples and their collection method are tabulated in **Table 2**.

TABLE 2: Type of blood samples for laboratory studies.

Type of specimen	*Collection method*	*Tube cap color*	*Additive added to collection tube*	*Description*	*Use*
Whole blood	Venipuncture	Yellow	Acid citrate dextrose (ACD)	Obtained by using collection tube without anticoagulant. After the tube has been filled with blood, immediately invert the tube 8–10 times to mix and ensure adequate anticoagulation of the specimen	• Hematology tests • For centrifugation to use the plasma portion
Clotted blood	Venipuncture	Light blue	3.2% sodium citrate	• No anticoagulant added • Citrate prevents blood from clotting by binding calcium	Coagulation studies

Contd...

Contd...

Type of specimen	***Collection method***	***Tube cap color***	***Additive added to collection tube***	***Description***	***Use***
Serum	Venipuncture	Red top	Serum tube with clot activator or gel	• Clot activator promotes blood clotting with glass or silica particles. Gel separates serum from cells • Clotted blood is allowed to stand for 20–30 minutes and then centrifuged. The upper portion is termed serum which does not contain fibrinogen	• Biochemistry tests • Serological tests • Immunology tests
Plasma	Venipuncture	Dark green-top	Sodium heparin	• Prevents clotting by inhibiting thrombin and thromboplastin • Whole blood containing anticoagulant is centrifuged and the upper portion is termed plasma which contains fibrinogen	• Coagulation studies • Plasma chemistries
Capillary blood	Fingerstick			A combination of venous, arterial blood, and tissue fluid obtained by a skin puncture	• For blood sugar testing • Used in children and infants, or where venipuncture cannot be performed • To obtain small blood volumes for laboratory testing as it minimizes pain

INDICATIONS

The typical indication for blood sampling is the need for a venous blood sample for blood-grouping crossmatching or various laboratory studies.

CONTRAINDICATIONS

There is no absolute contraindication for blood sampling. But, it can be relatively contraindicated in few clinical conditions wherein some other site can be preferred, or certain specific precautions can be taken. The relative contraindications include:

- Local site infection or hematoma
- Extremely edematous limb
- Local site burns or injured extremity
- Venous thrombosis or phlebitis
- Intravenous (IV) catheter distal to a prospective venipuncture site which may affect the laboratory results, if there are ongoing IV fluids or drugs

- Arteriovenous graft or fistula on the limb
- Ipsilateral mastectomy

In any of the above situations, there is always a potential to use any other site, e.g., the opposite arm for venipuncture.

Please note coagulopathy is not a contraindication per se for sampling, but the puncture site must be compressed adequately for a longer time after venipuncture.

EQUIPMENT

Before performing the procedure, the following equipment should be available at the bedside.

- *Aseptic solution/material for skin cleansing:* Alcohol swabs, 1% chlorhexidine, or povidone-iodine
- Tourniquet, preferably single use
- *Syringes with needle:* An appropriately sized hypodermic needle and syringe that fits comfortably into the most prominent vein with little discomfort is the most common means of blood sampling. Too large gauge needle for the vein will tear the vein and cause bleeding (hematoma); too small needle will damage the blood cells during sampling and may cause errors in laboratory tests that require whole blood cells, hemoglobin, or free plasma. Blood collection for transfusion requires a larger gauge needle than is used for drawing blood.
- Clean gloves
- Vacutainers, blood collection tubes, and blood culture bottles, as appropriate
- Ice packs/cold chain boxes
- *Sharps container within arm's reach and clearly visible*: To ensure safe disposal of sharps
- Bandages or gauze for dressing

  Certain optional equipment may be used to increase the success rate of procedure including:

  - Vein-finder devices such as ultrasonography device or infrared vein viewer
  - Topical anesthetics such as lidocaine gas-injector, mixture of lidocaine, epinephrine, tetracaine, or lidocaine/prilocaine cream.

SELECTION OF VEIN/RELEVANT ANATOMY

In routine, direct puncture of a superficial vein is the most common method of blood sampling. Any vein on the nondominant arm and hand may be used for venipuncture but the median cubital and the cephalic veins are the preferred veins. If upper extremity veins are inaccessible, leg veins like the greater saphenous vein, dorsal digital veins or sometimes, even the femoral vein may be used for blood sampling. The external jugular veins should preferably be avoided for the sole purpose of blood sampling.

Relevant Anatomy (Fig. 1)

The cephalic vein is located on the lateral (radial) side of the arm, while the basilic vein is located on the medial (ulnar) side. These veins extend through and branch within the antecubital fossa, creating the large antecubital and proximal forearm veins. While doing venipuncture, caution must be taken to avoid arterial puncture since the brachial artery lies just deeper to the basilic vein in the upper arm.

POSITIONING

- Patient should be comfortably seated with back supported or may be made supine, if they are anxious, moribund, have low Glasgow Coma Scale (GCS) score or have a history of vasovagal reaction.
- Position the arm below the heart level

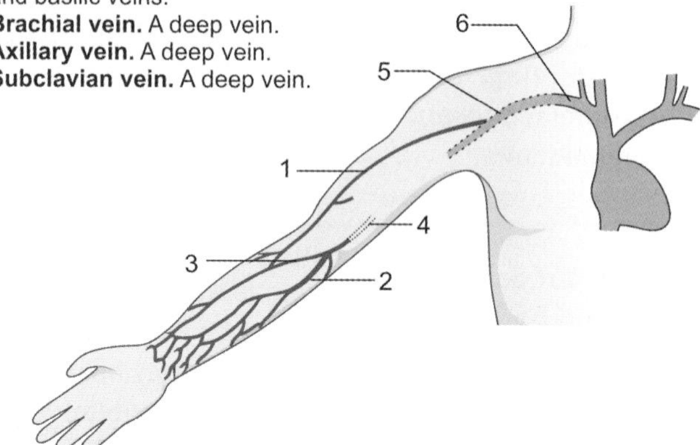

Fig. 1: Anatomy of veins in the arm.

- Support the supinated forearm on a comfortable surface

PROCEDURE

Aseptic Technique

- Closed systems for blood sampling are safer options than open systems and hence are preferable.
- The use of vacuum extraction tube systems as closed systems for blood collection reduces the risk of direct exposure to blood and makes it easier to take multiple samples from a single venipuncture.
- Disinfect your hand with handrub and wear disposable gloves before the procedure

Identification and Preparation of the Site

- Identify a suitable vein
- Apply a tourniquet ensuring optimum pressure
- Ask the patient to make a fist
- Palpate the vein with your index finger to locate a large-diameter vein which should be immobile and has good turgor. You can tap a potential site with your fingertips to help distend and make the veins more prominent. A vein-finder device may be used if a suitable vein is not readily seen or palpated.
- After identifying a suitable cannulation site, remove the tourniquet
- Cleanse the skin site with antiseptic solution in a circular motion from inner to outer beginning at the needle-insertion site.
- Wait for the antiseptic solution to dry completely: 30 seconds to 1 minute for chlorhexidine; 1.5–2 minutes for povidone-iodine; if applying povidone-iodine, wipe it off with alcohol and allow the alcohol to dry.
- After this, do not touch the skin over puncture site with any nonsterile item.

Obtaining the Blood Sample

- Palpate with your gloved finger to locate the middle of the target vein

- Apply gentle traction to the vein distally using the thumb of your nondominant hand to prevent the vein from moving. Traction may not be necessary for larger veins of the forearm or antecubital fossa.
- Inform the patient before the prick
- Needle direction should be proximally in the direction of venous blood flow along the midline of the vein, the bevel facing up at a shallow angle of about 10–30° to the skin.
- Blood will appear in the needle hub (called a blood flash) when the needle tip enters the lumen of the vein. Once the blood flash is seen, stop advancing the needle, lower the needle to better align it with the vein, and advance it into the vein an additional 1–4 mm, to ensure that it stays in position during blood collection.
- If no flash appears in the hub after 1–2 cm of insertion, withdraw the needle slowly. As you withdraw the needle tip back into the lumen, the flash may now appear if the needle had initially crossed the vein. If a flash still does not appear, withdraw the needle almost to the skin surface, change direction, and try again to advance the needle into the vein.
- *Any rapid localized swelling signifies blood extravasation*: Immediately stop the procedure, remove the tourniquet and the needle, and apply pressure to the puncture site with a gauze for 1–2 minutes.
- Keep the needle motionless and start withdrawing the blood sample. If using vacuum tubes, push each tube fully into the tube holder, taking care to avoid dislodging the needle from the vein. If using a syringe, pull back on the plunger gently to avoid excessive negative pressure causing collapse of the vein or damaging the blood cells.
- After completion of the blood collection, remove the needle in one motion and immediately apply pressure with a folded gauze to the puncture site.
- Deploy safety cover over the exposed needle and dispose of the sharp devices into a sharp container. Do not recap nonsafety needles prior to disposal.
- If syringe was used to collect the blood, transfer samples to collection tubes and bottles; insert the needle directly into the top of the vacuum tubes or remove the needle and attach a vacuum tube holder to the syringe. Do not push blood into vacuum tubes, rather allow the vacuum to draw the blood into the tube. Then gently invert the tube 6–8 times to mix the contents; do not shake the tubes.
- When multiple blood tests are to be done, blood should be allocated to the collection tubes in a proper sequence: first cultures, then plain tubes, followed by tubes with anticoagulant, and then others.

Aftercare

- Dress the site with gauze, tape, or a bandage
- The puncture site must always be rechecked after a few minutes post-procedure to look for any local site bleed or hematoma.
- Do not flex the elbow after antecubital venipuncture; this might actually cause hematoma formation.

TRANSPORT PRECAUTIONS

The storage and transportation of blood samples contribute to preanalytic errors, beyond the preparation and sampling procedure itself, which can significantly affect the laboratory results.

- The samples must be labeled for patient identification with patient name and identification. Barcode labels are methods of choice for reliable patient identification.

- Appropriately filled request forms indicating the required laboratories must accompany the sample.
- Most laboratories recommend storing and transporting blood samples at temperatures of between 4 and 25°C.
- For short-term storage or shipping serum or plasma samples, cooling packs can be used. Arterial samples should also be transported in icepacks for appropriate results.
- Prolonged exposure of samples to fluorescent light can damage the blood components, so blood samples should be covered and protected from strong light at all times.
- For transportation, adhering to specialized health and safety regulations is mandatory to prevent infections.

Cold chain is used for keeping and distributing blood specimens in good condition. The cold chain consists of a series of storage and transport links, designed to keep the samples at the correct temperature until they reach the testing laboratory. A typical cold chain system is shown in **Flowchart 1**.

Flowchart 1: Cold chain system.

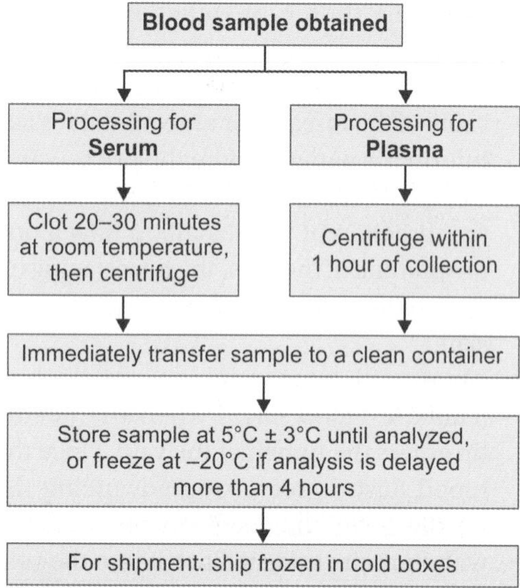

COMPLICATIONS

Complications are not usual with venipuncture. Some reported complications are included in **Box 2**.

BOX 2: Complications of venipuncture.

- Local infection
- Skin irritation/allergy
- Excessive pain
- Damage to the vein
- Bleeding/ooze from the site
- Hematoma
- Arterial puncture
- Nerve damage
- Vasovagal syncope
- Needlestick injuries leading to blood-borne infections in healthcare workers (HCWs)

SOURCES OF ERRORS

Potential errors can occur during the collection and handling of blood samples including inaccurate identification of specimens, incorrect anticoagulant use, and collection in inappropriate vacutainers. Erroneous laboratory results may occur due to technical issues with blood sampling which must be considered while taking samples:

- Blood stasis due to prolonged tourniquet placement can cause artifactually abnormal laboratory results such as hemolysis and hyperkalemia.
- Extending constriction or tourniquet times may lead to hemoconcentration leading to changes in various other laboratory parameters.
- "Pumping the fist" to enhance blood flow leads to erroneous increase in potassium and magnesium level due to muscle activity
- Povidone-iodine used for skin cleaning might cause erroneous hyperkalemia, hyperphosphatemia, or hyperuricemia, if not wiped off with alcohol.

Some special situations are shown in the **Box 3**.

BOX 3: Special situations.

- For blood cultures, venipuncture is to be done, and the sample should not be collected from central lines, unless for special situations
- Venous sample is preferred over arterial sample
- For blood cultures, larger volume of blood increases the chance of getting a positive culture
- For patients with urinary catheter, culture should be taken from the drainage port after sterilization

BOX 4: Take home message.

- The vein to be punctured should be localized and area cleaned with 70% alcohol or chlorhexidine and allowed to air dry before venipuncture.
- Do not apply torniquet for >1–2 minutes; do not clench the patient's fist repeatedly to visualize the vein.
- Do not collect the blood from the vein which is receiving an IV infusion; avoid collecting blood from an IV catheter.
- Amount of blood to be taken into an additive tube/vial should be exactly as is actually required for that tube/vial.
- Do not pour blood into the vial/tube through the needle with pressure.
- Do not shake the vial/tube vigorously after pouring the blood into it.
- Follow the following sequence when collecting blood into vacutainers: Plain tube (no additive)—citrated tube—heparin tube—EDTA tube—fluoride tube.
- Do not keep the blood sample in a freezer or a refrigerator; keep it at room temperature and send it to the laboratory as soon as possible or else, maintain the cold chain.

CONCLUSION

Blood sampling is one of the most commonly performed day-to-day nursing procedures. Meticulous collection technique and appropriate sample handling is crucial in reaching a correct diagnosis. Following the recommendations by the WHO along with the institutional, SOPs will ensure the safety of the procedure with minimal errors. Refer to **Box 4** for the take home message.

FURTHER READING

1. Bayot ML, Tadi P. Laboratory Tube Collection. 2023 Aug 8. In: StatPearls [Internet]. Treasure Island (FL): StatPearls Publishing; 2025.
2. Lippi G, von Meyer A, Cadamuro J, Simundic AM. Blood sample quality. Diagnosis (Berl). 2019;6(1):25-31.
3. MSD Manual. (2023). How To Do Venous Blood Sampling. [online] Available from https://www.msdmanuals.com/en-in/professional/critical-care-medicine/how-to-do-peripheral-vascular-procedures/how-to-do-venous-blood-sampling [Last accessed February, 2025].
4. Nigam PK. Preanalytical Errors: Some Common Errors in Blood Specimen Collection for Routine Investigations in Hospital Patients. J Clin Diagn Res. 2011;5(3):659-61.
5. Nybo M, Cadamuro J, Cornes MP, Gómez Rioja R, Grankvist K. Sample transportation - an overview. Diagnosis (Berl). 2019;6(1):39-43.
6. Srikanth KK, Lotfollahzadeh S. Phlebotomy. In: StatPearls [Internet]. Treasure Island (FL): StatPearls Publishing; 2025.
7. WHO Guidelines on Drawing Blood: Best Practices in Phlebotomy. Geneva: World Health Organization; 2010. 3, Blood-sampling systems.

CHAPTER

34 Nursing Care of the Terminally Ill

Nandhakishore Jampala, Ganshyam Jagathkar

"Dying can be a peaceful event or a great agony when it is inappropriately sustained by life support."

—Roger Bone

INTRODUCTION

Despite advances in medical treatment, death is inevitable and common in health care. Nurses have a special role in helping patients and their families during this time. Apart from providing standard care, it is also the responsibility of every nurse to provide utmost support and care to the patients who are dying.

UNDERSTANDING END-OF-LIFE CARE

End-of-life care (EOLC) is more than just medical treatment. It is about looking after a person's physical, emotional, and spiritual needs at their terminal phase of life. It is about the quality of dying. Without proper care, instead of a "good death", the patient may needlessly experience a lonely end. A "good death" means a peaceful and respectful transition that honors the patient's wishes. The manner in which death is managed may affect the survivors for the rest of their lives. EOLC is an integral part of nurse's role. Good EOLC can ease suffering and help families find peace. On the other hand, poor care can cause more pain and make it harder for loved ones to cope with their loss.

RECOGNIZING WHO NEEDS END-OF-LIFE CARE

In the intensive care unit (ICU), identifying signs that a patient is approaching the end of life can be complex due to the acute nature of their condition. However, subtle changes in vital signs, responsiveness, or overall deterioration may indicate that the end is near. It is crucial for nurses and the healthcare team to be attentive to these signs and communicate them sensitively to the patient and their family. An appropriate plan of care and support should be implemented and regularly reviewed which also includes care after death. All the nurses should act with compassion and empathy in providing this.

THE 6 C'S OF NURSING TERMINALLY ILL

1. *Competence:* The nurses should have enough knowledge, skills, and expertise required to deliver a high-quality care to the terminally ill patient, with the support of the multidisciplinary team (MDT). Nurses must possess specialized training in palliative and EOLC, including pain management, symptom control, and psychosocial support. Competent nursing care ensures that patients receive the most appropriate and effective interventions to

enhance their quality of life during this challenging time.

2. *Courage:* The nurses should have the courage to express their view that a patient may be transitioning to EOLC and should have the courage to advocate as per the patient and family needs. Nurses must be prepared to confront difficult situations and make tough decisions when necessary. Courageous nursing care involves advocating for patient's wishes, maintaining dignity, and providing support even in the face of uncertainty and loss.
3. *Communication:* Open and transparent communication with patients and their families is vital in enabling and supporting patients to consider what is important to them. It involves open and honest communication with the patient, their loved ones, and key members of the treating team. This collaborative approach ensures that everyone is informed and involved in decision making regarding the patient's care and treatment preferences. Encouraging discussions about goals of care and palliative options allows for a proper understanding of the patient's wishes. Clear communication fosters trust, enables decision making, and ensures that the patient's wishes are respected throughout their care.
4. *Compassion:* It involves understanding and empathizing with the patient's physical and emotional needs, providing comfort, and reduce suffering. Nurses show compassion by being present at the bedside, listening attentively, and offering support to both the patient and their loved ones throughout the end-of-life journey.
5. *Commitment:* Nurses must commit to upholding ethical principles, promoting patient-centered care, and advocating for the rights and preferences of their patients. This commitment extends beyond the bedside and encompasses ongoing professional development, collaboration with interdisciplinary teams, and active involvement in quality improvement initiatives.
6. *Care/Connection:* Building meaningful connections with terminally ill patients and their families is essential in nursing care. The emphasis is on improving quality of life by promoting comfort, respect, dignity and supporting the dying person and his family.

The basic steps of caring for the terminally ill are summarized in the **Figure 1**.

- *Priority 1 (recognize):* The possibility of patient dying should be recognized early and then decisions are made, and actions

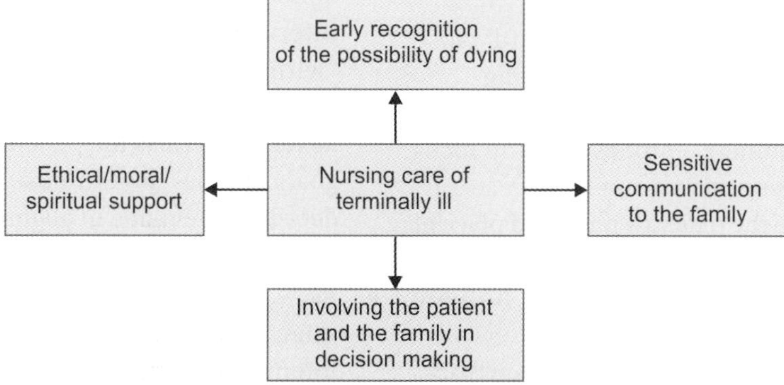

Fig. 1: Priorities of nursing care for terminally ill.

are taken in accordance with the person's needs and wishes, and these are regularly reviewed.

- *Priority 2 (communicate):* Sensitive communication between nursing staff and both the dying person and their family members is crucial.
- *Priority 3 (involve):* The dying person and their family members should be involved in decisions about treatment and extent of care to be given.
- *Priority 4 (support):* The needs of families and other significant individuals related to the dying person should be actively identified, respected, and addressed to the fullest extent possible.
- *Priority 5 (plan and execute):* Once the decision of transition to EOLC is made, it is crucial to implement a comprehensive plan that addresses the patient's physical, emotional, and spiritual needs. This plan should be regularly reviewed and adjusted based on changes in the patient's condition, ensuring that the patient's dignity is maintained even after death.

RESPONSIBILITIES OF THE NURSE IN EOLC

The nurse should:

- Inform the family about the patient's deterioration and address any questions they may have.
- Make the patient's family and close relatives involve in decision making
- Clearly communicate the care plan to family members, emphasizing the focus on promoting patient comfort
- Determine the patient's preferred place of care/death
- Conduct a comprehensive holistic assessment
- Provide due respect to patient's wishes/ priorities

Decision Making

Approximately 80% of critical care patients lack the capacity to make decisions about their terminal care, especially regarding life-sustaining treatments. Surprisingly, only about 10% of patients who die in critical care units have made any prior statements regarding their end-of-life preferences. Shared decision making involving patients and their loved ones is crucial, especially in complex and sensitive situations such as EOLC. It can help in the following:

- *Reduced confusion and conflict:* Involving patients and their close ones in decision-making processes helps ensure that everyone understands the situation, the options available, and the rationale behind the chosen course of action. This clarity reduces confusion and minimizes the potential for conflicts arising from misunderstandings or disagreements.
- *Respect for patient preferences:* Shared decision making respects the autonomy and preferences of the patient. It acknowledges that the patient is the central figure in their care and allows them to express their values, priorities, and wishes regarding their treatment and EOLC.
- *Support for complex decisions:* Complex decisions such as whether "not to escalate interventions", "do not resuscitate", or "withdraw life-sustaining treatment" require careful consideration of medical factors, as well as the patient's values and goals. Nurses should ensure that these decisions are made in alignment with the patient's wishes and best interests.
- *Reduced complicated grief:* Complicated grief, characterized by prolonged and intense emotional distress following a loss, can be mitigated. Being part of the

decision making allows them to be more prepared and involved in the process, thereby reducing the likelihood of experiencing complicated grief later on.
- *Improved quality of end-of-life care:* This personalized approach to care enhances the quality of life for the patient and ensures that their end-of-life wishes are respected and honored.

Choice of Preferred Place of Care

The choice of preferred place of care depends on various factors, including:
- The patient's current medical condition and whether critical care support is still needed.
- The cause of dying and the anticipated duration of the dying process
- Consideration of organ donation, if applicable
- Any previously expressed wishes or preferences of the patient regarding their care and place of death

Decision regarding futility and withdrawal of treatment should be made through a best interest process which would involve key members of the MDT. The nurse is in a pivotal position as having developed a therapeutic relationship with the patient and family, this allows the nurse to act as an advocate and convey the wishes or concerns to members of the MDT on their behalf.

SYMPTOM MANAGEMENT

The principles of symptom management at the end of life remain same regardless of the environment. These principles involve conducting a thorough assessment of all the patient's needs. The key symptoms to be considered and addressed at EOLC are:
- *Pain:* Pain management is paramount in EOLC. It involves assessing the type, severity, and location of pain and providing appropriate pharmacological and nonpharmacological interventions to reduce discomfort. Opioids (fentanyl and morphine) are the first-line agents to be considered. Nonsteroidal anti-inflammatory drugs (NSAIDs) and paracetamol can also be used.
- *Agitation, delirium, or distress:* Patients at the end of life may experience agitation, delirium, or distress due to various factors such as underlying illness, medications, or psychological distress. Management includes identifying the underlying causes and providing supportive care, reassurance, and medication to alleviate symptoms. Usually, benzodiazepines (midazolam) and antipsychotics (haloperidol and olanzapine) are used. Consider environmental changes to promote calmness.
- *Breathlessness:* Breathlessness, or dyspnea, is a common symptom in patients nearing the end of life, often associated with respiratory conditions or advanced disease. Management strategies may include positioning, oxygen therapy, medications such as opioids or benzodiazepines, and nonpharmacological interventions like relaxation techniques.
- *Nausea and vomiting:* Nausea and vomiting can significantly impact the quality of life for patients in EOLC. Management involves identifying the cause, providing antiemetic medications, adjusting oral intake, and implementing other supportive measures.
- *Upper respiratory tract secretions:* Excessive secretions in the upper respiratory tract can cause distress for patients and their families. Management may include suctioning, positioning,

medications to reduce secretions, and providing mouth care to maintain comfort.

- Extubating a patient as a part of EOLC requires caution due to potential distressing symptoms such as obstructive breathing and it may be distressing for both the patient and their family. Positioning the patient laterally can help improve airway patency, facilitate drainage of excess secretions, and reduce audible stridor.
- If positioning alone is insufficient to control secretions, suctioning may be necessary. Reassure the family that the patient is unlikely to be aware of the secretions as he or she is unconscious.
- Additionally, reducing or stopping intravenous fluids is prudent as patients nearing death typically do not require the same level of hydration or nutrition. This approach aims to optimize comfort and dignity for the patient and provide support for their loved ones during this challenging time.
- All necessary medications should be prescribed and made available in a form or route suitable for the patient's needs. In palliative care, there is typically a preference for the least invasive yet most effective route possible. The intravenous route is often discouraged unless absolutely necessary. What is crucial is that each patient receives a medication regimen tailored to their unique needs and symptoms.
- In EOL situations, the importance of nutrition and feeding may shift from sustaining life to maintaining comfort and quality of life. Providing appropriate nutrition can contribute to the patient's comfort and well-being, even if the goal is no longer to prolong life.
- It is important to weigh the potential risks and benefits of providing nutrition and hydration in the context of the patient's overall condition and prognosis. In some cases, aggressive feeding interventions may cause more harm than good, leading to discomfort or complications.

PSYCHOLOGICAL SUPPORT

Once the decision has been made to transition from curative care to promoting a comfortable death, the nurse's role is to ensure that the patient's death occurs in a dignified manner. This involves developing an individualized plan of care that encompasses basic care, symptom control, and psychological, social, and spiritual support.

One consideration would be to move the patient into a single room. If this is not possible, the curtains need to be drawn around the bed space to ensure privacy and dignity or the patient should be shifted to an isolation room inside the ICU, to create a space for the family to grieve and pay their last respects. Attention should also be given to any monitoring equipment. Where possible, these may be removed, or the alarms silenced.

Communicating the news of the death in a timely and sensitive way to the family is paramount. The body should be laid out in a culturally appropriate manner, with input from the family as needed. Timely and accurate verification and certification of death should be ensured.

Memory making is an important aspect of EOLC, providing family members with opportunities to create ever-lasting memories of their loved ones. This may include offering time and resources for activities such as creating handprints, preserving locks of hair, assembling memory boxes, or engaging in other meaningful rituals or traditions. These things can offer comfort and solace to grieving families in the wake of their loss.

AFTER DEATH CARE

After a patient's death, the EOLC process continues beyond the individual's passing. Sensitivity, cultural appropriateness, and logistical support are crucial in addressing the needs of the family. It is essential to ensure that the deceased person is transferred out from the hospital promptly and with dignity. This includes facilitating necessary arrangements and providing emotional support to the family during this difficult time.

CONCLUSION

Nurses have a big responsibility in caring for people at the end of life. With compassion and skill, they can make a difficult time a little bit easier for everyone. By focusing on comfort, communication, and support, nurses help ensure that every person's final moments are as peaceful and dignified as possible. Creating a peaceful and dignified environment for the patient's final moments is a fundamental aspect of nursing care. While providing care for a terminally ill patient, the nurse should also take into account about the established ethical principles and procedural practices, along with sociocultural and legal aspects unique to that country.

FURTHER READING

1. Bhatnagar S, Biswas S, Kumar A, Gupta R, Sarma R, Yadav HP, et al. Institutional end-of-life care policy for inpatients at a tertiary care centre in India: A way forward to provide a system for a dignified death. Indian J Med Res. 2022;155(2):232-42.
2. Hodo A, Buller L. Managing care at the end of life. Philadelphia: Lippincott Williams and Wilkins; 2012.
3. Macaden SC, Salins N, Muckaden M, Kulkarni P, Joad A, Nirabhawane V, et al. End of life care policy for the dying: consensus position statement of Indian association of palliative care. Indian J Palliat Care. 2014;20(3):171-81.
4. Mani RK, Amin P, Chawla R, Divatia JV, Kapadia F, Khilnani P, et al. Guidelines for end-of-life and palliative care in Indian intensive care units' ISCCM consensus Ethical Position Statement. Indian J Crit Care Med. 2012;16(3):166-81.
5. Myatra SN, Salins N, Iyer S, Macaden SC, Divatia JV, Muckaden M, et al. End-of-life care policy: An integrated care plan for the dying: A Joint Position Statement of the Indian Society of Critical Care Medicine (ISCCM) and the Indian Association of Palliative Care (IAPC). Indian J Crit Care Med. 2014;18(9):615-35.
6. Rajagopalan RE. End of life care: New paradigms in management. Postgrad Med. 2002;16:51-6.
7. Truog RD, Campbell ML, Curtis JR, Haas CE, Luce JM, Rubenfeld GD, et al. Recommendations for end-of-life care in the intensive care unit: A consensus statement by the American College of Critical Care Medicine. Crit Care Med. 2008;36:953-63.

SECTION 6

Infection

Section Editor: *Kapil Sharad Borawake*

35. Infection Control
Kapil Sharad Borawake, Swarna Deepak Kuragayala

36. Needlestick Injury
Asif Ahmed, Amit Kumar Sharma

37. Sterilization, Disinfection, and Waste Disposal
Pramod Sood, Inderpreet Kaur

CHAPTER

35 Infection Control

Kapil Sharad Borawake, Swarna Deepak Kuragayala

INTRODUCTION

As per estimates of the World Health Organization (WHO) >1.4 million people suffered from complications secondary to infections during their hospital stay. The usual hospital-acquired infections (HAIs) are ventilator-associated pneumonia, catheter-associated urinary tract infection (CAUTI), central line-associated bloodstream infection (CLABSI), surgical site infections (SSIs), etc. They usually occur in intensive care unit (ICU) settings ranging from 15 to 20% and may lead to complications in up to 40% of ICU population. Due to multidrug-resistant (MDR) hospital flora, most of the HAIs require usage of higher antibiotics which results in development of further antimicrobial resistance secondary to selection pressure. This results in tremendous increase in healthcare cost, morbidity, and mortality. Appropriate infection control measures play a major role in prevention of morbidity and mortality secondary to HAIs.

INTENSIVE CARE UNIT-ACQUIRED INFECTIONS

Hospital-acquired infections are distinguished from community-acquired infections usually by a cutoff time of 48 hours from admission. But one needs to understand that the causative microbes may not always belong to ICU flora and may be imported by the patient as a part of his normal flora.

SURVEILLANCE OF INFECTIONS IN INTENSIVE CARE UNIT

Surveillance plays a major role in the infection control. The control should be exerted at various levels including patients, healthcare workers (HCWs), medical equipment, and infrastructure. It has been observed that there is significant decrease in incidence of HAIs in hospitals which have institutional surveillance programs as against hospitals which do not have them.

There are various concepts of surveillance programs which can be applied in hospital.

Regular collection, analysis, and circulation of all information of HAIs in a specific patient care area or entire hospital are considered as total surveillance. Target oriented surveillance is focused on specific objectives like the control of the spread of multidrug-resistant organisms (MDROs) or reduction of the incidence of CAUTIs. Surveillance can also be infection specific limited to particular out break or resistance pattern in microbiological isolates. A general outline of infection control surveillance is given in **Figure 1**. The actual tools for such surveillance are given in **Figure 2**.

CRITICAL CARE BUNDLES

Critical care bundles are structured pathways to improve the patient outcomes by following clearly defined, easy to follow,

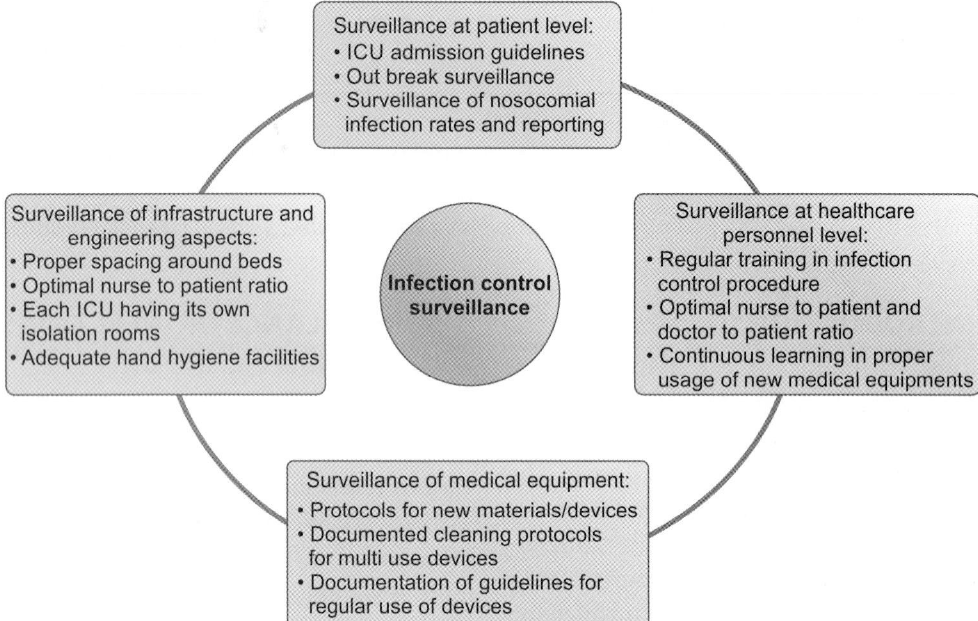

Fig. 1: Components of infection control surveillance in intensive care units (ICUs).

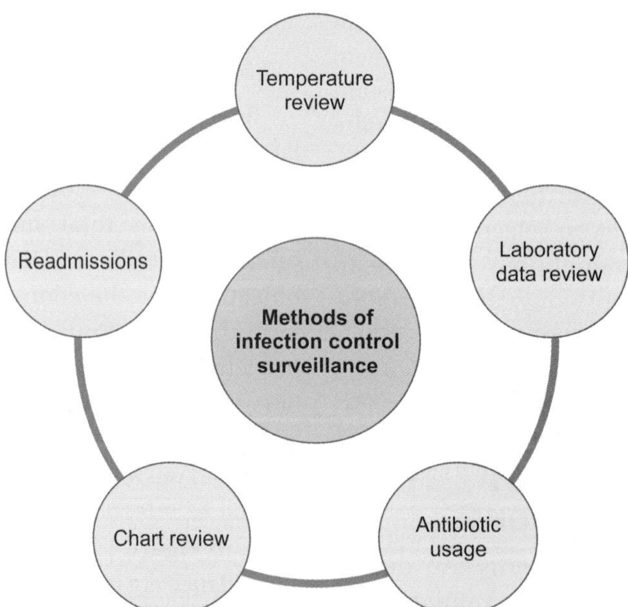

Fig. 2: Various methods/tools that can be used for infection control surveillance in hospital.

and checklist-based steps of evidence-based practices. They are important part of infection surveillance in ICUs.

"Bundle approach" has been shown to have a significant benefit in improvement of patient's outcomes by reduction in HAIs.

The HCW should be rigorously trained in regularly and religiously following the respective bundles.

Among them, few important bundles are discussed here.

Central Line Bundle

The sequence of steps that help in prevention of CLABSI is given in **Box 1**.

Ventilator Bundle

The sequence of steps that help in preventing development of ventilator-associated pneumonia in patients who are on mechanical ventilation is given in **Box 2**.

PREVENTION OF CATHETER-ASSOCIATED URINARY TRACT INFECTION

- Use urinary catheter only definite indications (not for incontinence).
- Use proper technique, using strict asepsis, hand hygiene, and gloves while inserting a catheter.
- A catheter should always drain into the collection bag, all kinks, obstruction should be avoided, and the collection bag should be always at a lower level to prevent backflow.
- There is no indication for using systemic antibiotics for prevention of infections while catheterizing a patient. The catheter site should be cleaned with normal saline and no advantage of using antiseptic solutions.
- There is no advantage in time bound changing of urinary catheter.
- To avoid long-term catheterization, external catheters, intermittent catheterization, suprapubic catheters, etc., are used. Many of these methods need further validation.

PREVENTION OF SURGICAL SITE INFECTION

From the nursing point of view, the important recommendations are:

- Preoperative parenteral antibiotic to be given in certain surgeries as per the guidelines. The timing of the antibiotics should be such that antibiotic reaches bactericidal concentration in blood before the skin incision.
- There is no role of intraoperative or post-operative antibiotics as a prophylaxis.
- The patient should take a bath on the preoperative day.
- Alcohol based solution are to be used as preoperative dressing.
- Blood sugar target should be <200 mg/dL to prevent SSI.

BOX 1: Steps of bundle can be followed for preventing central line-associated bloodstream infection (CLABSI).

- Review daily about the need for central line
- Mandatory hand hygiene while handling the intravascular line
- Inspection of insertion site every day
- Care of catheter-site
- Scrub the insertion hubs with alcohol for at least 15 seconds before use

BOX 2: Steps to prevent ventilator-associated pneumonia.

- Elevation of head end of the patient's bed by 30–40°
- 1–2% chlorhexidine mouth wash 6th hourly
- Subglottic suction of secretions every 2nd hourly
- Sedation vacation every day
- Peptic ulcer prophylaxis
- Deep venous thrombosis prophylaxis
- Assessment of weaning readiness every day
- Spontaneous breathing trial every day

- Blood transfusions for the purpose of SSI prevention, supplemental oxygen in a patient without any hypoxemia, intraoperative iodophor irrigation, and plastic adhesive drapes none have been proven to prevent SSI.

APPROACHES FOR PREVENTION AND CONTROL OF INFECTIONS IN ICU

- Identification of potential sources of infections and subsequent control of transmission. This can be achieved with cleaning, sterilization, and continuation of different medical equipment along with proper documentation.
- Strict guideline-based practice in patients requiring antibiotics both as empiric therapy and surgical prophylaxis
- Strategies to ensure judicious usage of higher antibiotics
- Strategies to prevent development of MDROs
- Isolation practices
- Standard precautions

ISOLATION PRACTICES

As per evidence, >50% patients who are admitted in ICUs have been already colonized with microbes which can cause HAIs during their subsequent course of hospital stay. These microbes include resistant organisms such as methicillin-resistant *Staphylococcus aureus* (MRSA), vancomycin-resistant enterococi (VRE), extended-spectrum beta-lactamases (ESBL), *Escherichia coli*, and MDROs. The routes of transmission can be direct contact, droplets, or airborne. Patients who are either carrier or colonizer of resistant microbes are to be isolated to prevent transmission to other patients.

With regards to the patients who are designated be on contact precautions needed to be handled by wearing gown and gloves along with mandatory practice of hand hygiene.

NEGATIVE AND POSITIVE PRESSURE ISOLATIONS

More than 12 exchanges per hour along with negative pressure ≥2.5 Pa are set in isolation rooms for airborne infections. Severely neutropenic patients are to be housed in rooms set at >12 air exchanges per hour with a positive pressure >2.5 Pa to prevent airborne pathogens coming inside the room. Note that negative pressure isolations prevent airborne infections from spreading from the isolated patient to others. This is meant for patients infected with a highly contagious disease. Positive pressure isolation on the other hand prevents the isolated patient from being infected from others. This is meant for an immunocompromised patient highly susceptible to infections.

STANDARD PRECAUTIONS (TABLE 1)

They are designed to decrease the risk of transmission of microbes from both known and unknown sources of infections in the healthcare setting. Standard precautions can be applied universally to all patients irrespective of their diagnosis. They are to be applied when faced with contact of any of the following: Blood or body fluids, mucous membranes, or nonintact skin.

As hand transmission is one of the very important routes of spread of microbes in hospital settings, proper hand hygiene is extremely important in halting this route of spread. Incidence of HAIs was proven to come down by 25–50% by improving the compliance of handwashing by 1.5–2 folds.

TABLE 1: Standard precautions.

Component	*Clinical application*
Hand hygiene	To be done after direct contact with body fluid, blood, secretions along with contaminated items, immediately before and after removal of gloves
Mask/eye protection/ face shield	To protect mucous membranes
Gloves	To be worn for anticipated contact with secretions, body fluids, and contaminated items along with mucus membranes
Gowns	To prevent soiling of skin and clothes during procedures and activities which are likely to generate splash of body fluid secretions or blood
Patient care equipment	Contaminated linen, devices, or clothing needed to be handled to prevent exposure of mucus membranes to environmental microbes
Sharp objects	• Not to recap needles which are used • Not to remove needles with hand which were used from disposable syringes. • Not to break or bend used needles with hand • Used needles and sharp objects have to be placed in puncture proof containers

RESTRICTION OF ANTIBIOTIC USAGE

As discussed earlier, injudicious usage of antibiotics plays a major role in evolution of MDROs in the healthcare settings.

Various approaches to improve the optimal usage of antibiotics are implementation of hospital antibiotic policy, restriction of reserve antimicrobials for routine use, antibiotic cycling, and de-escalation of antibiotics as per definitive culture sensitivity report. Regular training infection control nurses and pharmacists of the hospitals to identify the gaps in antibiotic policy are essential. Programs like antibiotic stewardship may help in proper treatment of infections as well as prevention of misuse of antibiotics and emergence of resistance. The antibiotics should be used in proper indications, proper doses, and for proper duration.

Hospital infection control committee (HICC)/infection prevention control committee (IPCC) should comprise of clinical microbiologists, intensivists, physicians, infectious disease experts, nursing heads, administrative heads of the hospital, operation theatre/central sterile supply department (OT/CSSD), housekeeping/sanitation personnel, clinical pharmacologist, store heads, and biomedical engineers. Infection control team comprising of microbiologist, infection control officer and infection control nurse takes measures for infection prevention and control daily.

CONCLUSION

Infections acquired in the ICUs are one of the very important reasons for increased morbidity, mortality, and healthcare cost. It is estimated that HAIs account for up to 15–40% of hospital admissions.

Attrition of healthcare personnel, sparsity of structured ICUs and incomplete training in infection control practices make prevention of HAIs in developing countries a difficult task. A good knowledge of local epidemiology, microbial prevalence, and judicious usage of antibiotics as well as understanding of concepts of infection control is essential. Infection control in a hospital or ICU should always be a part of everyday flow of work driven by HCWs.

FURTHER READING

1. Eggimann P, Pittet D. Infection control in the ICU. Chest. 2001;120:2059-93.
2. Ganguly NK, Arora NK, Chandy SJ, Fairoze MN, Gill JP, Gupta U, et al. Rationalizing antibiotic use to limit antibiotic resistance in India. Indian J Med Res. 2011;134:281-94.
3. Goldmann D, Larson E. Hand-washing and nosocomial infections. N Engl J Med. 1992;327:120-2.
4. Haley RW, Culver DH, White JW, Morgan WM, Emori TG, Munn VP, et al. The efficacy of infection surveillance and control programs in preventing nosocomial infections in US hospitals. Am J Epidemiol. 1985;121:182-205.
5. Mukhopadhyay C. Infection control in intensive care units. Indian J Respir Care. 2018;7:14-21.
6. Pittet D, Harbarth S. The intensive care unit. In: Bennett JV, Brachman PS (Eds). Hospital Infections, 4th edition. Boston, MA: Little, Brown and Co.; 1998. pp. 381-402.
7. World Health Organization. Prevention of Hospital-acquired Infections: A Practical Guide, 2nd edition. Geneva: World Health Organization; 2002.

CHAPTER 36

Needlestick Injury

Asif Ahmed, Amit Kumar Sharma

INTRODUCTION

A needlestick injury (NSI) is an accidental skin-penetrating wound caused by a hollow-bore needle contaminated with another person's blood or body fluid. As defined by the US National Institute for Occupational Safety and Health, these are injuries caused by hypodermic needles, blood collection needles, intravenous (IV) cores, and needles used for connecting IV delivery systems.

Healthcare workers (HCWs) using the above are at high risk of exposure to such occupational hazard, which gets complicated by blood borne infections because of the injury.

As per the World Health Organization (WHO), about 3 million healthcare professionals are exposed to the risk of these blood borne pathogens and two-thirds of these are hepatitis B virus (HBV), hepatitis C virus (HCV), and human immunodeficiency virus (HIV) infections. Many of these do go unreported. NSI has remained a major safety challenge for the healthcare community, as it has both direct as well as indirect implications. Over the years, the focus has been on primary prevention for reducing the incidence of NSI thereby decreasing the transmission of infections. Despite the availability of safety-conscious protected needles and hospital guidelines for proper handling and disposal, NSIs continue to happen due to the unsafe practices, noncompliance to established protocols, and negligence among HCWs.

IMPACT

The prevalence of NSIs among HCWs worldwide is 44.5%, whereas it has been reported to be as high as 90.5% in Indian settings. The most common causes of NSIs among HCWs globally are hypodermic needles (55.1%), IV cannulas (23%), and suture needles (19.6%). The higher prevalence of NSIs caused by hypodermic needles can be attributed to their ubiquitous use in all the areas. A significant number of HCWs who reported exposure to blood, were the nurses. 30% of all NSIs in the hospital are reported from the emergency room and intensive care unit.

Needlestick injury can directly or indirectly cause financial burden on the healthcare system. It has been reported that the cost implication of NSI could be in the range of 175–350 USD per HCW. In a hypothetical cohort, the cost per HCW per year per NSI could be saved to the tune of INR 47,661. Every NSI is itself a source of stress, causing significant impact on the physical and mental well-being of the exposed personnel. Fear of contracting infection or seroconversion, undergoing multiple tests and visits to hospital and facing restrictions, thereafter, including side effect of the drugs could be a harrowing experience for an already work-loaded HCW.

The major risk of NSI is exposure to body fluids and transmission of microorganisms but only few are of clinical importance. From the earlier times when HIV infection was a concern, the focus has now shifted to HBV and HCV infections. HIV affects the immune system, while hepatitis B and C primarily affect the liver.

Human Immunodeficiency Virus

Human immunodeficiency virus is one of the pathogens that can spread through NSIs. Without postexposure therapy, the probability of seroconversion is 0.3% following NSI from an HIV source that has been verified, but it could be higher too. Possibility of seroconversion increases with the depth of the puncture wound, visible blood on needle, and from needles used for intra-arterial and IV injections.

Hepatitis B Virus

Based on the active viral load, as determined by the hepatitis B e-antigen (HBeAg) status of the patient, the risk of developing clinical hepatitis ranges from 1 to 31% (31% if HBeAg is positive and 1–6% if HBeAg is negative).

Hepatitis C Virus

In HCWs who are exposed, there is a 1.8% chance of HCV seroconversion following a NSI. Unfortunately, the effectiveness of post-exposure prophylaxis (PEP) in reducing the risk of infection in this case, is not well substantiated.

Failure to follow universal precaution protocols, in patients where exposure to blood and body fluids is high, along with self-ignorance and negligence can increase the risk of NSI and subsequent infections.

ASSESSMENT FOLLOWING INJURY

The prerequisite for starting PEP after NSIs includes detailed history and physical examination of site of injury followed by laboratory investigation of source and exposed personnel.

History should include complete medical details including prior exposure to body fluids, past infections, sexual history, and details of previous immunizations and boosters. Physical examination should be done to know the baseline status, as it might help later if infection develops in future.

Laboratory investigation in the source patient includes testing for HIV, hepatitis B, and hepatitis C. In exposed HCW, laboratory investigation includes serological profile at the time of exposure and later at 6 weeks, 3 months, and 6 months duration.

The vaccination status should be enquired for tetanus and if the patient has not received a tetanus booster in the last 10 years, then it should be administered.

The exposure can be classified as mild, moderate, or high based on the category of exposure.

Superficial wound that is limited to epidermis or a subcutaneous injection with low caliber needle considered is mild exposure. Percutaneous injection with large caliber needle is considered moderate exposure whereas percutaneous injection with high caliber needle (>18 G) with visible blood stains on the needle signify high exposure category.

TREATMENT AND MANAGEMENT

After NSI happens, one should not panic. The exposed site should be thoroughly washed with running water and soap. The nature of exposure should be evaluated including the type of body fluid, needle involved as well as amount of blood present. The HIV, HBV, and HCV status of the source of exposure should be assessed, as stated earlier. Necessary incidence and exposure report form should be completed. Appropriate management for a positive exposure should be initiated as soon as possible.

On exposure to HIV positive patients, PEP is recommended. Medication regimen is started as soon as possible after occupational exposure to HIV and continued for 4-week duration. New recommendation is to include three antiretrovirals in PEP medication regimens for all occupational exposures to HIV.

Close follow-up by experts should be provided for exposed personnel and it includes counseling, baseline, and follow-up HIV testing, and monitoring for drug toxicity.

Follow-up appointments should begin within 72 hours of an HIV exposure. It is recommended that if a newer fourth-generation combination HIV p24 antigen-HIV antibody test is utilized for follow-up HIV testing of exposed HCW, HIV testing may be concluded at 4 months after exposure. If a newer testing platform is not available, follow-up HIV testing is typically concluded at 6 months after an HIV exposure.

On exposure to hepatitis B positive patients, PEP depends on patient's viral load, HCW vaccination status and anti-HBs level. For HCWs vaccinated with hepatitis B vaccine, postvaccination anti-HBs level is evaluated. If it is above 10 mIU/mL, then no further treatment is required. If anti-HBs titer is <10 mIU/mL, hepatitis B immunoglobulin should be administered.

For HCW not vaccinated against hepatitis B, and exposed with hepatitis B surface antigen (HBsAg) positive patient, they should promptly receive HBV immunoglobulin, followed by a rapid active immunization schedule beginning 2 weeks after. If the source is HBsAg negative there is no need to administer hepatitis B immune globulin, nevertheless, HCWs are strongly advised to get the hepatitis B vaccine.

In cases where the patient's clinical status is uncertain, HCWs should be provided with hepatitis B immune globulin and active vaccination within 14 days.

On exposure to HCV positive patients, no treatment has been shown to prevent infection for exposed HCWs. Testing for HCV antibodies, HCV ribonucleic acid (RNA) levels, and alanine aminotransferase (ALT) levels should begin immediately after the event. Repeat testing is done 2–8 weeks later. If infection occurs, the HCW should be referred to experts for management.

PREVENTION

It is crucial for HCWs to prioritize NSI prevention as the problem persists and is quite often encountered. Implementing primary prevention strategies can greatly decrease the occurrence of NSIs and help in reducing the spread of blood borne pathogens. One of the initial steps in preventing NSIs is to accurately assess its prevalence rate, which can be challenging due to various factors such as reporting, lack of standardized reporting methods, absence of central surveillance systems, and gross under-reporting of incidents.

A critical part of all safety and preventive program is a risk management strategy, with an aim to prevent NSI, and it should be the responsibility of all HCWs. A stepwise approach should include identification and removal of the risks, exploring safer and better alternatives, and implementation of administrative measures and policies. Some of these actions could be use of alternative drug administration routes, noninvasive skin closure techniques as an alternative to suturing, and utilization of needle-free IV access system. Avoiding manual transfer of sharps to avoid exposure and proper disposal can minimize the risk further **(Fig. 1)**.

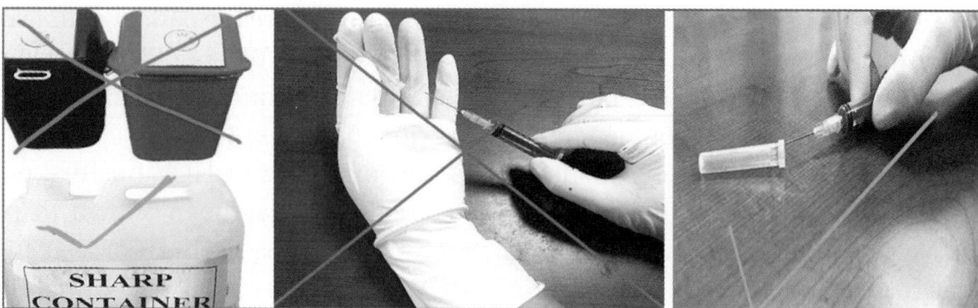

Fig. 1: Safe disposal and correct use of devices.

The other important measures being, setting up of workplace safety program, and it includes standard operating procedures and protocols for safety of sharps and sharp management. It should also include an induction and training program with refresher courses along with a monitoring mechanism having regular audits for ascertaining the compliance. Making vaccinations mandatory for HCWs and supported by use of personal protective equipment can reduce the risk of disease transmission.

CONCLUSION

Despite the increasing concerns, the prevalence of NSI has not decreased and continues to be a major challenge for HCWs. Therefore, a protocolized approach encompassing increased awareness, ownership and involvement, proper reporting, setting up of protocols with proper implementation and monitoring, to decrease NSI and its complications, resulting in betterment of the healthcare personnel.

FURTHER READING

1. André D, Zanetta G, Jianmin L. (2022). Diagnoses of HIV infection in the United States and dependent areas, 2020. [online] Available from https://stacks.cdc.gov/view/cdc/121127. [Last accessed February, 2025].
2. Arora G, Hoffman RM. Development of an HIV Postexposure Prophylaxis (PEP) Protocol for Trainees Engaging in Academic Global Health Experiences. Acad Med. 2017;92(11):1574-7.
3. Bamford A, Tudor-Williams G, Foster C. Post-exposure prophylaxis guidelines for children and adolescents potentially exposed to HIV. Arch Dis Child. 2017;102(1):78-83.
4. Bouya S, Balouchi A, Rafiemanesh H, Amirshahi M, Dastres M, Moghadam MP, et al. Global Prevalence and Device Related Causes of Needle Stick Injuries among Health Care Workers: A Systematic Review and Meta-Analysis. Ann Glob Health. 2020;86(1):35.
5. Ghanei Gheshlagh R, Aslani M, Shabani F, Dalvand S, Parizad N. Prevalence of needlestick and sharps injuries in the healthcare workers of Iranian hospitals: an updated meta-analysis. Environ Health Prev Med. 2018;23(1):44.
6. Joukar F, Mansour-Ghanaei F, Naghipour M, Asgharnezhad M. Needlestick Injuries among Healthcare Workers: Why They Do Not Report their Incidence? Iran J Nurs Midwifery Res. 2018;23(5):382-7.
7. Lee JM, Botteman MF, Nicklasson L, Cobden D, Pashos CL. Needlestick injury in acute care nurses caring for patients with diabetes mellitus: A retrospective study. Curr Med Res Opin. 2005;21(5):741-7.
8. Lee WC, Nicklasson L, Cobden D, Chen E, Conway D, Pashos CL. Short-term economic impact associated with occupational needlestick injuries among acute care nurses. Curr Med Res Opin. 2005;21(12):1915-22.
9. Mannocci A, De Carli G, Di Bari V, Saulle R, Unim B, Nicolotti N, et al. How much

do needlestick injuries cost? A systematic review of the economic evaluations of needlestick and sharps injuries among healthcare personnel. Infect Control Hosp Epidemiol. 2016;37(6):635-46.

10. Muller WJ, Chadwick EG. Pediatric Considerations for Postexposure Human Immunodeficiency Virus Prophylaxis. Infect Dis Clin North Am. 2018;32(1):91-101.
11. Samaranayake L, Scully C. Needlestick and occupational exposure to infections: a compendium of current guidelines. Br Dent J. 2013;215(4):163-6.
12. Vilar-Compte D, de-la-Rosa-Martinez D, Ponce de León S. Vaccination Status and Other Preventive Measures in Medical Schools. Big Needs and Opportunities. Arch Med Res. 2018;49(4):255-60.

CHAPTER 37

Sterilization, Disinfection, and Waste Disposal

Pramod Sood, Inderpreet Kaur

INTRODUCTION

Sterilization and disinfection are basic components of hospital infection control activities. Everyday in any hospital various procedures are being performed. The hospitals also generate waste materials. It is estimated that the each bed in a hospital in an average generate 1–2 kg of waste. The medical devices, surgical instruments, and linen of the patients have a chance of transmission of infection from patient to patient; from patient to other healthcare personnel; or from patient to the environment. Improperly sterilized devices may cause increase in the rate of infections and even sometime outbreaks of infections. Sterilization and disinfection are the basic components of infection control in any hospital. The hospitals are also required to dispose their wastes, in a category-wise method.

STERILIZATION

Sterilization is a process by which all living microorganisms including viable spores are either destroyed or removed from an article, surface, or medium. Results in reduction of $\geq 10^6$ log colony-forming unit (CFU) of microorganisms and their spores.

Sterilizers

There are various types of sterilizers, which are as follows:

- Steam sterilizer (autoclave)
- Flash sterilization
- Ethylene oxide (ETO) sterilizer
- Plasma sterilization
- Dry heat sterilizer (hot air oven)

Steam Sterilizer

It functions similar to pressure cooker and follow general gas laws:

- Water boils when its vapor pressure equals that of the surrounding atmosphere.
- When the atmospheric pressure is raised, the boiling temperature is also raised.
- At normal pressure, water boils at 100°C but when the pressure inside closed vessel increases, the temperature at which water boils also increases.

Mechanism of action: Moist heat destroys microorganisms by irreversible coagulation, denaturation of enzymes, and structural proteins.

Components of steam sterilizer (autoclave):

- Pressure chamber
- Lid
- Electrical heater

Types of steam sterilizer:

- Horizontal type—used in central sterile supply department (CSSD), large size laboratories, and for biomedical waste treatment.
- Vertical type—used for small size laboratories.

Flash Sterilization

- It is used at emergency or during unplanned procedures.

- It involves fast sterilization (134°C for 3–10 minutes) of surgical instruments in an unwrapped condition in steam sterilizer located close to operation theater.
- This practice should only be restricted for emergency situation, e.g., instrument has been contaminated and needs to be replaced in surgical field immediately.
- It is not suitable for porous and cannulated instruments, implants, and suction tubing.
- As the instruments are not packed, they remain wet following sterilization; therefore, there is a high risk of recontamination.

Ethylene Oxide Sterilizer

It is one of the widely used gaseous chemical sterilant in CSSD.

Mechanism of action: ETO has broad microbial action including spores, causes alkylation of cell components such as cell proteins, DNA, and RNA.

Sterilization cycle by ETO is as follows:

- Preconditioning
- Sterilization
- Aeration (degassing)

Plasma Sterilization

Plasma means a gaseous state consisting of ions photons and free radicals. Plasma sterilizer is a special device used to create the plasma state (commercial brands, such as Sterrad). It has following steps:

- Vacuum
- Chemical sterilant
- Gas plasma
- Excess gas removal
- Cycle duration
- Sterilization control

Filtration

Acts by removing microorganisms, not by killing, the Centers for Disease Control and Prevention (CDC) considers filtration as a sterilization method. There are two types of filter:

1. Depth filters
2. Membrane filters—has two wider applications—air and water filtration
   i. Filtration of air:
      a. Surgical mask (3-ply) mask and respirators
      b. High-efficiency particulate air (HEPA) filters
      c. Ultra-low particulate/penetration air (ULPA) filters
   ii. Filtration of liquid

Radiation

- Ionizing radiation include cobalt 60 gamma rays or electron accelerators
- Nonionizing radiation include infrared and ultraviolet radiations

Incineration

Incineration is used for treatment of biomedical waste materials. It burns the waste by providing a very high temperature 870–1,200°C and converting the waste into ash, flue gas, and heat.

Microwave

It is used in hospitals for disinfection of soft contact lenses, dental instruments, dentures, and urinary catheters.

The general practice of sterilization methods for various categories is summarized in **Table 1**.

DISINFECTION

Disinfection is a process that destroys or removes most if not all pathogenic organisms

TABLE 1: Approaches to disinfection and sterilization of medical devices.

Device classification	*Devices*	*Spaulding process classification/time*	*Processes*	*EPA product classification*
Noncritical (touches intact skin and not mucous membrane)	Stethoscope, bedpans, blood pressure cuffs, and patient furniture	• *Low-level disinfection:* Kills most bacteria, some viruses and fungi. Cannot reliably kill resistant microorganism (tubercle bacilli and bacterial spores) • Time—10 minutes or less	• Chemical disinfectants; ethyl or isopropyl alcohol, sodium hypochlorite • Hydrogen peroxide, quaternary ammonium germicidal detergent	Hospital disinfectant without label claim for tubercular activity
Semicritical [touches intact mucous membranes (except dental)]	Flexible, endoscopes, laryngoscopes, endotracheal tubes, and cervical diaphragms	• *High-level disinfection:* Destroys all microorganisms except high numbers of bacterial spores • Time—20 minutes or more	Wet pasteurization or chemical disinfectants. Heat sterilization preferred for between patient processing of heat stable instruments. Follow by rinsing with sterile water	Sterilant/ disinfectant
	Thermometers, hydrotherapy tanks	• *Intermediate level disinfection:* Inactive tubercle bacilli, vegetative bacteria, most viruses, and fungi. Does not necessarily kill bacterial spores. • Time—10 minutes or less	Chemical disinfectants sodium hypochlorite ethyl or isopropyl alcohol, phenolic and iodophor solutions	Hospital disinfectant with label claim for tuberculocidal activity
Critical (enters sterile tissue or vascular system)	Implants, scalpels, needles, cardiac and urinary catheters	• Sterilization • Time-prolonged contact (hours)	Purchase as sterile. Sterilize by steam under pressure. If heat liable, use ethylene oxide gas or chemical sterilants	Sterilant/ disinfectant

but may not destroy bacterial spores. Results in reduction of $\geq 10^3$ log CFU of most microorganism but not spores.

The sterilization practices for surgical instrument and other critical care items are carried out in CSSD.

Central Sterile Supply Department

An integrated place in hospital that performs sterilization of medical devices, equipment, and consumables; that are used in operating theater (OT) of the hospital and also for other aseptic procedures.

The processing area of CSSD consists of four unidirectional zones, i.e., decontamination area > packaging area > sterilization area > sterile storage area:

1. *Decontamination area:* Items are collected and then decontaminated/cleaned by either manual wash or by automated machines (ultrasonic washer and washer disinfector).
2. *Packaging area:* Items (medical devices) are enclosed in materials or a container designed to allow the penetration and removal of sterilant during sterilization and then to protect device from contamination and other damage following sterilization and until time of use.
3. *Sterilization area:* The packed medical devices received from packaging area are subjected to sterilization process by steam sterilizer and ETO sterilizer.
4. *Sterile storage area:* After sterilization the sterilized items are stored in this area. It has an issue counter to supply the items to OTs and various other areas of hospital.

CLEANING AND REPROCESSING OF PATIENT CARE EQUIPMENT

The general practice of cleaning and reprocessing of the critical patient care items are summarized in **Table 2**, and those of semicritical patient care items in **Table 3**, and those of noncritical patient care in **Table 4**.

TABLE 2: Cleaning and reprocessing of critical patient care items.

Objects	*Mode of processing*
Catheters (cardiac, arterial, and urine)	Sterile and single use
Needles	Disposable and single use
Implantable devices	Sterile and single use
Surgical instruments	Heat sterilization in autoclaves
Arterial pressure transducers	Sterile by heat/low temperature/ethylene oxide
Diagnostic ultrasound	Sterilization/high-level disinfection (HLD) as per instructions
Heart–lung oxygenator surfaces	Heat/low temperature sterilization
Hemodialysis and plasmapheresis	Heat/low temperature sterilization
Neurological test needles	Disposable, sterile by heat/steam/sterilize by ethylene oxide (ETO)

TABLE 3: Cleaning and reprocessing of semi-critical patient care items.

Items	*Methods*
Anesthetic equipment (airways, endotracheal tubes, etc.)	Sterilization/high-level disinfection (HLD)
Respiratory equipment	HLD
Laryngoscope and its blade	HLD with liquid germicides/ disinfectants
Endoscopes	Heat sterilization/ low temperature sterilization/HLD
Nebulizer and nebulizer cups	Clean and disinfectant
Respiratory therapy equipment	HLD
Resuscitation accessories	Heat disinfectant/wash with detergent and hot water

TABLE 4: Cleaning of noncritical patient care items.

Items	*Methods*
Ambu bag and mask	Clean with detergent, dry, and thermally disinfectant
Blood pressure apparatus and cuffs	Disinfect the cuff with 70–90% alcohol
Cloth appliances	If reusable, clean with detergent and water, dry and disinfect with 70% alcohol
Doppler	Head of Doppler should be wiped out with 70% alcohol
Bed and bed rails	Low-level disinfection (LLD)
Gowns	Single use in case of disposable, if reusable use 0.5% bleaching powder, dry in sun/cloth drier
High-touch surface	Clean with 70–90% alcohol twice a day
Intravenous (IV) stand and monitoring pumps	Clean with detergent and water and dry
Stethoscope	Clean the bell with 70–90% alcohol
Thermometer	After every use wipe with 70–90% alcohol
Trolleys	Wipe with 70–90% alcohol
Walls and wash basin	Clean with detergents and water
Surgical mask	Disposable/discard as per recommendation

FURTHER READING

1. Mathur P. Hospital Acquired Infections: Prevention and Control, 1st edition. Philadelphia (PA): Lippincott Williams & Wilkins: 2010.
2. Mohapatra S. Sterilization and disinfection. In: Prabhakar H (Ed). Essentials of Neuroanesthesia, 1st edition. Amsterdam, Netherlands: Elsevier; 2017. pp. 929-44.
3. Rutala WA, Waber DJ. New disinfection and sterilization methods. Emerg Infect Dis. 2001;7(2):348-53.
4. Sastry AS, Bhat S. Essentials of Medical Microbiology, 3rd edition. New Delhi: Jaypee Brothers Medical Publishers (P) Ltd.; 2021. pp. 250-7.
5. Sopwith W, Hart T, Garner P. Preventing infections from reusable medical equipment; a systemic review. BMC infect Dis. 2002;2:4.

SECTION

7

Soft Skills

***Section Editor:** Ajith Kumar AK*

38. Communication for Nurses
Ganesh KM, Ajith Kumar AK

39. Documentation in Intensive Care Unit: Nursing Guideline
Swapnil Thulung

40. Nursing Standards and Quality Indicators
Devi Prasad Samaddar, Parul Samadder

CHAPTER 38

Communication for Nurses

Ganesh KM, Ajith Kumar AK

"For the sick it is important to have the best"

–Florence Nightingale

INTRODUCTION

Communication can be defined as a two-way process of exchanging information from one individual or group to another. Good communication between nurses and patients and between nurses and doctors should become integral to patient care to achieve good outcomes. Admission to the hospital brings a great deal of anxiety and apprehension to the patient and their family members. Effective communication from the healthcare providers can help address most of their concerns. Communication is critical not only to patient-centered care but also to re-ensure high-quality care in the intensive care unit (ICU). Along with providing bedside care to the patients, nurses have the best opportunity to interact with patients and their families, and effective communication has been related to improved physical and psychological outcomes by easing the pain and fears in patients and their relatives. A well-informed relative also can help convey information to the patient.

COMMUNICATION TECHNIQUES

Verbal Communication

Most often, the information is shared orally; it may usually involve the diagnosis, the procedures being performed, or treatment options, especially for the terminally ill. It is always prudent to give the patient all the necessary information about the illness, but in some cases; being compassionate by holding the information and discussing it with relatives before letting the patient know is also encouraged. More emphasis should be given to closed-loop communication, asking if they understood the matter, and repeatedly cross-checking what they have understood. Moreover, a personalized and tailored approach with time well spent on listening to the concerns will allow for better understanding and addressing the most relevant areas. On some occasions, one can use a translator either on a smartphone or a person who is well-versed in a particular language to overcome the language barrier.

Nonverbal Communication

This is an often overlooked form of communication. During conversation, cues such as tone, body language, and facial expression are all employed to create a certain impression. Most often unintentional, but these can have a significant negative impact on certain aspects of conversation than the actual words used, which the patients and the relatives perceive as dishonesty by the healthcare provider, which in turn can influence their response or reaction in further conversations. At the same time, such cues can be effectively used to influence a conversation positively. The healthcare provider should also be receptive to nonverbal cues from the patient indicating pain, distress, and/or anxiety. Sometimes, a simple act of holding the patient's hand and maintaining eye contact can alleviate the anxiety.

COMMUNICATION STRATEGIES

Communication strategies need to be developed to assist information sharing with both patients and their relatives.

Effective strategies for improved communication:

- Introduce yourself
- Be honest and tell the truth
- Use simple language and avoid medical jargon
- Dress appropriately
- Make time
- Instil confidence
- Work as team
- Admit uncertainty about prognostic prediction
- Accept the lack of trust
- Employ educational tools

An introduction should include the name, position, and role played in the care of the patient, which will help the patient and relatives understand the depth of information provided. The patient and their relatives expect healthcare providers to present themselves in a certain way (dress, jewelry, hair, and others). They are entitled to the truth and honesty, which will also avoid errors in the information provided by different team members. Allotting a separate time to counsel the family members allows them to understand the level of commitment in the care and to clear doubts regarding the illness. Using simple language and explaining the due course in a language they understand makes them feel confident about the care their patient is receiving; repetition and allowing them to ask questions and express feelings should also be encouraged. On rare occasions, the relatives and the patients lose faith in the treating team. In such instances, offering a referral for a second opinion or to another facility should also be encouraged. Actively handing over or doing bedside rounds instils confidence in the patients that the healthcare providers are interested in them as persons, important information is not being hidden from them, and they feel they are involved in their care.

COMMUNICATION TOOLS

The AIDET is a communication framework for healthcare professionals which is shown to improve outcomes **(Fig. 1)**.

The acronym for AIDET is given in **Table 1**.

This is a simple and effective way to incorporate the fundamental patient communication elements into every conversation. This helps the healthcare

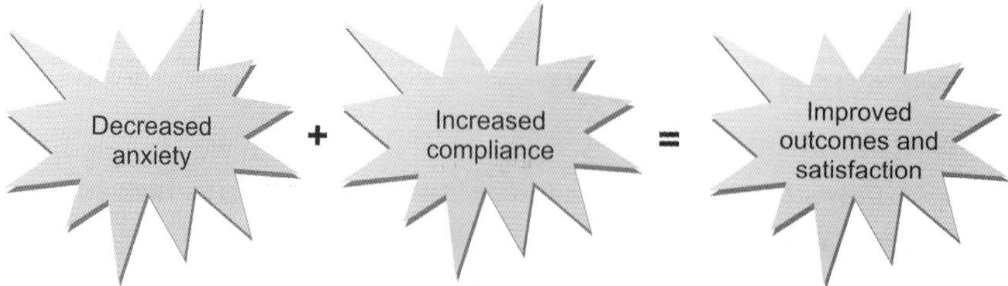

Fig. 1: Formula for better outcomes.

TABLE 1: AIDET acronym.

A	Acknowledge	Greet by name, make eye contact, and acknowledge family members
I	Introduce	Introduce by name, position, skill set, and qualification
D	Duration	Give an accurate time of expectation of test results, arrival of physician, or the time for an update regarding the progress
E	Explanation	Explanation of the further course of action, answer any questions, and let them know as to how to contact you (call button)
T	Thank you	Thank the patient for choosing your hospital, thank the relatives for their cooperation

workers to understand the needs of the patients and their families and exceed the level of care.

LISTENING AND EMPATHIZING

Listening is an important element of communication; it is a way of acknowledging the patient and family's needs. There are two types of listening: Active and passive. In active listening, the person not just listens to the conversation but also responds to it by paraphrasing the conversation, thereby confirming the needs, and establishing mutual understanding, and by giving feedback and/or reply. In passive listening, on the other hand, the person only listens to the conversation without responding or replying. This can have a negative impact and reduce the communication to a one-way conversation.

Empathy in simple words could mean the ability to understand one's feelings. Empathizing with the patients and their families also has a good impact on the outcome; it is a way of saying, "We are there for you."

ISBAR COMMUNICATION TOOL

The acronym for ISBAR is given in **Table 2**.

TABLE 2: ISBAR acronym.

I	Introduce
S	Situation
B	Background
A	Assessment
R	Recommendation

The ISBAR tool is very effective in communicating with colleagues (nurses) and physicians. The model helps in standardizing communication. It is very helpful in handing over in a systematic way. This is endorsed by the World Health Organization (WHO).

Nurses play a very important role in communicating the issues being faced by the patient to the concerned physician. The key aspects of ISBAR are first, Introduce yourself and the name of the patient along with room number, explain as to why you are calling the intensivist (Situation), state in brief the admission diagnosis, medical history and summary of the treatment for the situation (Background), brief the intensivist about the current condition of the patient that is the vital signs (Assessment), and communicate what you feel needs to be done and ask for the Recommendation from the intensivist.

The ISBAR tool is very effective in handing off the patient to the next shift staff without missing any valuable information. This tool has reduced errors in patient care and improved the quality of continuing care.

TABLE 3: SPIKES acronym.

S	Setting up
P	Perception
I	Invitation
K	Knowledge
E	Emotions with empathy
S	Strategy

BREAKING BAD NEWS

Breaking bad news about the prognosis of the patient often becomes very stressful for the intensivist. Nurses can help the treating team of doctors by being a part of the discussion of the outcomes when the patient's condition deteriorates since the family will know the nurses well. Empathy is useful in such situations. The SPIKES tool of breaking bad news is often used, and the acronym is given in **Table 3**.

The SPIKES tool is a standard communication tool for breaking bad news and will be helpful when initiating these difficult conversations. The first step is Setting up an interview, a stage for optimal conversation by preparing oneself as to what to say and have an appropriate care plan, next is to question the patient or family as to what their Perception of the disease or test is and empathic communication will ease the process of perception of the disease trajectory. Often, the patient or their family will be in denial, and coping with this mechanism is an important aspect of breaking bad news. After an understanding of the perception of the course, permission to reveal further details is sought for (Invitation). The sharing of bad news is based on the level of understanding by the patient and their family and their willingness for full disclosure. One should avoid using technical terms and instead show them trends of laboratory results, radiology or trends of the clinical deterioration, which can make the abstract concept clear to them (Knowledge). As the conversation around bad news is associated with Emotions and sometimes leads to dramatic breakdowns resulting in crying and sobbing, which creates a sense of awkwardness; this can be overcome by interacting with them with Empathy. The final step is to prepare a care plan and ask them if they understand the information provided; frequent clarification during the discussion of the treatment plan will help establish a level of understanding and the likelihood of continuation of the care plan. This is likely to reduce the agony and distress associated with the fear of losing the dear one.

THERAPEUTIC COMMUNICATION

In the late 1800s, Florence Nightingale was one of the first to endorse the importance of communication between nurses and patients. Therapeutic communication in nursing consists of an exchange between nurse and patient using verbal and nonverbal cues, in which a conscious effort is made to help patients understand their clinical condition and also allows the patient to express their fears and feelings in a mutually respective way. The main goal of this way of communication is to help the patients and their families to get through the emotional and psychological stress. Thus, the quality of communication is directly related to compliance, continuity of care, and improved outcomes as this approach is patient-centered.

CONCLUSION

Admission to the ICU can be frightening to both the patient and their family. Effective communication can help ease stress, improve mental and psychological well-being, and ultimately improve outcomes. Nurses play a pivotal role in this aspect of patient care as they are always by the bedside and spend the majority of the time with the patient and their families. With their smile and warm touch, the patient and their family can overcome the burden of stress associated with ICU admission to many extents. *C*ommunicate with *C*are and *C*ompassion to avoid *C*onflict should be the *4C* mantra of communication in the ICU to improve the outcomes of our patients.

FURTHER READING

1. Burgess A, van Diggele C, Roberts C, Mellis C. Teaching clinical handover with ISBAR. BMC Med Educ. 2020;20(Suppl 2):459.
2. https://nightingale.edu/blog/therapeutic-communication/
3. Huron consulting group; Strudergroup.com
4. Rosenzweig MQ. Breaking bad news: a guide for effective and empathetic communication. Nurse Pract. 2012;37(2):1-4.
5. Vincent JL. Communication in the ICU. Intensive Care Med. 1997;23:1093-8.

CHAPTER 39

Documentation in Intensive Care Unit: Nursing Guideline

Swapnil Thulung

INTRODUCTION

Nursing documentation in intensive care units (ICUs) plays a vital role in ensuring patient safety, continuity of care, and legal compliance. ICU environments are complex, with critically ill patients requiring intensive monitoring, rapid intervention, and seamless interdisciplinary communication. Documentation serves as a tool to record care provided, reflect clinical reasoning, and communicate patient status effectively among healthcare professionals. This chapter explores the principles of ICU nursing documentation, emphasizing clarity, accuracy, timeliness, comprehensiveness, confidentiality, and technological integration. Recommendations to address challenges and enhance practices are also provided.

IMPORTANCE OF DOCUMENTATION

Documentation is a critical aspect of nursing practice in the ICU. Accurate and thorough documentation serves several purposes, including the following:

- *Communication:* Facilitates effective communication among members of the healthcare team, ensuring continuity of care and patient safety
- *Legal protection:* Provides a legal record of the care provided, protecting both the patient and the healthcare provider in the event of litigation
- *Quality improvement:* Supports quality improvement initiatives by enabling analysis of patient outcomes, identification of areas for improvement, and evaluation of adherence to clinical guidelines
- *Reimbursement:* Forms the basis for reimbursement and billing processes, demonstrating the necessity and appropriateness of care provided

PRINCIPLES OF DOCUMENTATION

Effective documentation in the ICU adheres to the following principles:

- *Accuracy:* Information should be factual, objective, and precise to ensure accurate interpretation by all team members. Avoid assumptions or subjective interpretations.
- *Timeliness:* Document promptly after providing care or observing an event. Delayed documentation can lead to inaccuracies and compromise patient care.
- *Clarity:* Use clear and concise language. Avoid jargon or abbreviations that may be misunderstood.
- *Completeness:* Document all relevant information, including assessments, interventions, responses to treatment, and patient education.
- *Legibility:* Ensure that documentation is legible and easy to read. Use standard

abbreviations and symbols where appropriate.

- *Confidentiality:* Maintain patient confidentiality at all times. Avoid sharing sensitive information with unauthorized individuals.

DOCUMENTATION REQUIREMENTS

Intensive care unit nursing documentation should include the following components:

- *Admission assessment:* Comprehensive assessment data collected upon the patient's admission to the ICU, including vital signs, neurological status, cardiovascular status, respiratory status, gastrointestinal status, renal status, and any other pertinent findings
- *Interventions:* Documentation of all interventions performed, such as medication administration, procedures, assessments, and therapies
- *Response to treatment:* Evaluation of the patient's response to interventions, including changes in vital signs, symptoms, and other clinical indicators
- *Monitoring:* Continuous monitoring data, including vital signs, cardiac rhythm, oxygen saturation, invasive hemodynamic monitoring, and any other relevant parameters
- *Fluid and medication administration:* Documentation of all fluids, medications, and blood products administered, including dose, route, time, and any associated adverse reactions
- *Clinical assessments:* Ongoing assessments of the patient's physical and mental status, including neurological assessments, pain assessments, and assessments related to the primary reason for ICU admission

LEGAL AND ETHICAL CONSIDERATIONS

Nurses must be aware of legal and ethical considerations related to documentation in the ICU. Key considerations include the following:

- *Accuracy and honesty:* Document factual information accurately and honestly. Avoid altering documentation or falsifying records.
- *Confidentiality:* Protect patient confidentiality by ensuring that documentation is accessible only to authorized individuals. Avoid sharing patient information in public or nonsecure environments.
- *Legal standards:* Adhere to institutional policies and procedures to ensure compliance with legal requirements governing nursing documentation in your jurisdiction.

DOCUMENTATION REVIEW AND AUDITS

Regular review and audit of nursing documentation are essential for maintaining quality and accuracy. Nurses should participate in documentation audits and quality improvement initiatives to identify areas for improvement and ensure adherence to documentation standards.

DOCUMENTATION FORMATS

Intensive care unit nursing documentation may be completed using electronic health records (EHRs) or paper charts. Regardless of the format used, documentation should be organized and structured for easy retrieval and review. Common formats include the following:

- *Narrative notes:* Free-text descriptions of patient assessments, interventions, and responses to treatment. Narrative notes allow for flexibility but require careful organization to ensure clarity and completeness **(Table 1)**.

- *Flow sheets and checklists:* Structured forms for recording vital signs, assessments, and interventions. Flow sheets and checklists provide a standardized format for documentation and promote consistency among healthcare provided. ICU flow sheet may include in the **Table 2**:

Patient information:

- *Name:* (Patient's name)
- *UHID:* (0007777)
- *Date of admission:* (Date)
- *Diagnosis/reason for admission:* (Diagnosis)

Interventions: Interventions are shown in **Box 1**.

Fluid and output: Fluid and output are given in **Table 3**.

TABLE 1: Narrative notes.

Date and time	*Nurse's name*	*Narrative notes*
11-02-2024 08:00	Sonia S	Patient admitted to ICU following emergency surgery for ruptured abdominal aortic aneurysm. Vital signs stable
		Neurological assessment: Alert and oriented ×3
		Cardiovascular assessment: Heart rate 82 bpm, regular rhythm. Blood pressure 120/80 mm Hg
		Respiratory assessment: Breath sounds clear bilaterally. SpO_2 98% on room air
11-02-2024 14:00	Neeta K	Patient complained of incisional pain (8/10 on pain scale). Administered morphine 2 mg IV as ordered
		Patient's pain decreased to 4/10 following medication administration
11-02-2024 16:00	Ruth A	Physician performed bedside ultrasound to assess for abdominal fluid accumulation. No significant findings noted
		Patient tolerated procedure well without complications
11-02-2024 20:00	Ananya P	Patient developed sudden onset of dyspnea and tachypnea. Respiratory distress observed. Oxygen saturation dropped to 88%
		Initiated oxygen therapy via nonrebreather mask at 15 L/min. Respiratory therapist notified

TABLE 2: Vital signs.

Time	*Temperature (°C)*	*Heart rate (bpm)*	*Respiratory rate (bpm)*	*Blood pressure (mm Hg)*	*Oxygen saturation (%)*
08:00 AM	37.0	82	16	120/80	98
12:00 PM	37.2	88	18	118/78	96
04:00 PM	37.1	85	20	122/82	97
08:00 PM	37.3	90	22	118/76	95

Comments/notes:
- (Note 1)
- (Note 2)
- (Note 3)
- *Graphic charts*: Visual representations of trends in vital signs, laboratory values, and other clinical data. Graphic charts allow for quick identification of patterns and changes over time. The choice and type of chart used may vary from institute to institute. ICU graphic chart typically includes the following:

BOX 1: Interventions.

- *Medications*:
  - ☐ Administered medication as ordered
  - ☐ Documented patient response
- *Procedures*:
  - ☐ Completed procedure checklist
  - ☐ Documented any complications
- *Therapies*:
  - ☐ Implemented therapy plan
  - ☐ Monitored patient response

Assessments:
- *Neurological assessment*:
  - ☐ Alert and oriented ×3
  - ☐ Glasgow Coma Scale (GCS): (Score)
  - ☐ Pupillary response: Equal and reactive
- *Respiratory assessment*:
  - ☐ Lung sounds: Clear bilaterally
  - ☐ Oxygen therapy: (Device/Rate)
  - ☐ SpO_2: (Value)
- *Cardiovascular assessment*:
  - ☐ Heart rhythm: Regular
  - ☐ Peripheral pulses: Present and equal bilaterally
  - ☐ Capillary refill: <2 seconds

Patient information:
- *Name:* (Patient's name)
- *Medical record number:* (MRN)
- *Date of admission:* (Date)
- *Diagnosis/reason for admission:* (Diagnosis)

Vital signs:
- *Heart rate (bpm)*
- *Respiratory rate (bpm)*
- *Blood pressure (mm Hg)*
- *Temperature (°C)*
- *Oxygen saturation (%)*

Clinical assessments:
- *Neurological assessment:*
  - Glasgow Coma Scale (GCS)
  - Pupillary response
  - Motor strength
- *Respiratory assessment*:
  - Breath sounds
  - Chest symmetry
  - Use of ventilatory support
- *Cardiovascular assessment:*
  - Heart rhythm
  - Peripheral pulses
  - Capillary refill
- *Gastrointestinal assessment:*
  - Bowel sounds
  - Abdominal distention
  - Stool output
- *Renal assessment:*
  - Urine output
  - Serum creatinine
  - Blood urea nitrogen (BUN)

TABLE 3: Fluid and output.

Time	*Intake (mL)*	*Output (mL)*	*Balance (mL)*
08:00 AM	500	200	+300
12:00 PM	750	300	+450
04:00 PM	600	250	+350
08:00 PM	800	400	+400

- *Skin assessment:*
  - Skin color
  - Skin turgor
  - Presence of pressure ulcers

Interventions:

- Medications (stat, routine, and infusions)
  - Administration times
  - Doses
  - Routes
- *Procedures:*
  - Timing
  - Type
  - Complications
- *Therapies:*
  - *Ventilator settings:*
    - Mode (e.g., assist-control, pressure support)
    - Tidal volume (mL)
    - Respiratory rate (breaths/min)
    - Positive end-expiratory pressure (PEEP) (cmH_2O)
    - Fraction of inspired oxygen (FiO_2)
    - Inspiratory time (sec)
    - Peak inspiratory pressure (PIP) (cmH_2O)
    - Plateau pressure (cmH_2O)

Monitoring:

- *Continuous monitoring:*
  - ECG
  - Pulse oximetry
  - Invasive hemodynamic monitoring
- *Specialized monitoring:*
  - Arterial blood gas (ABG)
  - End-tidal CO_2 ($ETCO_2$)
  - Central venous pressure (CVP)

Fluid balance:

- *Intake:*
  - Oral fluids
  - IV fluids
  - Enteral nutrition
- *Output:*
  - Urine output
  - Emesis
  - Drainage

Pain assessment:

- Pain scale
- Pain location
- Analgesic administration

Risk assessments:

- *Fall risk assessment:*
  - High, medium, low
  - Fall-prevention measures implemented
- *Pressure ulcer risk assessment:*
  - Braden Scale Score
  - Skin inspection findings
- *Venous thromboembolism (VTE) risk assessment:*
  - Risk assessment score
  - Prophylactic measures implemented (pharmacological/nonpharmacological)

Fast hugs bid:

- *Feeding:*
  - Enteral/nutritional support
- *Analgesia:*
  - Pain management
- *Sedation:*
  - Sedative administration
- *Thromboembolic prophylaxis:*
  - Anticoagulant therapy
- *Head-of-bed elevation:*
  - Positioning
- *Ulcer prophylaxis:*
  - Stress ulcer prophylaxis
- *Glucose control:*
  - Blood glucose monitoring/insulin therapy
- *Bowel regimen:*
  - Bowel management
- *Indwelling catheters:*
  - Catheter management
- *Daily awakening and breathing trials:*
  - Sedation vacation/spontaneous breathing trials

Family communication:
- Family meetings
- Updates provided

Comments/Notes:
- Any additional information
- Significant events
- Changes in condition

OVERVIEW OF A NURSING DOCUMENTATION IN ICU

Overview of a nursing documentation in ICU is given in **Table 4**.

ENHANCING ICU DOCUMENTATION PRACTICES

- *Training and education:* Continuous education ensures that nurses remain proficient in documentation best practices.
  - *Orientation programs:* Include comprehensive training on documentation during on-boarding.
  - *Ongoing workshops:* Address new technologies, legal updates, and common errors in documentation.

TABLE 4: Overview of a nursing documentation in ICU.

Date	***Patient name***	***MRN***	***Admission assessment***
(Date)	(Patient's name)	(Medical record number)	• Admitted to ICU due to acute heart failure exacerbation • History of hypertension and congestive heart failure • *Initial assessment findings:* Tachypnea, orthopnea, dyspnea at rest (8/10), bilateral crackles on lung auscultation • *Allergies:* None reported, Medications: Lisinopril 10 mg daily, Furosemide 40 mg twice daily
Vital signs		***Respiratory assessment***	***Cardiovascular assessment***
HR: (Heart rate) bpm		Respiratory rate: (Respiratory rate) bpm	BP: (Blood pressure) mm Hg
BP: (Blood pressure) mm Hg		Oxygen saturation: (Oxygen saturation) %	Heart sounds: (Heart sounds), S3 present
Neurological assessment			***Wound care documentation***
Alert and oriented to time, place, and person GCS 15/15			No wound care required
Pupils equal, round, and reactive to light			
Pain assessment and management			***Sedation status***
Pain level assessed using numerical rating scale (NRS): (Pain level)			*Sedation level:* Alert and responsive
Administered morphine 2 mg IV for pain relief			No sedation required

Contd...

Contd...

Nutritional status	***Intake and output (I&O)***
Regular dietary intake, reduced appetite due to dyspnea	• *Intake:* Oral intake including fluids and medications • *Total intake:* 1,000 mL in the last 24 hours
Encouraged small, frequent meals	• *Output:* Urine output monitored every 1 hour • *Last 24 hours output:* 900 mL
Diagnostic test results	***Nursing care plan***
Laboratory: BNP elevated [BNP (BNP level) pg/mL]	Improve gas exchange by maintaining oxygen therapy
Chest X-ray: Pulmonary edema, bilateral infiltrates	Monitor fluid balance closely
Echocardiogram: Reduced ejection fraction [EF (EF Level)%]	Administer medications as prescribed (e.g., diuretics)
Cardiac enzymes: Elevated troponin levels	Assess for signs of worsening heart failure
Daily progress notes	
• Patient remains dyspneic, requiring oxygen therapy • Initiated diuretic therapy (Furosemide) to manage fluid overload • Encouraged mobility and positioning to improve ventilation and reduce respiratory distress	

    - *Simulation exercises:* Practice real-life scenarios to reinforce accurate and timely documentation.
- *Standardization:* Standardized documentation practices improve consistency and reduce variability.
    - *Templates and protocols:* Use predefined templates for ICU-specific scenarios, such as sepsis protocols or ventilator management.
    - *Standardized terminology:* Employ recognized terminologies, such as SNOMED CT or ICD-10 codes, to describe diagnoses and interventions.
- *Leveraging quality improvement metrics:* Documentation should reflect nursing-sensitive indicators to evaluate and improve care quality.
    - *Outcome monitoring:* Include metrics such as central line-associated bloodstream infection (CLABSI) rates or pressure injury prevalence.
    - *Audit systems:* Regularly audit documentation to identify gaps and implement corrective actions.
- *Interdisciplinary collaboration:* Encourage team-based documentation to reflect comprehensive care.
- *Shared notes:* Foster collaboration by allowing physicians, therapists, and nurses to contribute to shared care plans.
- *Feedback loops:* Regularly review documentation quality through team discussions.

CONCLUSION

Intensive care unit nursing documentation plays a critical role in ensuring comprehensive and high-quality care for patients in the ICU. Through thorough and accurate documentation, nurses facilitate communication among healthcare providers, track patient progress, monitor responses to treatments and interventions, and identify potential complications or changes in the patient's condition. Furthermore, ICU nursing documentation serves as a valuable resource for continuity of care, providing essential information for healthcare providers during shift changes, hand-offs, and interdisciplinary team meetings. It also supports evidence-based practice, quality improvement initiatives, and research efforts aimed at enhancing patient outcomes and optimizing healthcare delivery in the ICU setting.

FURTHER READING

1. American Association of Critical-Care Nurses (AACN). (2016). AACN standards for establishing and sustaining healthy work environments: A journey to excellence. [online] Available from https://www.aacn.org/nursing-excellence/standards/aacn-standards-for-establishing-and-sustaining-healthy-work-environments [Last accessed February, 2025].
2. American Thoracic Society. (2017). Recommendations for a Standardized ICU Set of Interventions. [online] Available from https://www.thoracic.org/ [Last accessed February, 2025].
3. Centres for Medicare & Medicaid Services (CMS). (2020). Discharge planning. 2020. [online] Available from https://www.cms.gov/ [Last accessed February, 2025].
4. College of American Pathologists. (2017). Laboratory General Checklist. [online] Available from https://www.cap.org/ [Last accessed February, 2025].
5. Institute for Healthcare Improvement (IHI). (2020). How-to-guide: Prevent harm from high-alert medications. [online] Available from http://www.ihi.org/resources/Pages/Tools/HowtoGuidePreventHarmfrom HighAlert Medications.aspx [Last accessed February, 2025].
6. Institute for Safe Medication Practices (ISMP). (2014). Guidelines for standard order sets. [online] Available from https://www.ismp.org/ [Last accessed February, 2025].
7. Joint Commission. (2018). Comprehensive Accreditation Manual for Hospitals. [online] Available from https://www.jointcommission.org/ [Last accessed February, 2025].
8. National Institute for Health and Care Excellence (NICE). (2019). Head injury: Assessment and early management. [online] Available from https://www.nice.org.uk/guidance/ng176 [Last accessed February, 2025].
9. NANDA International. (2018). Nursing diagnoses: Definitions and classification. 2018. [online] Available from https://www.nanda.org/ [Last accessed February, 2025].
10. Wound, Ostomy and Continence Nurses Society (WOCN). (2016). Guideline for prevention and management of pressure injuries. [online] Available from https://www.wocn.org/ [Last accessed February, 2025].

CHAPTER 40

Nursing Standards and Quality Indicators

Devi Prasad Samaddar, Parul Samadder

INTRODUCTION

Nurses remain in the forefront of clinical management; therefore, their role in improving care, patients' outcome, and satisfaction is pivotal. The first and most of the subsequent interactions of the patients and their relatives are generally with the nursing staff; hence, knowledge, judgement, skill, attitude, approach, and temperament of nursing staff are primarily important to decide patients' outcome and also cast a deep impression on the care takers' (i.e., the patient or the patients relatives) mind, about the institution's ability to provide quality of care. Nurses' approach focused on quality is most essential to achieve the ultimate goal of successful outcomes and patients' delight. This quality also needs to be measured by some parameters. The parameters can be preventive care and early recognition of adverse events, complications or errors, and also ultimate outcomes. An in-depth understanding among the nursing staff about the total quality, standards, and indicators is only basic to the quality-oriented service being provided to the end users.

BACKGROUND

Credit goes to Florence Nightingale who identified nurses' role in improving quality in health care. She initiated measurement of patients' outcome by using statistical tools. Reports were generated by her to establish a correlation between patients' outcome and environmental factors. Since 1970, American Nurses Association contributed effectively in developing quality assurance and introducing Donabedian's model which depends on structure, process, and outcome for the comprehensive evaluation of quality offered by nurses in health care. They also linked physical number of nurses providing the service, with safety, quality of care, and outcome of the patients.

Joint Commission International (JCI) introduced concept of identification, measurement, and best practices model in quality and patient safety throughout the world. At national level, Indian accreditation bodies such as Quality Council of India (QCI), National Accreditation Board for Hospitals (NABH), and Consortium of Accredited Healthcare Organizations (CAHO) have taken initiatives to set standards and indicators which are also applicable in general to nursing care. In spite of all these, a recent international review highlighted that a widely accepted set of quality indicators (QIs) specific to the nursing care in the intensive care units (ICUs) are not available which deserve serious attention.

QUALITY

The American Nurses Association (ANA) has defined quality as "The degree to which the nursing services for healthcare consumers, families, groups, communities, and populations increase the likelihood of desirable outcomes which is consistent with the evolving nursing knowledge."

The definition mainly focuses on under-mentioned components:

- Nursing interventions
- Desirable outcomes
- Evidence-based practice.

Although the outcome (e.g., survival, weaned off ventilator, discharged from the ICU, etc.) is the most important parameter, the process followed and the knowledge-based care are also equally important. Dr Juraon, renowned architect of quality, projected process-oriented approach as big "Q" while a narrower and only result-monitored approach was termed as small "q" **(Fig. 1)**. For example, while inserting a urinary catheter, if resource availability and process (infection control principles and processes) adherence are ensured then it is expected that incidence of catheter-associated urinary tract infections (CAUTIs) will be lesser. Compliance to CAUTI prevention bundle is, therefore, advocated as a process-focused approach (Q) to reduce the resultant incidence of CAUTI. Monitoring of CAUTI incidence alone without the process is small q **(Fig. 1)**. The same concept is also applicable for other quality parameters (indicators) used in health care.

STANDARDS

Standards are the prerequisites for the promotion of safe, effective ethical and competent care delivered by the nurses. Nursing excellence guidebook has 7 chapters, 48 standards, and 216 objective elements. These chapters cover: (1) Nursing resource management (NRM), (2) nursing care of patients (NCP), (3) management of medications (MOM), (4) education, communication, and guidance (ECG), (5) infection control practices (ICPs), and (6) empowerment and governance (EG). The 7th chapter is dedicated to nursing quality indicators (NQIs). Standards express the broad-based expectation from the nurses on any aspect of care. For example, in chapter 3, MOM standard number 3 mentions—"The monitoring of patients after medication administration is supervised by responsible person". These standards offer a common platform for evaluating quality of care and should be applicable irrespective of the size, role, and complexity of the healthcare set up. National Quality Forum (NQF), via its voluntary consensus standards process, endorsed 15 national standards to be used in evaluating the nursing-sensitive care. These standards are now known as the NQF 15 **(Table 1)**.

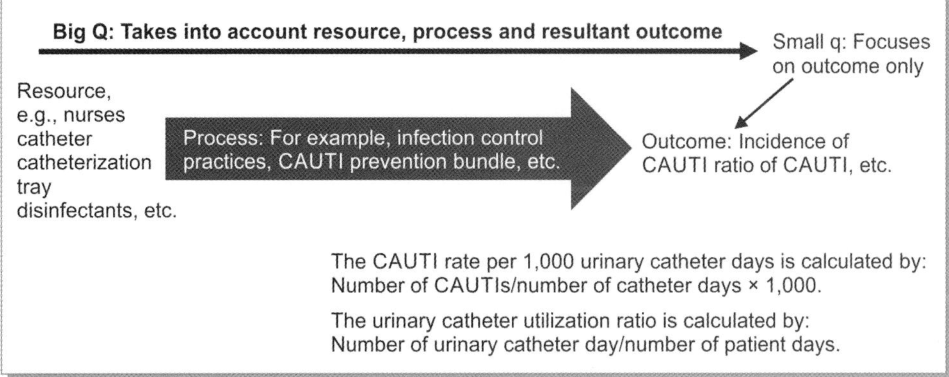

Fig. 1: Approach to quality control: Q vs q. (CAUTI: catheter-associated urinary tract infection)

TABLE 1: Relevant indicators for adult ICU.

Indicators	***NDNQI indicators, USA***	***NABH***	***CAHO***
Patient related:			
Patient falls	Yes	Yes (standard NQI-2)	
Patient falls with injury	Yes		
Fall needing medical attention		Yes (standard NQI-2)	
Pressure ulcer prevalence	Yes	Yes (standard NQI-2)	Yes
Medication errors		Yes (standard NQI-2)	Yes
Accidental delining		Yes (standard NQI-2)	
Extravasation		Yes (standard NQI-2)	
Restraint prevalence	Yes	Yes (standard NQI-2)	
Nosocomial infections: • Urinary catheter-associated urinary tract infection (CAUTI) • Central line catheter-associated bloodstream infection (CLABSI) • Ventilator-associated pneumonia (VAP)	Yes	Yes	Yes
Surgical site infection			Yes
Process related:			
Waste disposal compliance		Yes	
Needlestick injury incidence		Yes, including personal health and safety (standard NQI-2)	Yes
Hand hygiene compliance		Yes (standard NQI-2)	Yes
Compliance to pain assessment		Yes (standard NQI-2)	
Percentage/score-based satisfaction of patient		Yes (standard NQI-2)	
Work force and administrative elements:			
Skill mix: Percent of total nursing hours supplied by experienced nurses	Yes		
RN satisfaction survey options	Yes	Yes	
Voluntary nurse turnover	Yes	Attrition rate	Attrition rate
Nurse vacancy rate	Yes		
Nursing hours per patient day	Yes	Adequate resource	
Induction and in-service training	RN education/ certification	Yes, including PPE use, infection control practices, code blue, disaster, barrier nursing, fire and nonfire emergencies	

Contd...

Contd...

Indicators	*NDNQI indicators, USA*	*NABH*	*CAHO*
Resource for infection control practices		Yes	
Incidence reporting system, collect feedback/receive complaints, process of analysis along with corrective and preventive actions		Yes	
Error prevention, reporting, addressing mechanism		Yes	
Quality audit and review process			

(CAHO: Consortium of Accredited Healthcare Organizations; ICU: intensive care unit; NABH: National Accreditation Board for Hospitals; NDNQI: National Database of Nursing Quality Indicators, USA; PPE: personal protective equipment)

WHAT IS NURSING QUALITY INDICATOR?

Quality indicators are standardized, evidenced-based measures of healthcare quality that can be used with readily available hospital inpatient administrative data to measure and track clinical performance and outcomes. Nursing excellence guidebook chapter 7 has quoted various indicator such as patient's fall, hospital-acquired decubitus ulcer, and medication error which are relevant to the nursing services. Nurses quality indicators are the key to the care excellence. Indicators should be used as screening tool to identify potential deficiency in care and may be classified as structure/ resource, process, and outcome. Indicators are necessary to match with the radical shift in roles of healthcare professionals, and meet the expectations of consumers and technological advancements in health care. It helps in fixing accountability, transparency, and improving quality.

Common nursing quality indicators: **Table 1** highlights very common indicators generally used to monitor the quality of care provided by the nurses. It is not an exhaustive list but a summarized approach to important indicators. For ease of understanding, it is segregated into patient, process, and administrative subheadings. However, there is wide variation in the selection of indicators for the nurses, by various authors in the published literature. A recently published review highlighted, in a very vivid manner, the gap present in identifying the QIs specific to nurses and particularly in ICU setup. Most published literatures have considered nurses number as a parameter and correlated the same with the patients' outcome. Apart from this, multiple other indicators are available to relate patient safety, adverse events, infections, complications with mortality, and survival. The review quoted 13 published literatures where different indicators were used without maintaining uniformity in selection of the indicators **(Table 2)**.

MEDICATION ERRORS

Approximately 7,000–9,000 Americans die due to a medication error annually. Medication error has the potential to exert life-threatening impact on the patients' outcome. Therefore, focused attention is desirable on this error and associated indicators. Wrong doses (46.9%) were the most common type of medication error. Poor training, deficient knowledge, and negative attitude were the frequent causes for the

TABLE 2: Categorization of quality indicators identified in the included studies.

Category of outcome variables	Subcategory of outcome variables	QIs identified	Studies identified												
			Kendall-Gallagher and Blegen, 2009	*Chio et al., 2008*	*Robert et al., 2000*	*Dang et al., 2002*	*Amaravid et al., 2000*	*Alonso-Echanove et al., 2003*	*Whitman et al., 2002*	*Bracco et al., 2001*	*Valentin et al., 2006*	*Tarnow–Mordi et al., 2000*	*Garcia and Fugulin, 2012*	*Metnitz et al., 2008*	*Stone et al., 2007*
Primary QIs	Setting related	Mortality (adjusted and unadjusted, observed and expected—SMR)/fatal outcome		X			X			X		X		X	
	Setting related	30-day mortality													X
	Patient-related use of health care	ICU LOS				X	X			X	X	X		X	
	Patient-related use of health care	Hospital LOS				X	X							X	
	Setting related	Cost					X			X					
	Patient-related use of health care	Readmission								X		X			
Secondary QIs — Infections	Patient-related safety	UTI	X												X
		Central venous catheter-associated infections, BSI/CLABSI	X					X	X						X
		BSI	X		X										

Contd...

Contd...

Category of outcome variables	Subcategory of outcome variables	QIs identified	Studies identified												
			Kendall-Gallagher and Blegen, 2009	Chio et al., 2008	Robert et al., 2000	Dang et al., 2002	Amaravid et al., 2000	Alonso-Echanove et al., 2003	Whitman et al., 2002	Bracco et al., 2001	Valentin et al., 2006	Tarnow–Mordi et al., 2000	Garcia and Fugulin, 2012	Metnitz et al., 2008	Stone et al., 2007
Secondary QIs – Infections		Postoperative septicemia				X	X								
		Postoperative infection					X								
		Postoperative pneumonia					X								
		VAP													X
Secondary QIs – Adverse events	Patient-related safety	Medication errors	X						X		X				
		Skin breakdown, pressure sores	X						X				X		X
		Falls	X						X						
		Reintubation				X	X								
		Extubation incidence/ unplanned extubation									X		X		
		Aspiration				X	X								
Secondary QIs – Complication after OR	Patient-related safety	Acute MI				X	X								
		Cardiac arrest				X	X								

Contd...

Contd...

Category of outcome variables	*Subcategory of outcome variables*	*QIs identified*	*Studies identified*												
			Kendall-Gallagher and Blegen, 2009	*Chio et al., 2008*	*Robert et al., 2000*	*Dang et al., 2002*	*Amaravid et al., 2000*	*Alonso-Echanove et al., 2003*	*Whitman et al., 2002*	*Bracco et al., 2001*	*Valentin et al., 2006*	*Tarnow–Mordi et al., 2000*	*Garcia and Fugulin, 2012*	*Metnitz et al., 2008*	*Stone et al., 2007*
Secondary QIs Complication after OR	Patient-related safety	Complications after procedure				X									
		Pulmonary insufficiency after procedure				X									
		Ventilation >96 hours				X									
		Renal failure				X	X								
		Platelets transfusion				X									
		Cardiac complications					X								
		Reoperation for bleeding					X								
		Surgical complications					X								
		Critical incidence								X					

Contd...

Contd...

Category of outcome variables		***Subcategory of outcome variables***	***QIs identified***	***Studies identified***												
				Kendall–Gallagher and Blegen, 2009	***Cho et al., 2008***	***Robert et al., 2000***	***Dang et al., 2002***	***Amaravid et al., 2000***	***Alonso–Echanove et al., 2003***	***Whitman et al., 2002***	***Bracco et al., 2001***	***Valentin et al., 2006***	***Tarnow–Mordi et al., 2000***	***Garcia and Fugulin, 2012***	***Metnitz et al., 2008***	***Stone et al., 2007***
Secondary QIs	Errors	Patient-related safety	Human errors related to venous lines and catheters								X					
			Human errors related to respiratory system								X					
			Human errors related to cardiovascular system								X					
			Human errors related to drug-related complications								X					
			Human errors related to neurological system complications								X					
			Human errors related to urinary system complications								X					
			Human errors related to gastrointestinal system complications								X					
			Human errors related to skin and muscular system								X X					
			Human errors related to management complications													

Contd...

Contd...

Category of outcome variables	Subcategory of outcome variables	QIs identified	Studies identified												
			Kendall–Gallagher and Blegen, 2009	Cho et al., 2008	Robert et al., 2000	Dang et al., 2002	Amaravid et al., 2000	Alonso–Echanove et al., 2003	Whitman et al., 2002	Bracco et al., 2001	Valentin et al., 2006	Tarnow–Mordi et al., 2000	Garcia and Fugulin, 2012	Metnitz et al., 2008	Stone et al., 2007
Secondary QIs	Patient-related perception	Patient satisfaction with pain management							X						
	Patient-related safety	Restraint application							X						
Secondary QIs – Sentinel/unintended events	Patient-related safety	Sentinel events related to medication (prescription, administration)									X				
		Sentinel events related to airway									X				
		Sentinel events related to indwelling lines (lines, catheters, drains, arterial lines, CVP lines, pulmonary artery catheters, Foley catheters, dialysis catheters, chest drain, nasogastric tubes)									X		X		
		Sentinel events related to equipment									X				

(CLABSI: central line-associated bloodstream infection; CVP: central venous pressure; ICU: intensive care unit; MI: myocardial infarction; QI: quality indicator; SMR: standardized mortality ratio; UTI: urinary tract infection; VAP: ventilator-associated pneumonia)

Source: Inclusion of table is with kind permission of the authors Ekaterini Lambrinou et al.

BOX 1: Incidence of medication error.

- Prescription error
- Transcription error
- Dispensing error
- Administration error
- Percentage of admissions with ADR
- Percentage of medication charts with which are prone to error
- Compliance rate to medication
- Prescription in capitals
- Percentage of patients receiving high-risk medications developing adverse drug event
- Percentage of contrast allergic reaction
- Number of patients on NG tube receiving nonenteric-coated drugs

(ADR: adverse drug reaction; NG: nasogastric)

occurrence of medication errors. Zirpe et al., based on a study conducted in tertiary care hospital in India, quoted an incidence of 6.11%. The authors stratified the incidence into transcription error (44.1%), prescription error (40%), and administration error (14%).

The CAHO, India has subgrouped medication error in multiple QIs **(Box 1 and Fig. 1)**.

IMPLEMENTATION

Each ICU should preselect the indicators as per need. The indicators should be owned, monitored, analyzed, and tracked on regular basis to get daily, monthly, and yearly report and the trend to identify the deviations. Implementation of QI is a multistep process and necessitates a team approach. Productive implementation deserves a process owner, data capturing methodology, proper storage of data, and drawing conclusion from the analysis of periodically collected data and the trend.

Data Capturing and Documentation

Cochrane review by Urquhart et al. (2009) failed to show any measurable benefit between electronic and paper documentation on the nursing care or patients' outcome. However, more recent reviews preferred electronic documentation over paper-based data acquisition. User-friendliness of software is essential to prevent unnecessary workload on the already stressed staff. Data in digital format is easy to access, read, monitor, and analyze for meaningful conclusions, decision making, and initiate data-dependent action plan.

Review

Regular review of data on monthly, quarterly, and annual basis for each indicator is essential to keep track of the incidence, trend monitoring, identify deviations, and compare with the benchmarks. Review helps in deciding the corrective measure to be taken for all unacceptable deviations. During such reviews, the results of the hospital can be compared with the national or international benchmarks. Sometimes, interdepartmental comparisons may also be made.

TARGET SETTING

Ideally, there should be a zero tolerance for infections and morbidity indicators, but achieving ideal target is not possible very often. Therefore, target setting should be done as part of the improvement cycle to at least reach near the target and then surpass the internal benchmarks and subsequently external benchmarks. Target setting for better process compliance such as hand hygiene/bundle compliance and other outcome parameters by controlling the influencing factors through process improvement should be part of the routine quality-oriented exercise.

PROCESS IMPROVEMENT

Continuous improvement is the core and fundamental concept of any quality

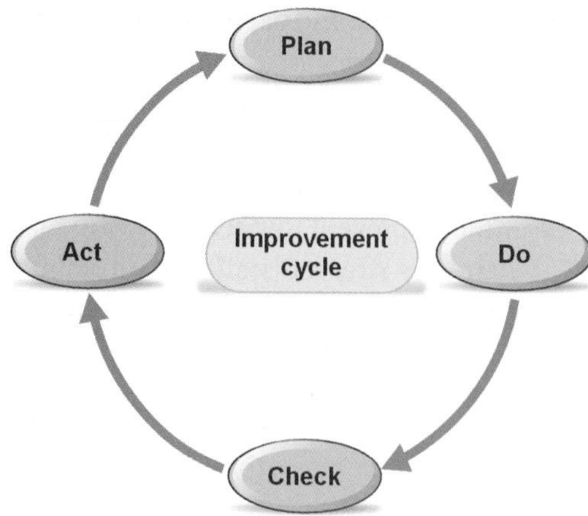

Fig. 2: Improvement cycle.

initiative. The team should take pride in maintaining and improving the QIs. Systemic improvement projects (SIPs) should be taken to address negative changes in performance indicators. SIP should incorporate the basic problem-solving steps such as:

- Identification and quantification of issues/gap in the performance
- Brainstorming
- Root cause analysis
- Prioritization
- Deciding corrective action plan
- Implementation of plan, monitoring of compliance to the plan
- Ultimate result (outcome indicator)

Conducting clinical audits to find deficiencies in process and rectification by repeated PDCA (Plan-Do-Check-Act cycle) approach are essential steps to ensure total and continuous quality improvement (TQM) **(Fig. 2)**.

ADDITIONAL INDICATORS

Each institution and its ICU setup is unique and could be having individualized issues, therefore, the team should prioritize the QIs and take additional indicators during the TQM journey, as per need. Flexibility in adopting quality as the way of life is important and reluctance to pursue quality-focused approach in apprehension of higher workload should be avoided.

CONCLUSION

Standards are the broad-based domain which include QIs as the pointers to the performance of the nursing services. Indicators could be related to the infrastructure/resource, process, and outcome. All the three components are interlinked but outcome ultimately depends on the process improvement and availability of adequate resource. Multiple basic and potential additional indicators are available. Nurses should identify the most suitable indicators for judging the performance of the team and the unit. Indicators should be owned and monitored to identify unacceptable deviations which suggest deterioration in the performance. Constant effort should be made to match the performance with the internal and external benchmarks. Improvement projects should be taken to address the root causes responsible for the negative deviation in the performance. PDCA cycle should be followed for the progressive improvement in care and holding on to the gain.

FURTHER READING

1. AHR Quality Indicators. Agency for Health Care Research and Quality (AHRQ). [online] Available from https://qualityindicators.ahrq.gov/measures/qi_resources [Last accessed February, 2025].
2. Alandajani A, Khalid B, Ng YG, Banakhar M. Knowledge and Attitudes Regarding Medication Errors among Nurses: A Cross-Sectional Study in Major Jeddah Hospitals. Nurs Rep. 2022;12(4):1023-39.
3. American Nurses Association. (2021). Nursing: Scope and standards of practice, 4th edition. [online] Available from https://wtcs.pressbooks.pub/nursingmpc/

chapter/9-2-quality-care/ [Last accessed February, 2025].
4. Custom Builder. (2011). Quality Management |Big Q and little q. [online] Available from https://www.custombuilderonline.com/blog/quality-management-big-q-and-little-q [Last accessed February, 2025].
5. De Groot K, Triemstra M, Paans W, Francke AL. Quality criteria, instruments, and requirements for nursing documentation: A systematic review of systematic reviews. J Adv Nurs. 2019;75:1379-93.
6. Efi E, Ekaterini L, Christiana K, Nicos M. Identifying validated nursing quality indicators for the intensive care unit: An integrative review. World Crit Care Nurs. 2018;12(2):28-39.
7. Michael JCJ. (2021). Nurses quality indicators. [online] Available from https://www.caho.in/files/CQE-7-Nursing-Quality-indicators_1.pdf [Last accessed February, 2025].
8. Montalvo I. (2007). The National Database of Nursing Quality Indicators (NDNQI). [online] Available from https://ojin.nursingworld.org/table-of-contents/volume-12-2007/number-3-september-2007/nursing-quality-indicators/ [Last accessed February, 2025].
9. National Accreditation Board for Hospitals and Health Care Providers (NABH). (2013). Guide book to standards for nursing excellence, 1st edition. [online] Available from https://www.nabh.co/Images/pdf/DRAFT-STANDARDS-FOR-NURSING-EXCELLENCE.pdf [Last accessed February, 2025].
10. National Health Care Safety Network (NHSN). (2025). Urinary Tract Infection (Catheter-Associated Urinary Tract Infection [CAUTI] and Non-Catheter-Associated Urinary Tract Infection [UTI]) Events. [online] Available from https://www.cdc.gov/nhsn/pdfs/pscmanual/7psccauticurrent.pdf [Last accessed February, 2025].
11. Urquhart C, Currell R, Grant MJ, Hardiker NR. Nursing record systems: Effects on nursing practice and healthcare outcomes. Cochrane Database Syst Rev. 2009;21(1):CD002099.
12. Zirpe KG, Seta B, Gholap S, Aurangabadi K, Gurav SK, Deshmukh AM, et al. Incidence of Medication Error in Critical Care Unit of a Tertiary Care Hospital: Where Do We Stand? Indian J Crit Care Med. 2020;24(9):799-803.

SECTION 8

Disaster Management

Section Editor: *Subramani Kandasamy*

41. **Disaster Management**
Subramani Kandasamy

CHAPTER 41

Disaster Management

Subramani Kandasamy

INTRODUCTION

Disaster is defined as an event that disrupts normal function and causes suffering and loss that exceeds the coping capacity of a region. In relation to health care, various organizations and departments will be involved in mobilizing the victims to the hospital. Intensive care units (ICUs) play a vital role in taking care of seriously ill patients amongst the survivors. The disaster may be a major one needing the whole or major area of the hospital being converted to ICU and may involve larger geographical areas including the whole world. The world has seen many pandemics in the recent past severe acute respiratory syndrome coronavirus 1 (SARS-COV-1) 2003 and H1N1 in 2009 and 2017. Though disaster preparedness plans were formulated and published, more than 50% of the institutions across the US were not prepared for the coronavirus disease 2019 (COVID-19) pandemic. During the COVID-19 pandemic, about 5% of the infected patients needed ICU care. Major hospitals will have policies for such admission surges as mandated by accreditation agencies like the National Accreditation Board for Hospitals (NABH).

HOSPITAL INCIDENT COMMAND SYSTEM

A central command system headed by the head of the institution, often the medical superintendent, is important to coordinate the disaster response.

Disaster planning consists of the four phases of comprehensive emergency management:

1. *Mitigation:* In healthcare, these include structural hardening and nonstructural measures such as laws, guidelines, and surveillance preventive measures to reduce vulnerabilities.
2. *Preparedness:* This involves capabilities to manage the impact of hazards and includes drills and exercises, education, and stockpiling supplies.
3. *Response:* A response is an action to reduce adverse actions during the disaster such as triage, treatment, and management of patient flow.
4. *Recovery:* Actions to restore areas affected by the disaster to predisaster operations such as normal surgical schedules and billing procedures.

Disaster preparedness can be aimed at all hazards or hazard specific. All hazard preparedness is a preparation for any hazard and can be tailored/calibrated according to the type of hazard, should an event occurs. A hazard-specific approach may be more effective for the specific hazard. For example, anticipate another wave of COVID-19 or preparedness for disasters like earthquake or flooding in geographical areas prone to such events. Hazard vulnerability analysis (HVA) is a useful tool to assess and prepare for hazards considering the occurrence of a disaster, its severity, current level of preparedness, and ability to respond. As there are many unknown variables, a general level of preparedness should be in place.

Emergency department (ED) and ICU would be most vulnerable with sick patients. The operating room (OR) may be in cases of surge related to mass casualties, for example road traffic accident with a pile up on highways or natural disaster like a landslide or earthquake or floods. ICU would be impacted more compared to the patients who are admitted to the ED or the OR as the patients from these areas would be triaged, stabilized, and if necessary operated and transferred to the ICU for more definitive care. It is difficult to determine the length of stay in ICU and therefore difficult to plan. Critical services may have to move out of their boundaries and become a service without boundary.

Building capacity forms an important step in critical care. Most of the units in busy centers already run to full capacity (accepted as 80% bed occupancy). This allows strain-free flow of work, yet maintaining satisfactory economics. Situations may arise from time to time when 100% beds are full. Hospitals should have facility to increase the capacity by 20% (up to 120%) of existing capacity to deal with unexpected situations like a disaster. The disaster may overwhelm the 120% also. In low- and middle-income countries, the ICUs are located in the bigger cities, and in a disaster situation, these hospitals would be overwhelmed. When it comes to building capacity, it involves four factors referred as 4 S's—*space, staff, stuff, and support.*

1. *Space:* The typical recommendation is provision of 120% of the need to manage the surge.

   Disasters may overwhelm existing bed capacity, and non-ICU areas may need to be converted to critical care area. Specifically in pandemics, need for isolation, quarantine, negative and positive pressure rooms, donning, and doffing areas demand more space. One radical measure to meet the demand is the cancellation of elective surgeries, which will increase the number of beds available in the whole hospital. This way, areas like postanesthesia care units (PACU) or the OR recovery rooms and the ORs can be repurposed for ICU care. As these areas have facilities for ventilation, monitoring, etc. It is a rapidly up-scalable measure while these facilities are being installed in other areas of the hospital if more capacity is needed. Treating emergencies in patients who may be infected and emergencies who are not infected also has to be balanced in this method.
2. *Staffing:* Intensive care involves a multidisciplinary team, and the preparedness should involve the team as listed below. Staffing can be affected in a pandemic, and the staff are affected too or if they were deemed exposed without appropriate protection and quarantined. In a study published by Arabi YM et al., ICU staff were strained because of infection and burnout.
   a. *Critical care physicians:* They are an essential part of the clinical services who have the skills to treat critically ill patients. The clinical lead should be in consultation with his colleague intensivist and should take the leadership. He should be the nodal contact person for the administrators, the hospital command system, and other support systems within and outside the ICU. India still has an insufficient intensivist workforce and the pool is building up. Pooling up staff

from departments like anesthesia/emergency medicine would help to improve workforce. Services of retired intensivists can also be utilized to improve the service.

b. *Critical care nursing:* The role of nurses in disaster management is vital. Senior nurses should take a leadership/administrative role in coordinating with departments and services to ensure smooth running. In the event of surge in admissions, the following steps may be followed to maintain patient care.
   i. Change in the nurse–patient ratio from 1:1 to a higher ratio like 1:2 or even higher if necessary. This could become challenging for infection control measures if the disaster is a pandemic.
   ii. Deputing nurses from non-ICU areas. The non-ICU nurses can be used to perform indirect patient care such as medicine preparation, while the ICU nurses perform direct patient care. They can be simultaneously trained "on the job" and can subsequently undertake direct patient care.
   iii. Using nurse practitioners, nurse anesthetists, physician assistants, and paramedics (critical care). There are many common skill sets in this group and it would be easier to integrate with the ICU nursing.
   iv. Use of electronic medical records (EMRs)
   v. Medication delivery
   vi. Use of non-ICU staff will involve upskilling and adding new competencies, education, and possible licensing in certain countries.

c. *Respiratory therapists (RT)*: RT form an important group of allied medical specialty in the ICU. Their role can be expanded from regular work. Students in their later years of training can be deputed to work alongside qualified RTs.

d. *Dieticians*: Nutrition forms an important aspect of care of the critically ill and should be streamlined with adequate input from dieticians.

e. *Physio and occupational therapists*: Inflammation, immobilization, and polypharmacy are common in ICU patients, leading to muscle wasting and weakness. This is an important group, especially for patients who spend a long time in the ICU.

f. *Psychiatrists and psychologists*: This team may be necessary more in the post ICU phase of hospitalization. They may also have a role in counseling the relatives.

3. *Stuff*:
   a. *Equipment*: Essential equipment such as mechanical ventilators, multiparameter monitors, and pumps will be needed in repurposed areas and may be difficult to procure due to high demand if the disaster like a pandemic involving many geographical areas or due to supply chain disruptions. Use of anesthesia workstations, and transport ventilators may circumvent the issue to a small extent.
   b. *Disposables*: Masks, gowns, etc. may be in short supply till production is ramped up. Policy of reduce, reuse, and recycle.

4. *Support*:
   a. *Laboratory, diagnostic, and imaging services*: The volume of samples increases exponentially and the

contribution of these service is unparalleled.

b. *Pharmacy*: Their role would be to ensure adequate stock piling of sedative, antiseptic, antimicrobials, intravenous fluids, access cannulas, airway equipment, and other commonly used medications.
c. *Facilities*: The facilitation department may have an important role in managing the increased footfall in the hospital. They should also ensure supply of adequate food/snacks for the hospital personnel.
d. *Information technology (IT) and communication*: EMR, virtual medical care, etc. should be provided by the IT department. If there are strict visitation policies for relatives, if privacy allows, IT can be used to arrange a virtual meet to see the patient. Communication being an important aspect of critical care, the technology should be used to maintain communication with the family at all times.

Additional support will be necessary from the disciplines as listed here.

- Trauma and ED
- Perioperative services
- Obstetrics, neonatal, and pediatric
- Security
- Administration and finance

DISASTER EXERCISES

Regular exercise is necessary to maintain awareness and preparedness for disasters.

EDUCATION AND TRAINING

This is necessary for the existing intensive care staffs as we saw with the COVID-19 pandemic. The disease was totally new, and treatment protocols were introduced as more and more evidence was available. Teaching and training in ICU become very important for non-ICU staff at all levels and disciplines. In the presence of pandemics, it ideally should happen virtually in the form of lectures or recorded on demand content.

GUIDELINES AND RESEARCH

As it happened in the COVID-19 pandemic, a group should be formed to formulate guidelines as new evidence emerges. This could be at the international [World Health Organization (WHO)] or national level (ICMR). Research should be initiated to add to the scientific literature.

PROTECTION OF STAFF

Apart from provision of personal protective equipment of the highest quality, adequate rest is necessary to prevent burnout. Vaccinating staff should be the priority.

PATIENTS NOT AFFECTED BY PANDEMICS

Provision has to be in place to treat this group of patients who attend with an emergency and also effectively to protect them from infection.

RECENT DEVELOPMENTS/ NOVEL IDEAS

- *Telemedicine*: With the advancement of IT, virtual patient care has become possible across continents even from remote areas. The technology is also affordable and was useful in the COVID-19 pandemic.
- *Electronic medical record*: This reduces the work on documentation, and the data collected will be useful if artificial intelligence (AI) is used.
- *Artificial intelligence*: AI using EMR with vital parameters obtained from patient

monitor, ventilator, etc. will be useful and may be the way forward. Hypotension prediction index is a proprietary software (Baxter health care), which analyses the data from patient monitors and can predict hypotension 15 minutes before the event. This is an example of AI.

- *Protocols*: Formulation of protocols will help to standardize treatment across the board and would be very useful when non-ICU staff are caring for patients.
- *Finance*: Public hospitals will need enhanced funding by the government. Private hospitals would have to meet their own funding. The corporate social responsibility (CSR), a business model where corporates have responsibility for the society ensured funding in the form of equipment, cots, etc. during the COVID-19 pandemic. These may be also supported by contributions from individuals and staff of various organizations.

THE FUTURE

Disaster management for the future can be planned based on experiences in the past. With the experience of managing the COVID-19 pandemic, the worst this generation of physicians have seen, many systems have been placed across the globe. These systems will be helpful in managing any pandemic.

FURTHER READING

1. Arabi YM, Myatra SN, Lobo SM. Surging ICU during COVID-19 pandemic: an overview. Curr Opin Crit Care. 2022;28(6):638-44.
2. Covid Guidelines India. [online] Available from https://indiacovidguidelines.org/ [Last accessed February, 2025].
3. Harris G, Adalja A. ICU preparedness in pandemics: Lessons learned from the coronavirus disease-2019 outbreak. Curr Opin Pulm Med. 2021;27(2):73-8.
4. Hossain T, Ghazipura M, Dichter JR. Intensive Care Role in Disaster Management Critical Care Clinics. Crit Care Clin. 2019;35(4): 535-50.
5. IICA. Business response to COVID 19 through CSR Indian Institute of corporate affairs. [online] Available from https://iica.nic.in/images/CSR_COVID_Publication.pdf [Last accessed February, 2025].
6. Murthy S, Leligdowicz A, Adhikari NKJ. Intensive Care Unit Capacity in Low-Income Countries: A Systematic Review. PLoS ONE. 2015;10(1):e0116949.
7. Wax RS. Preparing the Intensive Care Unit for Disaster. Crit Care Clin. 2019;35(4):551-62.
8. WHO. (2021). Critical preparedness, readiness and response actions for COVID-19: Interim guidance. [online] Available from https://www.who.int/publications/i/item/critical-preparedness-readiness-and-response-actions-for-covid-19 [Last accessed February, 2025].
9. WHO. Safe Hospitals in emergencies and disasters. [online] Available from https://www.nabh.co/Images/PDF/Fire_safety_WHO.pdf [Last accessed February, 2025].

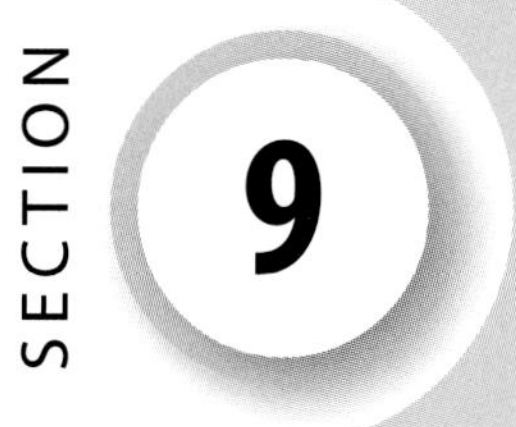

Brain Death and Organ Donation

Section Editor: *Bharat G Jagiasi*

42. **Brain Death**
Bharat G Jagiasi, Anand Srivastava

CHAPTER 42

Brain Death

Bharat G Jagiasi, Anand Srivastava

INTRODUCTION

As organ donation is picking up across the globe, a time has come to identify persons with brain death who can be potential organ donors. Critical care nursing plays a pivotal role in managing patients with life-threatening conditions, and identification of brain death. The American Association of Neurology has made a position statement where brain death is defined as "irreversible cessation of all functions of the entire brain, including the brainstem, which has been determined by the demonstration of complete loss of consciousness (coma), brainstem reflexes, and the independent capacity for the ventilatory drive (apnea), in the absence of any factors that imply possible reversibility."

ORGAN DONATION

There are two types of organ donations: Living organ donations and deceased organ donations.

Living Organ Donation

This is when you retrieve an organ from a healthy living person and transplant it into the body of someone who is suffering from end-stage organ failure. This is commonly done in the case of a liver or a kidney failure (because the liver can grow back to its normal size and a donor can survive on one kidney).

Living donors are classified as either a near relative or a distant relative/friends, etc.

A near relative is spouse, son/daughter, brother/sister, parents, grandparents, and grandchildren.

Those other than near relative can be distant relatives and friends who will need the permission of the State Authorization Committee to donate organs. If the hospital refuses to entertain such cases, the patient may send a legal notice to the hospital for not following the Transplant Act.

Deceased Organ Donation

When we talk about pledging your organs for donation or about organ donation after death, we are talking about Deceased Organ Donation. This is an organ donation from a person who has been declared brain stem dead by a team of authorized doctors at a hospital.

A person is said to be brain stem dead when there is an irreversible loss of consciousness, absence of brain stem reflexes, and irreversible loss of the capacity to breathe.

A lot of people think that whenever and however they die, their organs can be donated. That is not true. In India, organ donation after death is only possible in the case of brain stem death.

Donation after cardiac death is common in the West, but in India it is rare for donations to take place after cardiac death.

Although it is possible for organs such as the liver and the kidney to be easily donated from a living donor to a recipient, we should work toward an environment where everyone donates their organs after their deaths (if they can), so no living person should have to donate an organ to another.

Organ donation following circulatory determination of death (DCDD) has contributed significantly to the donor pool in several countries. In India, majority of deceased donations happen following brain death (BD). While existing legislation allows for DCDD, there have been only few reports of kidney transplantation following DCDD from India.

BRAIN DEAD

The awareness of brain death as an entity and promotion of organ donation were initially taken up by private and nongovernmental organizations (NGOs) and institutions, such as the MOHAN (Multi-Organ Harvesting Aid Network) foundation.

Eventually governmental organizations took lead of these programs and established a network of pyramidal organizations under National Organ Transplantation Program (NOTP).

The National Organ and Tissue Transplant Organization (NOTTO) was also established with an aim to oversee the entire program under the leadership of the Ministry of Health, Government of India. Despite these eventual changes, India is significantly lagging behind many, in both brain death declarations and organ donations.

Whereas about 500,000 potential recipients are waiting to be transplanted each year in the country, only about 8,000 deceased donor transplantations are actually happening per year. It is imperative that the political, administrative, and medical community analyze this glaring gap and evolve corrective measures, to promote this program toward saving more lives of recipients in waiting.

DEATH

Complete and irreversible cessation of spontaneous cardiac and respiratory function is defined as death.

In 1959, Mollart and Goulon first coined the term "Coma dépassé," meaning a state beyond coma, for brain death.

Similarly in 1968, Harvard Medical School (in 1968) defined it as Apneic Coma, in the absence of elicitable brain stem reflexes for a period of 24 hours as confirmed by an EEG.

Finally in 1981, Universal Definition of Death Act (UDDA) by USA, defined death as:

- Irreversible cessation of circulatory and pulmonary function
- Irreversible cessation of all brain functions including brain stem

The concept and understanding of brain death was first accepted after the Sydney Declaration in 1968, and many countries started their program from the early 1970s by setting the legal framework necessary to establish brain death, followed by organ donation.

In India, the Transplantation of Human Organs Act (THOA) 1994 and the subsequent amendments in 2011 and rules in 2014 form the legislative foundation for brain death and organ donation.

This act established a transparent and robust system to support the much-needed cause of organ transplantation in India. The primary legislation related to organ donation and transplantation in India, Transplantation of Human Organs and Tissues Act (THOTA), was passed in 1994 and is aimed at regulation of removal, storage, and transplantation of human organs for therapeutic purposes and for prevention of commercial dealings in human organs.

Some of the main provisions of the Act are as follows:

- Brain stem death identified as a form of death. Process and criteria for brain stem death certification defined
- Allows transplantation of human organs and tissues from living donors and cadavers (after cardiac or brain stem death)
- Regulatory and advisory bodies for monitoring transplantation activity and their constitution defined

BRAIN DEATH CERTIFICATION

Brain death is defined as the irreversible loss of all functions of the brain, including the brainstem.

The three essential findings in brain death are:

1. Coma
2. The absence of brainstem reflexes
3. Apnea

An evaluation of brain death should be considered in patients who have suffered a massive, irreversible brain injury from an identifiable cause.

The THOA 1994 defines brain stem death in India, as opposed to the whole brain dead in many countries like the United States.

Prerequisites:

- *Identification of history or physical examination findings that provide a clear etiology of brain dysfunction:* The determination of brain death requires the identification of the proximate cause and irreversibility of coma.

  Etiologies:

  - Severe head injury
  - Hypertensive intracerebral hemorrhage
  - Aneurysmal subarachnoid hemorrhage
  - Hypoxic-ischemic brain insults are potential causes of irreversible loss of brain stem function.

  The evaluation of a potentially irreversible coma should include, as may be appropriate to the particular case; clinical or neuroimaging evidence of an acute central nervous system (CNS) catastrophe that is compatible with the clinical diagnosis of brain death.
- Exclusion of any condition that might confound the subsequent examination of cortical or brain stem function:
  - Shock or hypotension
  - Hypothermia with temperature <32°C
  - Drugs are known to alter neurologic, neuromuscular function, and electroencephalographic testing, such as anesthetic agents, neuroparalytic drugs, methaqualone, barbiturates, benzodiazepines, high-dose bretylium, amitriptyline, meprobamate, trichloroethylene, and alcohols.
  - Brain stem encephalitis
  - Neuromuscular disease like Guillain-Barré syndrome
  - Neurotoxic snake bites
  - Encephalopathy associated with hepatic failure, uremia, and hyperosmolar coma severe hypophophatemia

DEMONSTRATION OF COMA

The absence of brain stem reflexes:

- *Pupils:* No response to bright light size: Mid-position (4 mm) to dilated (9 mm) (absent light reflex—cranial nerve II and III)
- *Ocular movement:* Cranial nerve VIII, III, and VI, no oculocephalic reflex (testing only when no fracture or instability of the cervical spine or skull base is apparent). No deviation of the eyes to irrigation in each

ear with 50 mL of cold water (tympanic membranes intact; allow 1 minute after injection and at least 5 minutes between testing on each side)

- Facial sensation and facial motor response
- No corneal reflex (cranial nerve V and VII)
- No jaw reflex (cranial nerve IX)
- Pharyngeal and tracheal reflexes (cranial nerve IX and X)
- No response to stimulation of the posterior pharynx
- No cough response to tracheobronchial suctioning

DEMONSTRATION OF APNEA

- Objective test—apnea test: To demonstrate absence of respiratory center reflex, i.e., spontaneous breathing effort in response to hypercapnia
- A positive apnea test—no spontaneous respiratory effort to hypercapnia

Prerequisites of apnea test:

- Systolic blood pressure >100 mm Hg
- Euvolemic
- Normothermia (temperature >36°C)
- Normal PCO_2 (arterial PCO_2 >40 mm Hg)
- Normal PaO_2 (preoxygenate with 100% oxygen for at least 10 minutes to achieve PaO_2 >200 mm Hg)
    - Complete monitoring of patient and disconnect the ventilator
    - Deliver 100% O_2, 6 L/min, into the trachea by placing a cannula at the level of the carina. Look closely for any respiratory movements (abdominal or chest excursions that produce adequate tidal volumes).
    - Measure arterial PO_2, PCO_2, and pH after approximately 8 minutes and reconnect the ventilator. If respiratory movements are absent and arterial PCO_2 is ≥60 mm Hg (option: in carbon dioxide retainers 20 mm Hg increase in PCO_2 over a baseline PCO_2), the apnea test result is positive (i.e., it supports the diagnosis of brain death). If respiratory movements are observed, the apnea test result is negative (i.e., it does not support the clinical diagnosis of brain death).

Connect the ventilator, if during testing:

- The systolic blood pressure becomes <90 mm Hg (or below age-appropriate thresholds in children <18 years of age) or
- The pulse oximeter indicates significant oxygen desaturation
- Cardiac arrhythmias develop.

Immediately draw arterial blood sample and analyze arterial blood gas.

If PCO_2 is ≥60 mm Hg or PCO_2 increase is ≥20 mm Hg over baseline normal PCO_2, the apnea test result is positive (it supports the clinical diagnosis of brain death). If PCO_2 is <60 mm Hg and a PCO_2 increase is <20 mm Hg over baseline normal PCO_2, the result is indeterminate and a confirmatory test can be considered (not allowed in Indian law).

The general approach in diagnosing a brain death is summarized in **Flowchart 1**.

DOCUMENTATION

In India, as per Section 3 of THOTA, brain death can be certified by a team of four members:

Two doctors either:

- Neurologist
- Intensivist
- Anesthesiologist
- Physician who are nominated by appropriate authority, perform the test independently at least 6 hours apart, and if both tests are positive for brain death, the patient is declared as Brain Dead.

The complete process is also observed by a primary admitting doctor of the patient,

Flowchart 1: Diagnosing a brain death.

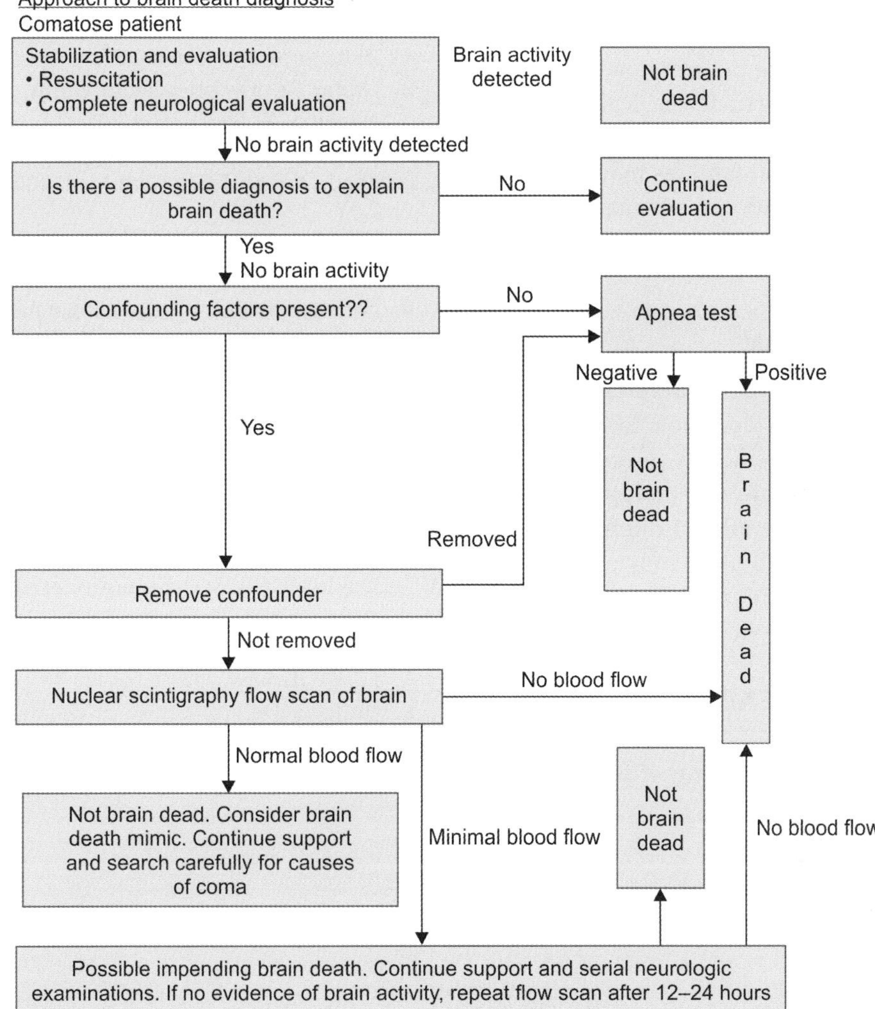

and the hospital head, who along with the two doctors complete the Form 10 and certify death.

The time of death is the end of second apnea test.

The medical record must include:

- Etiology and irreversibility
- Absence of motor response to pain, brainstem reflexes, and positive apnea test (done on two separate occasions at least 6 hours apart)
- Result of ancillary test if used
- Date and time of death

NURSING CONSIDERATIONS

- Critical care nurses are at the forefront of recognizing signs of brain death promptly.
- Use the Brain Death Assessment flowchart to guide the assessment process.
- Rapid identification allows for timely evaluation, supporting accurate diagnosis, and determination of organ viability.

- Provide emotional support and information to families facing the decision of organ donation.
- Acknowledging the emotional burden on families during such a critical time fosters trust and understanding.
- Well-supported families may find solace in the altruistic act of organ donation, turning tragedy into a life-saving opportunity.

CONCLUSION

The importance of understanding brain death and organ donation in critical care nursing lies in the ability to provide timely and compassionate care, support grieving families, navigate ethical dilemmas, foster collaboration, and ultimately contribute to successful organ transplantation, saving lives and honoring the gift of donation.

FURTHER READING

1. Busl KM, Lewis A, Varelas PN. Apnea Testing for the Determination of Brain Death: A Systematic Scoping Review. Neurocrit Care. 2021;34(2):608-20.
2. Ganapathy K. Brain death revisited. Neurol India. 2018;66(2):308-15.
3. Gilder SS. Twenty-second world medical assembly. Br Med J. 1968;3:493-4.
4. Goila AK, Pawar M. The diagnosis of brain death. Indian J Crit Care Med. 2009;13(1): 7-11.
5. Machado C. Diagnosis of brain death. Neurol Int. 2010;2(1):e2.
6. National Organ Transplant Program. Director General of Health Services India. [online] Available from http://www.dghs.gov.in. [Last accessed February, 2025].
7. National Organ Transplant Program. Director General of Health Services India. [online] Available from http://www.dghs.gov.in. [Last accessed February, 2025].
8. Seth AK, Mohanka R, Navin S, Gokhale AG, Sharma A, Ramachandran B, et al. Organ Donation after Circulatory Determination of Death in India: A Joint Position Paper. Indian J Crit Care Med. 2022;26(4):423-40.
9. Uniform Determination of Death Act, 12 Uniform Laws Annotated (U.L.A.) 589 (West 1993 and West Supp. 1997.

SECTION 10

Formulas and Scores

Section Editor: *Diptimala Agarwal*

43. **Formulas and Scores Used in Intensive Care Unit**
Diptimala Agarwal, Vivek Badada

CHAPTER

43 Formulas and Scores Used in Intensive Care Unit

Diptimala Agarwal, Vivek Badada

- 1 teaspoon = 60 drops = 5 mL
- 1 tablespoon = 3 teaspoons = 15 mL
- 1 cup = 16 tablespoons = 240 mL
- 1 liter = 4 glasses, 4 cups

Tablets required = Dose ordered/tablet supplied (if the dose of furosemide ordered is 20 mg but the tablet strength is 40 mg):

$$X = 20/40 = 1/2 \text{ tablet}$$

- Critical care drugs administered intravenously must be infused using an infusion pump.
- If a pump is not available may be infused using microdrip tubing (60 drops per milliliter calibration) and a volume control set
- The flow rate of critical care drugs is usually based on drug weight (such as milligram, microgram, milliequivalent, or unit) per time unit (minute or hour), instead of the usual milliliter per hour flow rate.
- Smart infusion pumps have made weight-based IV therapy easy.
- The patient's weight, the medication dosage, amount of diluent, and desired length of time for the infusion can be programmed into the pump, and the pump will infuse the solution at the correct rate.
- The drug is titrated up or down by small increments using the keypad on the pump.
- The nurse must manually calculate the infusion rate (milliliter per hour) and the medication dosage that the patient is to receive in the specified amount of time (milligram per minute or microgram per minute)

$$\frac{\text{Desired dose} \times \text{Volume}}{\text{Available dose}} = \text{Dose}$$

Example: Administer heparin 10,000 units intravenous (IV) push. Available is heparin 5,000 units/mL. How many mL will you need to administer to achieve a 10,000 unit dose?

$$10{,}000 \times 1/5{,}000 = 2 \text{ mL}$$

CALCULATIONS IN μg/MINUTE

Four steps:

1. How much in your IV bottle/syringe (drug concentration or number of mL of fluid)
2. In which units your drug is measured (units/hour, mg/hour, or μg/kg/minute)
3. Patient's weight in kg if you want in per kg
4. Use the universal formula below and then divide your final answer by the patient's weight in kg to arrive at μg/kg/minute

$$\frac{\text{Total dose (mg)} \times 1{,}000\ \mu\text{g} \times \text{ordered mL} \times 1\ \text{hour}}{\text{Total volume (mL)} \times 1\ \text{mg} \times 1\ \text{hour} \times 60\ \text{minutes}} \div \text{Patient weight} = X\ \mu\text{g/kg/min}$$

Dopamine is infusing. The bottle states dopamine 1,000 mg (200 mg × 5 ampules), and it is mixed in 500 mL of D5W. The IV pump in your patient's room is set at 25 mL, and the patient weighs 80 kg (80,000 g). At how many μg/kg/minute is the patient's dopamine infusing?

$$\frac{1{,}000 \text{ mg} \times 1{,}000 \text{ μg} \times 25 \text{ mL} \times 1 \text{ hour}}{500 \text{ mL} \times 1 \text{ mg} \times 1 \text{ hour} \times 60 \text{ minutes}} \div 80 = 10.4 \text{ μg/kg/min}$$

CALCULATION OF IV DRIP RATES: IV INFUSION RATES FORMULA

Amount of fluid (mL) total time of infusion (min) × Drop factor (gtts/mL) = IV infusion rate (gtts/min)

Note: Drops are always rounded to the nearest whole number.

Macrodrip tubing administers a larger drop 15 gtts/mL

Microdrip tubing administers 60 gtts/mL

These are called drop factors. The drop factor is the number of drops contained in 1 milliliter.

Example:

Given:

- Amount of fluid: 3,000 mL
- Total time of infusion: 24 hours
- Administration set drop factor: 15 gtts/mL
- IV infusion rate: ? gtts/min

Step 1: Convert 24 hours into minutes
24 hours × 60 min/h = 1,440 minutes

Step 2: Use the formula above to calculate the IV infusion rate.

IV infusion rate = 3,000/1,440 × 15 = 32 drops/min

VOLUME DEFICIT/CORRECTION OF HYPERNATREMIA

The water deficit (in liters) = 0.6 × body weight × (1 - (140/serum sodium) is used in medicine and nutrition to estimate the volume (L) of water required to correct dehydration during the initial stages of fluid-replacement therapy.

MAINTENANCE FLUID RATE

It is calculated based on weight.

4 mL/kg/hour for the first 10 kg of body mass

2 mL/kg/hour for the second 10 kg of body mass (11–20 kg)

1 mL/kg/hour for any kilogram of body mass above 20 kg (>20 kg)

NITROGEN BALANCE

Nitrogen balance (grams/day) = protein intake (grams/day)/6.25 - urinary urea nitrogen (grams/day) - 4.

Nitrogen balance is simply the difference between nitrogen (N2) intake and output. If more N2 is given to the patient than excreted, then the patient is considered to be in positive NB or anabolic. If more N2 is being excreted than being given, the patient is considered to be in negative NB or catabolic.

SERUM OSMOLALITY

Serum osmolality = 2 (Na) + Glucose/18 + BUN/2.8

The normal serum osmolality should range from 275 to 295 mOsm/kg[2]

CREATININE CLEARANCE

Cockcroft–Gault Formula

Cockcroft–Gault creatinine clearance (CrCl) = [(140-age) × (Weight in kg) × (0.85 if female)]/(72 × Cr)

SODIUM DEFICIT

Sodium deficit is calculated by using the formula:

[Target Na level (135 mEq/L) - current Na level] × 0.6 × body weight (kg)

The calculated amount is given in addition to the 24 hours maintenance electrolytes and fluids. The serum Na level increase should not exceed 12 mEq/L in 24 hours.

Infusates:

- Na level 135–45 milliequivalent per liter (mEq/L)
- 3% saline = 513 mEq/L
- 0.9% saline = 154 mEq/L

POTASSIUM DEFICIT

Potassium deficit in mmol is calculated as follows:

$K_{deficit}$ (mmol) = ($K_{normal\ lower\ limit}$ – $K_{measured}$) × kg body weight × 0.4

Normal K 3.5–5.5 millimoles per liter (mmol/L)

For every 1 mEq/L decrease in serum potassium, the potassium deficit is approximately 200–400 mEq.

Patients with a potassium level of 2.5–3.5 mEq/L may need only oral potassium replacement.

If the potassium level is <2.5 mEq/L, IV potassium should be given.

RANSON CRITERIA AND SCORE

Criteria

Findings at admission:

- Age >55 years
- Serum glucose >200 mg/dL
- Serum lactate dehydrogenase >350 IU/L
- Serum aspartate transaminase >250 U/L
- White blood cell count >16,000 cells/mm^3

Findings obtained 48 hours after admission:

- Fall in hematocrit >10
- Rise in blood urea nitrogen >5 mg/dL
- Serum calcium >8 mg/dL
- PaO_2 >60 mm Hg
- Base deficit >4 mEq/L
- Estimated fluid sequestration >6 L

Score

Mortality increases with the number of criteria present as given in **Table 1**.

RIKER SEDATION-AGITATION SCALE

The Riker Sedation-Agitation Scale (SAS) is given in **Table 2**.

GLASGOW COMA SCALE

Glasgow Coma Scale (GCS) is used to objectively describe the extent of impaired consciousness in all types of acute medical and trauma patients. The scale assesses patients according to three aspects of responsiveness: Eye-opening, motor, and verbal responses.

The total coma score thus has values between 3 and 15; 3 being the worst and 15 being the highest **(Table 3)**.

EARLY WARNING SCORES

It was developed in 1990s. There is deranged physiological parameter in large number of patient populations many hours before the critical events such as sudden cardiac arrest, coma, or unplanned intensive care unit (ICU) admissions.

TABLE 1: Ranson criteria.

Number of criteria	*Mortality (%)*
0–2	1
3 or 4	15
5 or 6	40
>7	100

TABLE 2: Riker Sedation-Agitation Scale (SAS).

Score	*Term*	*Descriptor*
7	Dangerous	Pulling at endotracheal tube (ETT), trying to remove catheters, climbing over bedrail, striking at staff, thrashing side-to-side
6	Very agitated	Requiring restraint and frequent verbal reminding of limits, biting ETT
5	Agitated	Anxious or physically agitated, calms to verbal instructions
4	Calm and cooperative	Calm, easily arousable, follows commands
3	Sedated	Difficult to arouse but awakens to verbal stimuli or gentle shaking, follows simple commands but drifts off again
2	Very sedated	Arouses to physical stimuli but does not communicate or follow commands, may move spontaneously
1	Unarousable	Minimal or no response to noxious stimuli, does not communicate or follow commands

TABLE 3: The Glasgow Coma Scale score.

Score	*Best eye response (E)*
1	No eye opening
2	Eye opening to pain
3	Eye opening to verbal command
4	Eyes open spontaneously
Score	***Best verbal response (V)***
1	No verbal response
2	Incomprehensible sounds
3	Inappropriate words
4	Confused
5	Oriented
Score	***Best motor response (M)***
1	No motor response
2	Extension to pain
3	Flexion to pain
4	Withdrawal from pain
5	Localizing pain
6	Obeys commands
A coma score of 13 or higher correlates with a mild brain injury, 9–12 is a moderate injury, and 8 or less a severe brain injury	

Contd...

Contd...

The pediatric Glasgow Coma Scale			
Score	***Eye opening***	***Verbal response***	***Motor response***
6	–		Normal, spontaneous, obeys commands
5	–	Age-appropriate words, social smile, fixes, and follows	Localizes pain
4	Spontaneous	Cries, but consolable	Withdraws from pain
3	To voice	Persistently irritable	Flexion posture to pain
2	To pain	Restless agitated	Extension posture to pain
1	None	None	None

Deterioration can be prevented if regular physiological observations were linked to thresholds or triggers for seeking assistance, coupled with the development of rapid response teams (RRTs).

NATIONAL EARLY WARNING SCORE 2

The NEWS 2 is the latest version of the National Early Warning Score (NEWS), first produced in 2012 and updated in December 2017, which advocates a system to standardize the assessment and response to acute illness. It is due for review in 2023.

Simple aggregate scoring system in which a score is allocated to physiological measurements.

Six simple physiological parameters form the basis of the scoring system are as follows:
1. Respiration rate
2. Oxygen saturation
3. Systolic blood pressure
4. Pulse rate
5. Level of consciousness or new confusion
6. Temperature

The patient has new-onset confusion, disorientation, and/or agitation, where previously their mental state was normal—this may be subtle. The patient may respond to questions coherently, but there is some confusion, disorientation, and/or agitation. This would score 3 or 4 on the GCS (rather than the normal 5 for verbal response), and scores 3 on the NEWS system.

A score is allocated to each parameter as they are measured, with the magnitude of the score reflecting how extremely the parameter varies from the norm. The score is then aggregated. The score is uplifted by 2 points for people requiring supplemental oxygen to maintain their recommended oxygen saturation.

THE SEQUENTIAL ORGAN FAILURE ASSESSMENT SCORE

The Sequential Organ Failure Assessment (SOFA) score is a simple and objective score that allows for calculation of both the number and the severity of organ dysfunction in six organ systems (respiratory, coagulatory, liver, cardiovascular, renal, and neurologic), and the score can measure individual or aggregate organ dysfunction **(Table 4)**.

CURB-65 score: Used to predict the severity of pneumonia:
- C: Confusion (if present +1)
- U: bUn (if >20 mg/dL +1)
- R: Respiratory rate (if >30 + 1)

TABLE 4: The Sequential Organ Failure Assessment (SOFA) score.

SOFA score	*1*	*2*	*3*	*4*
Respiration:[a]				
PaO_2/FiO_2 (mm Hg)	<400	<300	<220	<100
SaO_2/FiO_2	221–301	142–220	67–141	<67
Coagulation:				
Platelets × $10^3/mm^3$	<150	<100	<50	<20
Liver:				
Bilirubin (mg/dL)	1.2–1.9	2.0–5.9	6.0–11.9	>12.0
Cardiovascular:[b]				
Hypotension	MAP <70	Dopamine ≤5 or dobutamine (any)	Dopamine >5 or norepinephrine ≤0.1	Dopamine >15 or norepinephrine >0.1
CNS:				
Glasgow Coma Score	13–14	10–12	6–9	<6
Renal:				
Creatinine (mg/dL) or urine output (mL/d)	1.2–1.9	2.0–3.4	3.5–4.9 or <500	>5.0 or <200

[a]PaO_2/FiO_2 ratio was used preferentially. If not available, the SaO_2/FiO_2 ratio was used
[b]Vasoactive mediations administered for at least 1 hour (dopamine and norepinephrine µg/kg/min)
(CNS: central nervous system; FiO_2: fraction of inspired oxygen; MAP: mean arterial pressure; PaO_2: partial pressure of arterial oxygen; SaO_2: peripheral arterial oxygen saturation)

B: Blood pressure (if <90 systolic or 60 diastolic +1).

FURTHER READING

1. Cheuvront SN, Kenefick RW, Sollanek KJ, Ely BR, Sawka MN. Water-deficit equation: systematic analysis and improvement. Am J Clin Nutr. 2013;97(1):79-85.
2. Cockcroft DW, Gault MH. Prediction of creatinine clearance from serum creatinine. Nephron. 1976;16:31-41.
3. Dickerson RN. Using Nitrogen Balance in Clinical Practice. Hosp Pharm. 2005;40(12):1081-5.
4. Dorwart WV, Chalmers L. Comparison of methods for calculating serum osmolality form chemical concentrations, and the prognostic value of such calculations. Clin Chem. 1975;21(2):190-4.
5. Holliday MA, Segar WE. The maintenance need for water in parenteral fluid therapy. Pediatrics. 1957;19(5):823-32.
6. Morgan RJM, Williams F, Wright M. An early warning scoring system for detecting developing critical illness. Clin Intensive Care. 1997;8:100.
7. Ranson JH, Rifkind KM, Roses DF, Fink SD, Eng K, Spencer FC. Prognostic signs and the role of operative management in acute pancreatitis. Surg Gynecol Obstet. 1974;139(1):69-81.
8. Riker RR, Picard JT, Fraser GL. Prospective evaluation of the Sedation-Agitation Scale for adult critically ill patients. Crit Care Med. 1999;27(7):1325-9.
9. Royal College of Physicians. National Early Warning Score (NEWS) 2: Standardising the Assessment of Acute-Illness Severity in the

NHS. Updated report of a Working Party. London: Royal College of Physicians; 2017.

10. Smithline N, Gardner KD Jr. Gaps—anionic and osmolal. JAMA. 1976;236(14):1594-7.
11. Teasdale G, Jennett B. Assessment of coma and impaired consciousness. A practical scale. Lancet. 1974;2(7872):81-4.
12. Vincent JL, Moreno R, Takala J, Willatts S, De Mendonça A, Bruining H, et al. The SOFA (Sepsis-related Organ Failure Assessment) score to describe organ dysfunction/failure. On behalf of the Working Group on Sepsis-Related Problems of the European Society of Intensive Care Medicine. Intensive Care Med. 1996;22:707-10.
13. Yıldızdaş HY, Demirel N, İnce Z. Turkish Neonatal Society Guideline on fluid and electrolyte balance in the newborn. Turk Pediatri Ars. 2018;53(Suppl 1):S55-64.

Index

Page numbers followed by *b* refer to box, *f* refer to figure, *fc* refer to flowchart, and *t* refer to table.

A

ABCDEF bundle checklist 180*t*
Abdomen 8
Abdominal distention 202, 303
Abscess formation 137
Activated partial thromboplastin time 21, 118, 119
Activity chart 10
Acute cardiopulmonary life support 27
Acute coronary syndrome 107, 110*t*
 management of 108
Acute decompensated heart failure
 management of 112
 severe 114
Acute kidney injury 142
 stages of 68
Acute pancreatitis 130
 medical management of 131*fc*
Acute respiratory distress syndrome 21, 30, 88
Adequate nutrition 190
 assessment 190*f*
Adequate support surfaces 192*b*
Adhesive gel pads 214*f*, 215
Adhesive small bowel obstruction 135
Adjunctive therapies 192
Adrenal
 androgens 150
 cortex 149, 150
 medulla 150
Advanced cardiac life support 53, 213
Adverse drug reaction 317
Aerosol therapy 125
Agitation 271
AIDET acronym 297*t*
Air 80*f*
 assisted lateral transfer systems 203, 204
 bubble 232*f*
 oxygen blender 79
Airway 6, 30, 108, 202
 adjuncts 167
 clearance 197*fc*
 compromise 202
 evaluation 157
 loss, high risk of 202
 lower 165
 management 165, 220
  steps of 166
 obstruction 165
 patency 157
 reflexes 147
 resistance 88
Alanine aminotransferase levels 285
Alarm 256
 fatigue 256, 258
  effects of 257
 management 258
Albumin 242, 246*t*, 247*t*
Aldosterone 61, 150
Alkalemia 61
Allen's test 69*f*
 modified 69
Allergies 205
Alpha cells 150
Alteplase 110
Altered mental status, acute onset of 178
Alveolar capillary membrane 124
Alveolar ventilation 125
Ambu bag 166*f*, 292
Ambu laryngeal mask airways 169
Amiodarone 229
Amitriptyline 333
Analgesia 14, 304
 epidural 228
Anesthesia 146
 epidural 234
Aneurysmal subarachnoid hemorrhage 333
Anion gap 57, 58
Anterior-lateral placement 217
Anterior-posterior placement 217
Antibiotics
 intravenous 137
 usage, restriction of 281
Anticholinergics 179
Anticoagulants, oral 118
Anticoagulation 99
Antidiuretic hormone 150
Antiplatelet agents 109
Antithyroid medications 154
Anuria 68, 181
Aortic regurgitation 114
Apnea 331, 333
 central 80
 demonstration of 334
Appendicitis, acute 130, 139
Arrhythmias 45, 47, 49-53, 218, 220*t*
Arterial blood gas 7, 117, 120, 121, 125, 171
 analysis 56
 monitoring 102
 values, normal 57*t*
Arterial cannula 252
Arterial carbon dioxide, partial pressure of 58
Arterial oxygen, partial pressure of 57, 344
Arterial waveform interpretation 70, 70*f*
Arteriovenous fistula 230
Artificial airway, suctioning of 196
Artificial intelligence 326
Aseptic non-touch technique 175
Aseptic solution 263
Aseptic technique 264
Aspiration pneumonia 172
Aspirin 109, 110
Assembling memory boxes 273
Assisted breath 93
Asymmetrical chest movements 166
Asystole 53
Atherosclerosis 49, 143
Atorvastatin 109
Atrial fibrillation 48-50, 186, 218, 219*f*
Atrial flutter 40, 48, 50, 218, 219*f*
Atrial rate 49
Atrioventricular blocks 47
Auscultation 7, 166
Automated external defibrillator 213, 214*f*
 use of 218
Axillary temperature 39

B

Back care 103
Barbiturates 333
Basic monitoring checklist 204*f*

Baxter health care 327
Bed elevation, head of 16, 25*f*
Bedside
  monitoring 35
  oral exam 172, 173
  oxygen monitoring 35
  percutaneous tracheostomy 253
  temperature monitoring 38
Bedsore 184
  classification of 186*f*
  common sites of 185*f*
  stages of 186*f*
Beer-Lambert law 35
Benzodiazepines 179, 181, 333
  short-acting 180
Bernoulli's principle 126
Best eye response 342
Best motor response 342
Best verbal response 342
Beta-adrenergic stimulation 61
Bicarbonate 57, 58
Bilevel positive airway pressure 80
Biological response modifier 235
Bisphosphonates 63
Bleeding 100, 102
Blocked nasal passages 80
Blood 225, 233
  collection needles 283
  component administration set 230*f*
  drop sample 43
  flash 265
  flow 69*f*, 143
  glucose monitoring 42, 304
  pressure 302, 344
    apparatus 292
    elevated 114
    noninvasive 21, 204*f*
    systolic 28, 67, 114, 117-119, 159, 334, 343
  product 233
    compatibility of 234*t*
    transfusion 233
  sample 264
    types of 261*f*
  stasis 266
  sugar 35
    level 121
  transfusions 280
  urea nitrogen 303
Bloodstream infection
  central line-associated 277, 279*b*, 316
  catheter-related 224
Board transfer 203
Body
  compartment 240*f*
    crystalloids 241*f*
  organ systems of 193*f*
  positioning 198
  surface area 21
Bone 63
  marrow
    aspiration 252
    biopsy 234
Bowel
  management 304
  movement 19
  obstruction 130, 132
    diagnostic assessment of 135*fc*
  regimen 304
  rest 137
  sounds 8, 303
Brachial artery 69
Braden scale 189
  score 304
Bradycardia 181
  severe 27
  symptomatic 221
Brain
  death 329, 331-333, 335, 335*fc*
    awareness of 332
    certification 333
  injury
    moderate 159
    severe 159
Brainstem
  death 333
  encephalitis 333
  reflexes 331
    absence of 333
Brainstorming 318
Breath
  basic types of 94*f*
  sounds 303
  types of 94
Breathing 6, 7, 30, 108, 157, 202
  circuit 92*f*
  exercises 126
  management 220
  reduced work of 79
Breathlessness 271
Bretylium, high-dose 333
Bronchodilators 126
Bronchoscopy 234
B-type natriuretic peptide levels 8
Burn-out syndrome 256, 258
Burns 157, 160
  center referral criteria 161
  facial 161
  first-degree 160
  fourth-degree 160
  partial thickness 160
  second-degree 160
  superficial 160
  third-degree 160

C

Caffeine 61
Calcium 239
  serum 57
Cannula site 102
Capillary blood 262
  glucose test 43
  system 261
Capillary refill time 66, 67, 303
Capnogram always, normal 42
Capnography 41
  waveform 42*f*
Carbon
  dioxide 35
    partial pressure of 57, 125
  monoxide poisoning 38
Carboxyhemoglobin 36
Cardiac
  arrest 213, 217
    confirmation of 217
  biomarkers 108
  critical care 107
  death 331
  examination 7
  muscle stabilization 61
  output 39, 54
  rhythms 66*f*
Cardiopulmonary
  function, optimization of 195*b*
  resuscitation 29*fc*, 37, 53
Cardiovascular
  assessment 303, 305
  depression 147
  disease 112*f*
  support 7
  system 8
Cardioversion 213, 218, 220, 220*t*
  complications of 218*b*
Care, preferred place of 271
Catheter 19
  management 304
Catheter-associated urinary tract infection 277, 309*f*
  prevention of 279
Catheter-related bloodstream infections 224
Cavity, abdominal 135
Central command system 323
Central line
  bundle 279
  removal 234
Central nervous system 333, 344
Central Sterile Supply Department 281, 288, 291
Central venous access 211, 229
  device 226, 252
    infusions 225

Central venous pressure 66, 72, 131, 316
measurement 73*f*
Cerebrospinal fluid 121
Cerebrovascular accident 88
Checking capillary refill 67*f*
Chemical sterilant 289
Chemotherapeutic agents 223
Chest
auscultation 7
drainage systems 126
expansion 7
physiotherapy 126, 127*f*, 196
symmetry 303
tubes 127
X-ray 127
Chloride 239
Choanal atresia 80
Cholecystitis, acute 130, 139
Chronic kidney disease 113, 236
Chronic obstructive pulmonary disease 37, 49, 53, 126, 185, 186
Circulation 6, 108, 157
assessment of 28
management 220
Cisatracurium 229
Clopidogrel 109, 110
Clotting 100
Coagulation 344
Cockcroft-Gault
creatinine clearance 340
formula 340
Cognitive behavior therapy 180
Cold chain system 266*fc*
Colistin 126
Collection
method 261, 262
tube 261, 262
Colloids 240*f*, 241*f*, 242, 246
movement 241*f*
Colon, preparation of 145
Coma 331-333
demonstration of 333
of unknown cause 120, 121, 121*t*
Commitment 269
Communication 4, 9, 198, 201, 269, 300, 326
strategies 296
techniques 295
tools 296
Compatible plasma 234
Complete blood count 117, 119-121, 142
Compound sodium lactate 243*t*
Computed tomography 117-121
scans 128
Confusion
assessment method 178*fc*
acute 155
Consciousness
level of 28, 53, 165, 343
loss of 331
Consortium of Accredited Healthcare Organizations 308, 310, 311
Continuous mandatory ventilation 93
Continuous monitoring 304
Continuous nursing assessment sheet 10
Continuous positive airway pressure 197
Continuous renal replacement therapy 98, 99, 142
Control mode pressure control ventilation 95*f*
Co-oximetry 36
Cor pulmonale 48
Core temperature monitoring method 39
Corneal epithelial defects 173
Corneal ulcers 173
Coronary artery
bypass graft 236
disease 236
Corticotropin-releasing hormone 149
Cortisol 150
Cough, poor 181
COVID-19 pandemic 326
C-reactive protein 131
Creatine kinase MB 108
Creatinine
clearance 110, 340
serum 303
Critical cardiac emergencies 213
Critical care 175*fc*, 223*b*
bundles 277
drugs 339
neurology 116
neurosurgery 116
nurses 83*f*, 335
nursing 3, 223, 325, 331
physicians 324
units 3
Cryoprecipitate 233, 234
Crystalloids 29, 240, 241*f*, 242
behavior of 240*f*
Cuffed endotracheal tube 170
CURB-65 score 343
Cyanosis 166

D

Daily awakening and breathing trials 304
Daily monitoring tools 10
Death 332
care 273
circulatory determination of 332
triad of 159*b*
Deep partial thickness burns 161
Deep sedation 179
Deep tissue injury 187, 188*f*
Deep vein thrombosis, prediction of 24
Defibrillation 213, 216, 218, 220, 220*t*
complications of 218*b*
Defibrillator 213
parts of 214
primary types of 213
setup 217
Dehydration 59
Dehydroepiandrosterone 150
Delirium 177-179, 181, 271
cause of 178
complications of 179
management of 179
prevention of 180
types of 177
Deoxyhemoglobin 35
Device 167, 290
classification 290
Dexamethasone 155
Dexmedetomidine 180, 182, 229
Dextran 242, 248*t*
Diabetes mellitus 112*f*
Diabetic chart 10
Diabetic emergencies 151
Diabetic ketoacidosis 151, 152, 154
Diagnostic alarm 256
Diagnostic endoscopy 234
Diarrhea, acute 130
Diazepam 182
Difficult mask ventilation 166
Digital led infrared thermometer 40*f*
Disability 6, 157, 202
Disaster
exercises 326
management 321, 323, 327
planning 323
Discomfort 218
severe 155
Disinfection 288, 289, 290*t*
Distal esophagus 38
Distress 271
Diverticular disease 138*fc*
Diverticulitis 130, 136
Dobutamine 114, 229, 344
Documentation 9, 300, 334
audits 301
formats 301
principles of 300

requirements 301
review 301
Donepezil 180
Dopamine 114, 149, 339, 340, 344
Double-lumen hemodialysis catheter 231*f*
Drilling machine 257
Drugs 229
de-escalation 20
infusion 224*f*
therapy 3
Dry heat sterilizer 288
Duodenal ulcer 136*fc*

E

Early warning score 9, 341
Echocardiogram 112*f*
Echocardiography 68
Edema, pulmonary 114
Ejection fraction 112
Elective cardioversion 221*b*
Electrical stimulation 192
Electrocardiogram 45, 109*t*, 117, 121
changes 108*t*
tracing 45, 45*f*
typical 107
Electrode
pads 215
placement 217
Electroencephalogram 121
Electrolyte 58
imbalances 56
relative concentration of 239*t*
values, normal 57*t*
Electronic
flow control device 225*f*
medical record 326
Emotional impact 104
Emotions 298
Empathy 298
Encephalopathy 333
End-diastolic pressure 70
Endocrine emergency 149, 151
Endocrine system 149
physiology of 149*t*
Endoscopic retrograde cholangiography 131
Endoscopic variceal ligation 142
Endotracheal suctioning, steps of 170
Endotracheal tube 21, 24*f*, 170, 342
insertion 170
End-tidal carbon dioxide 204*f*
phases of 41
Energy 220
level selection 220*t*
selection knob 214
Enoxaparin 110
Enteral nutrition 207
Enteral tube feeding 207
Enterococcus faecalis 172
Epidural catheter infusion set 230*f*
Epinephrine 114, 150, 229
Errors, sources of 266
Escherichia coli 280
Esophageal temperature 40
probe 40*f*
Esophagogastroduodenoscopy 135
Ethylene oxide sterilizer 288, 289
Etidronate 63
Euvolemic hyponatremia, cause of 60
Excessive parathyroid hormone 62
Expiration 96
trigger sensitivity 93*f*
Extended-spectrum beta-lactamases 280
External defibrillator, types of 213
Extracorporeal membrane oxygenation 101
initiation 101
maintenance 102, 103
nursing care 104
removal of 103
technology 104
weaning 103
Extubation 171
Eye
care 173, 174
opening 343
response 159

F

Face mask 166, 170, 171
Facial
motor response 334
sensation 334
Familial hypocalciuric hypercalcemia 62
Fatigue 104
Febrile nonhemolytic transfusion reaction 235
Feeding 13, 304
tubes 210
Femoral artery 69
Fentanyl 229
Fever, classification of 38, 39*t*
Fiberoptic
bronchoscopy 252
intubation 157
Fine needle aspiration 131
Fingerstick 262
Flaccid paralysis 60
Flash sterilization 288
Flexed wrist 64*f*
Flow
checklists 302
control devices 225
sheets 302
Fluid 239, 301, 303*t*
amount of 340
intravenous 239
management 237
rate 340
responsiveness 74
assessment of 73, 74
resuscitation 7, 160
warmer 225, 226*f*
Fondaparinux 110
Forehead temperature monitoring 40*f*
Fresh frozen plasma 142, 233, 234
Full thickness tissue loss 187, 188*f*
Functional residual capacity 125

G

Gait belts 203
Gallstones 139
Gamma aminobutyric acid 177
Gas 80*f*
exchange of 123
plasma 289
Gastric dilatation 22*f*
Gastroenterology 130, 140*t*
Gastrointestinal 133-135, 142
assessment 303
bleeding 130, 132
investigation of 133*fc*
loss 61
system 8
Gastroparesis 181
Gelatin 242
General nursing 163
considerations 113
principles 103
General oral health assessment index 172
Giddiness 155
Glasgow Coma Scale 6, 31*t*, 118-120, 159, 159*t*, 174, 202, 303, 341
score 263, 342*t*
Glucagon 150
Glucocorticoids 150
Glucometer 43*f*
use of 25*f*
Glucometry 44*f*
Glucose 43*f*, 239, 242*t*, 243*t*
control 304
serum 341
Glycemic control 18
Gonadotropin-releasing hormone 149

Grab bars 203
Graft versus host disease, transfusion-associated 235
Granulocyte concentrate 233
Growth hormone-releasing hormone 149
Guillain-Barré syndrome 333

H

Haemaccel 248*t*
Hand hygiene 281
compliance 310
Harris-Benedict equation 210*b*
Hazard vulnerability analysis 323
Head
burns 161
injury, severe 333
tilt 197
Head-of-bed elevation 304
Head-to-toe assessment 8
Healthcare
teams 4
workers 277, 283
Heart
abnormal rhythm of 45
block 221
disease, congenital 49
failure 48, 49, 66, 67, 107, 111, 114
acute decompensated 112, 113*f*, 114
classification of 112*t*
diagnosis of 111
hypoxia like 186
sign of 111*t*
stages of 111, 112*f*
symptoms of 111*t*
with preserved ejection fraction 114
with reduced ejection fraction 114
rate 28, 39, 66, 115, 117-119, 302
rhythm 66, 303
Heavy metal ingestion 179
Hematic products 145
Hemodialysis 100
catheters 230
different modes of 99*t*
intermittent 99, 142
prescription parameters 100, 100*t*
Hemodynamic 17
instability 218
monitoring 66, 75*fc*, 102
parameters 73
Hemorrhage 158
intracranial 110
Hemothorax 202
Heparin 110, 229
Hepatic failure 333
Hepatitis
B
immune globulin 285
surface antigen 285
virus 283, 284
C virus 283, 284
High cardiac output state 92*f*
High parathyroid hormone levels 63
High-flow nasal
cannula 79, 82
setup 80*f*
oxygen 79
High-flow systems 167
His bundle 45
Home message 267*b*
Hormone 149, 150
Hospital
incident command system 323
infection control committee 281
Hot air oven 288
Human immunodeficiency virus 260, 284
infections 283
Humidified high-flow nasal prong 79
Humidified temperature-regulated oxygen 82
Humidifier 79
Hydration, adequate 190, 190*f*
Hydroxyethyl starch 247*t*
Hyperactive delirium 177
Hyperbaric oxygen therapy 192
Hypercalcemia 62
cause of 62*t*
clinical features of 63*t*
Hyperglycemic hyperosmolar state 154
Hyperinflation, manual 195
Hyperkalemia 60
cause of 60*t*
Hypernatremia 58, 59*t*
correction of 59, 340
Hyperosmolar coma 333
Hyperosmolar hyperglycemic state 151, 153, 154*t*
Hyperplasia 62
Hypertension 112, 112*f*, 181
Hypertensive intracerebral hemorrhage 333
Hypertonic
fluid 241*f*
saline 126
solutions 241
Hypervitaminosis D 62
Hypervolemic hyponatremia, cause of 60
Hypoactive delirium 177
Hypocalcemia 63
cause of 63*t*
treatment 64
Hypodermic needles 283
Hypoglycemia 151, 178
pathophysiology of 151
Hypokalemia 61
cause of 61*t*
Hypokalemic periodic paralysis 61
Hyponatremia 59
cause of 60*t*
treatment of 59
Hypoparathyroidism 63
Hypophosphatemia 212
severe 333
Hypotension 67, 100, 114, 181, 155, 202, 333
Hypotensive reaction 236
Hypothalamus 149
Hypothermia 38, 333
different types of 39*t*
inadvertent 147
Hypotonic fluid 241
Hypotonic solutions 241
Hypovolemic hyponatremia, cause of 60
Hypoxic-ischemic brain 333

I

Immobility 181
Immunomodulation, transfusion-related 235
Impaired potassium excretion 60
Incentive spirometry 196
Incineration 289
Indwelling
catheters 304
lines 19
Infections 100, 102, 172, 275
acquired 277
control 4, 8, 224, 235, 277, 280
surveillance 278*f*
hospital-acquired 277
prevention 224, 280
control committee 281
surveillance of 277
Information 204
technology 326
Infusion 223, 223*b*, 230, 231
equipment 224
medication administration 232*b*
pump 339
rates formula 340
therapy 228
teams 223, 232

Initial nursing assessment 5
sheet 10
Injections 223-225, 231
common routes of 223*b*
Inotropes 3
Inspiration 96
Inspired oxygen, fraction of 80, 125, 167, 304, 344
Insulin 61
Intake-output chart 10
Intensive care 324
nursing 237
Intensive care unit 3, 5, 6, 12, 21, 30, 38, 45, 53, 85, 107, 117, 131, 144, 173-175, 177, 178*fc*, 179, 181, 193, 194, 194*t*, 198, 198*b*, 208, 237, 250, 277, 278*f*, 295, 300, 311, 316, 323, 339
delirium assessments 177
nursing 3
procedures 251*t*
list of 250*b*
Intercostal drainage systems 128
Interference 38
Interleukin 208
Intermittent percussive ventilation 197
Intermittent pneumatic compression 24*f*
Intermittent positive pressure ventilation 93
International normalized ratio 21, 118, 119, 121
Interstitial space 43*f*
Intra-abdominal drainage catheter 254
Intracellular potassium 60, 61
Intracerebral bleed 116
Intracranial bleed 118
Intracranial pressure 115, 121
Intraparenchymal bleed 116
Intrapleural pressure 126
Intravenous administration set 232*f*
Intravenous fluid 239
infusion containers, types of 239*f*
therapy 237, 238*fc*
types of 240
use of 237
Intravenous infusion set 225*f*
Intubation, steps of 170
Invasive arterial blood pressure 66, 68
Invasive hemodynamic monitoring 68
Invasive therapy 109
Ipratropium bromide 126
ISBAR
acronym 297*t*
communication tool 297
Ischemia
acute mesenteric 143
chronic mesenteric 143
intestinal 130, 143
Ischemic colitis 130, 137
treatment of 139*fc*
Isolation practices 280
Isotonic fluid 241*f*

J

Jet nebulizers 125
Joint Commission International 308

K

Keratitis 173
Kidney
disease, chronic 113, 236
failure 66, 331
injury, acute 142
Kussmaul's respiration 67, 152

L

Labetalol 229
Lactate 66, 67, 239
dehydrogenase, serum 341
Lactic acidosis, management of 68
Lagophthalmos 173
Laryngoscope 170
Latent tetany, sign of 64*f*
Lead positions 45*f*
Left ventricle 112*f*
Left ventricular 75
hypertrophy 112*f*
Levothyroxine, intravenous 155
Life-threatening
device malfunction, detection of 256
situations, detection of 256
Liver
failure 130, 331
acute 130, 132
function test 120, 121, 142
Living organ donation 331
Lorazepam 182
Low flow system 167
Low molecular weight heparin 21
Low-efficiency daily dialysis 98
Lumbar puncture 234, 252
Lung 128
computed tomography scan of 129*f*
disease 37
hyperinflation techniques 195
ultrasound of 128*f*
ventilator unit 90*f*

M

Macrodrip tubing administers 340
Magnetic resonance imaging 117, 120, 121, 158
Malignant 62
Malnutrition 61, 186
Manual electrode pads 215, 215*f*
Manual external defibrillator 213, 214*f*
Mask 166*f*, 292
choosing correct size of 169*t*
continuous positive airway pressure 80
size 169
Mean arterial pressure 70, 119, 344
Mechanical ventilation 3, 88, 89*t*
indications of 88
modes of 94
settings 96*t*
Medical devices
disinfection of 290*t*
sterilization of 290*t*
Medical record number 305
Medication 110, 205
administration 228, 228*b*, 301
error, incidence of 317*b*
errors 311
management of 309
Melatonin 150
Mental status 67
Mentation 68
Meprobamate 333
Mesh nebulizers 126
Metabolic acidosis 58
Metabolic alkalosis 58
Metabolic bone disease 212
Metacarpophalangeal joint 64*f*
Metformin 67
Methaqualone 333
Methemoglobin 36
Methemoglobinemia 38
Methicillin-resistant *staphylococcus aureus* 280
Microbial colonization 172
Microdrip tubing administers 340
Microorganisms, colony-forming unit of 288
Microwave 289
Midazolam 180, 181, 229
Mineralocorticoids 150
Minor brain injury 159
Minute ventilation demand 79
Mitigation 323

Mitral regurgitation 114
Mitral valve diseases 48
Mixed delirium 177
Mixed venous oxygen saturation 73
Mobilization 193, 197
  early 191*f*
Modified early warning score 28*t*
Moisture 189
Monitor rhythm 111
Morphine 229
Motion artefacts 38
Motor response 159, 343
Multidisciplinary team 268
Multidrug-resistant organisms, spread of 277
Multiorgan failure 139
Multiple endocrine neoplasia syndromes 62
Multiple punctures 57
Multi-wavelength pulse oximeters 37
Muscle cramping 100
Musculoskeletal system 8
Myocardial infarction 47, 53, 186, 316
  acute 107
  location of 109
Myocardial injury 218
Myocardial necrosis 108
Myxedema coma 154

N

Nail polish 38
Nasal cannula 167, 171
Nasogastric tube 21*f*, 22*f*, 81
  in situ 21*f*
  insertion 254
  malposition 21*f*
Nasopharyngeal airway 168
  placement of 169*f*
  sizing of 169*f*
Nasopharyngeal temperature 40
Nasopharynx 38
Nasotracheal tube 157
National Accreditation Board for Hospitals 308, 310, 311, 323
National Database of Nursing Quality Indicators 310, 311
National Early Warning Score 343
National Organ and Tissue Transplant Organization 332
National Pressure Ulcer Advisory Panel 184
National Quality Forum 309
Nausea 148, 271
Nebulizers 125, 291
Neck injuries 157
Needlestick injury 283
Needs end-of-life care 268
Negative pressure isolations 280
Nervous regulatory mechanisms, dysfunction of 184
Neurological assessment 8, 157, 303
Neuromuscular disease 333
Neuroparalytic drugs 333
Neurotoxic snake bites 333
Nitrogen balance 340
Nitroglycerin 115, 229
Nitroprusside 115
Nonconvulsive status epilepticus 121
Noncritical patient care items, cleaning of 292*t*
Noninvasive arterial blood pressure 66
Noninvasive machines, types of 83*f*
Noninvasive ventilation 21, 38, 79, 82, 84*f*, 85, 86, 125
  circuit components 82
  indications of 85
Nonrebreathing masks 167
Nonsteroidal anti-inflammatory drugs 21
Non-ST-segment elevation myocardial infarction 108
Nonverbal communication 295
Norepinephrine 114, 150, 229, 344
Nosocomial infections 172
N-terminal pro-B-type natriuretic peptide 112*f*
Nuisance alarm 257
Nurses
  expanded role of 3
  led eye care 175*fc*
  role of 101-103
Nursing
  care 81, 144, 146, 147
    plan 306
  considerations 107, 111, 114, 115, 335
  documentation 300
    overview of 305*t*
  perspectives 144
  quality indicator 309, 311
  resource management 309
  standards 308
Nutrition 103, 189, 207
  risk in critically ill score
    system 208*t*
    variables 208*t*
  therapy, types of 207
Nutritional supplements 207

O

Obesity 139
Ocular movement 333
Ocular surface disease 174, 174*t*
Oliguria 67, 68
Open fracture 202
Opioids 179
  analgesics, side effects of 148
Optical interference 38
Optical plethysmography 36
Oral airways, different sizes of 168*f*
Oral assessment guide 172
Oral bite block 167
Oral care 172, 173*t*
Oral cavity hosts 172
Oral polio vaccine 236
Oral temperature 39
Organ
  donation 329, 331, 332
  dysfunction 102
  support 77
Organophosphate 117
Oropharyngeal airway 167
Oscillation, high-frequency 197
Osmolality 239
  serum 340
Overdamped waveform 72
Oversedation 181
Oxygen 35
  blender 80*f*
  delivery
    capacities 167*t*
    systems 166
  saturation 7, 117-120, 125, 166, 302, 343
    level 30
  therapy 7
  topical 192
Oxygenation, inadequate 186
Oxyhemoglobin absorbs 35
Oxytocin 149, 150

P

Packaging area 291
Packed red cells 233
Paddles
  anterolateral placement of 217*f*
  anteroposterior placement of 217*f*
Pain 181, 218, 271
  assessment 304, 305
  management 148, 305
  severe abdominal 130
  thermometer 22*f*
Pamidronate 63
Pancreas 150

Pancreatitis 130
  acute 130
Paralysis 186
Parameter 96, 100
Parasternal short axis 68
Parathyroid 150
  gland
    adenoma 62
    destruction 63
  hormone 150
Parenteral nutrition 21, 207, 209
Parkland formula 161
  modified 161
Paroxysmal supraventricular tachycardia 50
Partial thromboplastin time 159
Passive leg raising
  technique 75*f*
  test 74
Peak inspiratory pressure 304
Peak systolic pressure 70
Pediatric glasgow coma scale 343
Pelvic
  fracture 202
  ulcer, perforated 130, 134, 137*f*
Percutaneous coronary intervention 110
Peripheral arterial oxygen saturation 344
Peripheral cannulae 227*f*
Peripheral devices 226
Peripheral line 234
Peripheral oxygen saturation 80
Peripheral pulsation monitoring 102
Peripheral pulse 67, 303
Peripheral temperature monitoring 39
Peripheral venous access 229
Peripherally inserted venous cannula 251
Peritoneal dialysis 99
Peritonitis 135
Personal protective equipment 311
Pharmacologic interventions 180
Pharmacy 326
Phlebostatic axis 71, 71*f*
Phlebotomy 260
Physician responsibilities 235
Physiotherapy 193, 194*t*, 198
  goals of 194
  role of 194
Pineal gland 150
Pivot disks 204
Plasma 262
  sterilization 288, 289
Plasmalyte 239, 245*t*
Plateau pressure 91*f*, 304
Platelet 233
  count 234
  refractoriness 235
  rich plasma 233
Pleura, ultrasound of 128*f*
Pleural biopsies 128
Pneumonia, ventilator-associated 172, 277, 279*b*, 316
Pneumothorax 127
Polymerase chain reaction 21
Positive pressure isolations 280
Positive-end expiratory pressure 21, 91*f*, 96, 304
  generation of 80
Positive-expiratory pressure 197
Post end-expiratory pressure 175
Postanesthetic ward 147
Post-exposure prophylaxis 284
Post-transfusion purpura 235
Post-traumatic stress disorder 181
Potassium 239
  deficit 341
  excretion 61
  intake 60, 61
  loss 61
  serum 57
Povidone-iodine 266
Prasugrel 109, 110
Premature ventricular contraction 52, 53
Pressure 92
  control 95
  injuries 184
  preset assist control 96
  regulated volume control 96
  support 96
    ventilation 96
  transducing system 71*f*
  trigger 92*f*
  ulcer 187*f*
    cause of 185*fc*
    risk assessment 304
    stages of 186
Pretransfer stabilization 202*t*
Pretransfusion monitoring 234
Prioritization 318
Prophylactic antibiotics 146
Propofol 182
Prothrombin time 118, 119, 121
Protocols 306, 327
  application of 13
Proton pump inhibitor 21, 134
Proximal interphalangeal joint 64*f*
Psychic overtones 63
Psychological support 272
Pulmonary arterial
  catheter 41*f*, 74*f*
  temperature 41
Pulmonary artery 38
  diastolic pressure 73
  occlusion pressure 73
  systolic pressure 73
Pulmonary critical care nursing 123
Pulmonary embolism 48
Pulse
  oximeter estimates 35
  oximetry 35
    types of 36
    use of 37
  pressure 70
Pulseless
  electrical activity 29
  ventricular tachycardia 29, 54
Pupillary examination 7
Pupillary response 303

Q

Quality 235
  control 308, 309*f*
  improvement 300
  indicator 311, 316
  initiatives 192

R

Radial artery 69
  puncture, site of 57*f*
Radiation 289
Ranson criteria 341, 341*t*
Ranson score 341
Rapid response teams, detection of 343
Reactive hyperemia cycle, failure of 185
Rebreathing, partial 167
Rectal temperature probe 39, 40*f*
Red blood cell 133, 234
Redistribute pressure 192*b*
Reduce heart rate 46
Refeeding syndrome 212
Reflectance pulse oximetry 36, 36*f*, 37
Regular atrial rhythm 48
Relaxation interventions 198
Releasing organ 149, 150
Renal assessment 303
Renal failure 67, 98
Renal function test 120, 121
Renal loss 61
Renal replacement therapy 98
  modalities, overview of 99
  indications of 98*b*
Renal system 8
Replacement fluids 237
Respiration 344

muscles of 124
rate 343
Respiratory acidosis 58
Respiratory alkalosis
acute 58
chronic mesenteric 58
Respiratory assessment 165, 303, 305
Respiratory depression 181
Respiratory distress 80
Respiratory effort 165
Respiratory failure 125
life-threatening effects of 66
Respiratory function 332
Respiratory physiotherapy 200
Respiratory rate 7, 28, 302, 304
Respiratory support 7
Respiratory system 123, 147
factors determining compliance of 89*f*
physiology of 124
Respiratory therapists 325
Respiratory tract, anatomy of 123
Respiratory zone 124
Resuscitation 6, 27, 159, 237
goals of 159
Reteplase 110
Rhythm 220
analysis 217
Ribonucleic acid levels 285
Richmond agitation sedation scale 23*t*, 179*t*
Right ventricle 112*f*
Right ventricular 75
Riker sedation-agitation scale 341, 342*t*
Ringer's solution 244*t*
Rivastigmine 180
Roll boards 203
Root cause analysis 318

S

Safe phlebotomy 260*t*, 261*b*
Sample, collection of 56
Sedation 15, 177, 181, 304
monitoring depth of 181
protocols 181
status 305
vacation 304
Sedative medications, clinical pharmacology of 181*t*
Seizure prophylaxis 8
Semiautomatic external defibrillator 214
Semicritical patient care items
cleaning of 291*t*
reprocessing of 291*t*
Sensory perception 189
Sepsis 66, 67, 236
Sequential organ failure assessment 208
score 343, 344, 344*t*
Serum aspartate transaminase 341
Setting up pressure transducing system 70
Severe acute respiratory syndrome coronavirus 323
Shock 28, 67, 114, 220
cardiogenic 30
delivery 218
distributive 30
hemorrhagic 29
hypovolemic 28
obstructive 30
sign of 114, 143
Shockable rhythms 216
Sickle cell anemia 38
Silver sulfadiazine 161
Simple face mask 167
Simulation exercises 306
Single and triple chamber chest drainage systems 128*f*
Sinus
bradycardia 47, 49
tachycardia 46, 49
Skin
assessment 304
burns 218
care 103, 189, 189*f*
cleaning 266
preparation of 145
Slow low-efficiency daily dialysis 99
Small bowel obstruction 135
Smallpox, vaccination of 236
Smart infusion pumps 339
Sodium 239
based disorders 58
chloride 244*t*, 245*t*
deficit 341
serum 57
Soft skills 293
Somatostatin 149
Spaulding process classification 290
Specimen, types of 261, 262
Spectrophotometer 35, 35*f*
Spikes acronym 298*t*
Spontaneous breathing trial 18, 73*f*, 304
Square wave test 72
Staphylococcus aureus 172
Starches 242
Static calibration 71
Static lung volumes 124*f*
Status epilepticus 116, 120, 120*t*
types of 120
Steam sterilizer 288
components of 288
types of 288
Sterile gauze dressings 227
Sterile storage area 291
Sterilization 288, 289
area 291
control 289
Sterilizer 288
Steroid supplementation 155
Stethoscope 292
Stomach 21*f*
Stones 63
Streptococcus mutans 172
Streptokinase 110
Stress 17
ulcer
prevention 17
prophylaxis 17, 304
Stroke 116, 117*t*
acute ischemic 117
neurological assessment of 8
volume 39
ST-segment elevation 108*f*
myocardial infarction 108, 110
Subarachnoid hemorrhage 116, 119, 119*t*
Subcutaneous injections 230
Sulfonamide, topical 161
Supraglottic airway 169
device 169, 169*t*
Supraventricular tachycardia 49, 218, 219*f*
Surgical site infection 277
prevention of 279
Synchronous intermittent mandatory ventilation 93, 95*f*, 96

T

Tachyarrhythmias 27, 46
Tachycardia 181
Tachypnea 7, 67, 165
Target mean arterial pressure 113
Telemedicine 326
Temperature 35, 302
management 8
monitoring 16, 38
Templates 306
Temporary pacemaker insertion 252
Tenecteplase 110
Tension pneumothorax 202
Therapeutic communication 298
Therapeutic endoscopy 234
Therapeutic touch 198
Thermal burns 160

Thermometer 292
Three-way stop cock 226*f*
Thromboembolic prophylaxis 304
Thromboembolism 218
Thrombolytic agents 110
Thrombophlebitis 22*f*
Thromboprophylaxis 15
Thrombotic thrombocytopenic purpura 234
Thyroid 150
  emergencies 154
  gland 149
  storm 154
Thyrotropin-releasing hormone 149
Ticagrelor 109, 110
Tidal volume 304
Tirofiban 110
Tissue 149, 150
Tobramycin 126
Total parenteral nutrition 22*f*
Tracheobronchial tree, anatomy of 123*f*
Transcutaneous oximetry 36
Transcutaneous pacing 213, 221
Transdermal loss 61
Transfer
  boards 204
  equipment, types of 203
  sheets 203
Transfusion
  associated circulatory overload 236
  complications of 235
  medicine 233
  therapy 228
Transmission pulse oximetry 36, 36*f*
Trauma 66, 157
Traumatic brain injury 158,159*t*
Trichloroethylene 333
Tricuspid valve 48
Triiodothyronine T3 150
Triple-lumen central venous catheter 227*f*
Troponin 8
Trousseau sign 64*f*
Tube cap color 261, 262
Tubular necrosis, acute 68
Tympanic membrane 38
  intact 334
  temperature probe 39, 40*f*

U

Ulcer prophylaxis 304
Ultrasonic nebulizers 126
Ultrasonography 128
Ultrasound 131, 142
  topical 192
Universal mercury thermometer 40*f*
Unstable angina 107, 108
Upper airway 165
  anatomy of 165
  obstruction 80, 165
Upper gastrointestinal bleed, management of 134*fc*
Upper respiratory tract
  anatomy of 123*f*
  secretions 271
Uremia 333
Urinary bladder 39
  temperature monitoring catheter 40*f*
Urinary catheterization 251, 279
Urinary system 8
Urinary tract infection 316
  catheter-associated 277, 309*f*
Urine output 17, 66, 68, 303

V

Vacuum 289
Vancomycin-resistant enterococi 280
Vascular access 99
  devices 224
Vascular injury 202
Vasoactive mediations 344
Vasodilators 3
Vasopressin 114, 149, 229
Vasopressor support 7
Vecuronium 229
Veins
  anatomy of 264*f*
  selection of 263
Venipuncture 261
  complications of 266*b*
Venous blood gas monitoring 102
Venous thromboembolism risk assessment 304
Ventilation 91, 123
  bag 170
  different modes of 94*t*
  indications of 88*t*
  mechanics of 90
  modes of 93
Ventilator
  asynchrony 181
  breath, types of 92
  bundle 279
  chart 10
  hyperinflation 195
  settings 304
Ventilatory breaths 91*f*
Ventilatory support, use of 303
Ventricular escape 47
Ventricular fibrillation 29, 53, 55, 216, 216*f*
Ventricular rate 49
Ventricular tachycardia 27, 52, 54, 55, 216, 216*f*
Verbal
  communication 295
  description scale 22*f*
  response 31, 159, 343
Vessel 109
Vibrating mesh nebulizer 126*f*
Viral infection transmission 236
Visual analog scale 23*f*
Visual infusion phlebitis scale 231*t*
Vital signs 302*t*, 303, 305
Vital, monitoring of 126
Vitamin
  deficiencies 179
  supplementation 64
Volume control
  breaths 93
  mode 95*f*
  ventilation 95
Vomiting 148, 271

W

Ward rounds 4
Waste disposal 288
Waveform
  capnography 42
    normal 42*f*
  shape 42
Weakness 60
Weaning process 103
Wedge pressure 73
Wells criteria 24, 24*t*
Wernicke's encephalopathy 212
White blood cell count 341
Wolff-Parkinson-white syndrome 219, 219*f*
World Health Organization 326
Wound
  care documentation 305
  management 191

X

Xanthines 61